An Approach to
Surgical Emergency

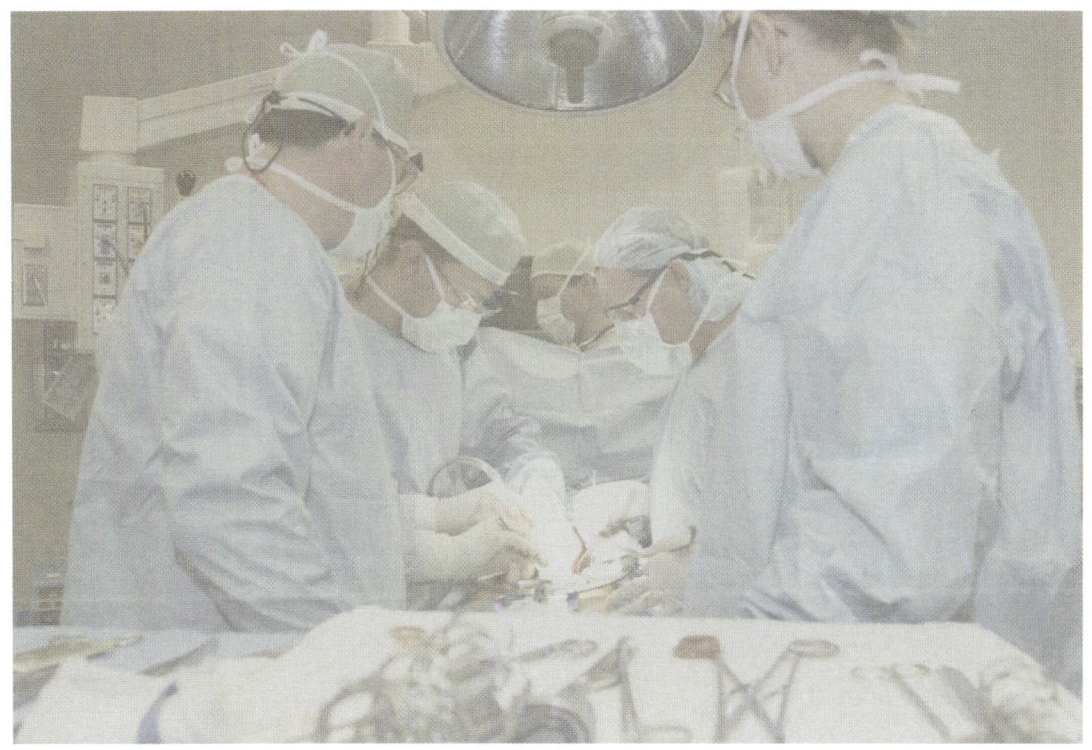

An Approach to
Surgical Emergency

UK Shrivastava MBBS MS FAIS DHA

Professor of Surgery
University College of Medical Sciences
Senior Consultant Surgeon to associated GTB Hospital, Delhi

Former Dean and Head, Surgical Discipline, Faculty of Medical Sciences
Chairman, Board of Research and Studies
University of Delhi

Sudipta Saha MBBS MS

Lecturer in Surgery
University College of Medical Sciences
Consultant Surgeon to associated GTB Hospital, Delhi

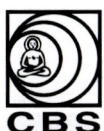

CBS Publishers & Distributors Pvt Ltd

New Delhi • Bangalore • Pune • Cochin • Chennai

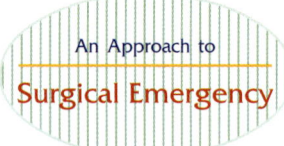

An Approach to
Surgical Emergency

First Edition: 2010

Published by Satish Kumar Jain and produced by Vinod K. Jain for

CBS Publishers & Distributors Pvt Ltd

Head off: CBS Plaza 4819/XI Prahlad Street, 24 Ansari Road, Daryaganj, New Delhi 110 002, India.

Website: www.cbspd.com

Ph: 23289259, 23266861/67   Fax: +91-11-23243014   e-mail: delhi@cbspd.com; cbspubs@vsnl.com; cbspubs@airtelmail.in.

Branches

- Bangalore: Seema House 2975, 17th Cross, K.R. Road, Banasankari 2nd Stage, Bangalore 560 070, Karnataka
  Ph: +91-80-26771678/79   Fax: +91-80-26771680   e-mail: bangalore@cbspd.com

- Pune: Shaan Brahmha Complex, 631/632 Basement, Appa Balwant Chowk, Budhwar Peth, Next To Ratan Talkies, Pune 411 002, Maharashtra
  Ph: +91-20-24464057/58   Fax: +91-20-24464059   e-mail: pune@cbspd.com

- Cochin: 36/14 Kalluvilakam, Lissie Hospital Road, Cochin 682 018, Kerala
  Ph: +91-484-4059061-65   Fax: +91-484-4059065   e-mail: cochin@cbspd.com

- Chennai: 20, West Park Road, Shenoy Nagar, Chennai 600 030, TN
  Ph: +91-44-26260666, 26208620   Fax: +91-44-45530020   email: chennai@cbspd.com

Printed at Paras Offset Pvt. Ltd., C-176, Naraina Industrial Area Phase-I, New Delhi

Foreword

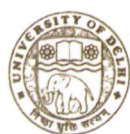

University of Delhi
दिल्ली विश्वविद्यालय

Professor Deepak Pental
Vice-Chancellor

December 16, 2009

It gives me immense pleasure to write the foreword for the book *An Approach to Surgical Emergency* authored by Prof. UK Shrivastava and Dr Sudipta Saha. Prof. Shrivastava is the senior-most Professor in the Department of Surgery at University College of Medical Sciences, Delhi. He has been Dean and Head of Surgical Discipline of Faculty of Medical Sciences of University of Delhi. Prof. Shrivastava has been a medical teacher for undergraduate and postgraduate students for more than thirty years in various universities.

His book *An Approach to Surgical Emergency* brings out his wealth of experience for the benefit of the surgical trainees and undergraduate medical students. The twenty-seven chapters cover the commonly encountered acute conditions and provide clear and concise approach to their management.

The book will be an excellent source of guidance for all those engaged in providing immediate surgical care to patients. The book is written in a lucid and easy to read manner and the concepts driven home will stay with the reader long after the words have faded from the memory.

I wish Prof. Shrivastava and his readers all the best.

Deepak Pental

University Road, Delhi-110 007, India. Phones: +91-11-27667011, 27667190 Fax: +91-11-27667049
email : vc@du.ac.in / dpental@gmail.com

Preface

Surgical emergency has always been a critical component in the field of medical discipline. The emergence of several investigative modalities has changed the scenario for accurate diagnosis and management of these cases. The introduction of focused abdominal sonogram in trauma (FAST), computerized tomography (CT), MRI/MRCP, Doppler scan, and especially laparoscopy, has really been a boon in the management of this field.

After gaining experience in the field of surgery for more than four decades around the globe, I felt the need of writing a book for surgical trainees, incorporating all the recent facts in the management of basic surgical emergencies. I alongwith my coauthor Sudipta Saha, have also been able to persuade a few of the experts to share their wisdom as contributors in this textbook. The book encompasses the basic concepts of surgical approach for all acute common surgical emergencies.

The text of the book comprises twenty-seven chapters of common surgical problems, having comprehensive source of core knowledge and skills for all those medical graduates and postgraduates striving to achieve a successful career as practising clinicians and surgeons.

UK Shrivastava

List of Contributors

Dua, Rakesh
Head
Department of Neurosurgery
Guru Teg Bahadur Hospital
and associated UCMS
Delhi

Gulati, Divesh
Senior Resident
Department of Orthopedics
University College of Medical Sciences and
associated GTB Hospital
University of Delhi
Delhi

Kumar, Sudhir
Professor and Head
Department of Orthopedics
University College of Medical Sciences and
associated GTB Hospital
University of Delhi
Delhi

Mahapatra, L.
Senior Resident, Department of Surgery
University College of Medical Sciences and
associated GTB Hospital
University of Delhi
Delhi

Mohta, Anup
Professor and Head
Department of Pediatric Surgery
Chacha Nehru Bal
Chikitsalaya associated with
Maulana Azad Medical College
Delhi Government
Delhi

Rai, Ashish
Specialist and Head,
Department of Burns and Plastic Surgery
Guru Teg Bahadur Hospital
and associated UCMS
Delhi

Rajaram, Shalini
Professor
Department of Obstetrics and Gynecology
University College of Medical Sciences and
associated GTB Hospital
University of Delhi
Delhi

Saha, Sudipta
Lecturer, Department of Surgery
University College of Medical Sciences and
associated GTB hospital
University of Delhi
Delhi

Satti, Dinesh
Resident Medical Officer
Department of Neurosurgery
University College of Medical Sciences and
associated GTB Hospital
University of Delhi
Delhi

Saxena, Ashok
Professor of Anaesthesiology
University College of Medical Sciences and
associated GTB Hospital
University of Delhi
Delhi

Sharma, Jai Prakash
Lecturer
University College of Medical Sciences and
associated GTB Hospital
University of Delhi
Delhi

Shrivastava, UK
Professor and Senior Consultant Surgeon
University College of Medical Sciences and
associated GTB Hospital
University of Delhi
Delhi

Sinha, Shagun
Senior Resident
Department of Obstetrics and Gynecology
University College of Medical Sciences and
associated GTB Hospital
University of Delhi
Delhi

Acknowledgements

I am indebted to all my colleagues for their contributions and I am sure the readers will find their expertise interesting and clinically useful in their future life.

I must thank my wife Dr. Meera Shrivastava, retired Additional Deputy Director-General, Central Health Services, for giving time-to-time valuable suggestions, guidance and encouragement in bringing out this book.

I express my gratitude and thanks to CBS Publishers & Distributors Pvt Ltd for their help and support in publishing the book.

UK Shrivastava

I would especially like to mention my lovely wife, Sushmita, whose patience and encouragement has enabled me to attempt such an enormous task.

I would like to express my sincere gratitude to my teachers Dr Anurag Srivastava and Dr Sunil Chumber; and thank Dr Lalatendu Mahapatra for providing me valuable assitance.

I would like to express gratitude to my wonderful parents who have been unfailing in their support throughout my journey in this challenging profession of medicine and surgery.

Sudipta Saha

Contents

1

Acute Abdomen

Acute abdomen means painful abdomen and it refers to some kind of pathological condition of intra-abdominal organs. It could be inflammatory, bowel obstruction, intestinal ischemia, strangulation, infarction or perforation. Roughly around 25% of patients attending emergency department suffer from acute abdomen. It is important to remember that some non-surgical conditions like that of endocrine metabolic origin (uremia, diabetic crisis), hemato-logical origin (acute porphyria, sickle cell crisis, acute leukemia) and also toxins (like spider poisoning) can also present as acute abdomen.

Abdominal pain of surgical importance would be either visceral or parietal in nature. Visceral pain is generally vague and poorly localized depending on its origin from foregut, midgut or from hindgut (Fig. 1.1), whereas the parietal pain is clearly localized to

its segmental nerve root origin, supplying the area of perietal peritoneum.

Causes of Acute Abdomen

There are numerous conditions, inflammatory or non-inflammatory, involving the intra-abdominal organs responsible for causing acute abdomen. The list of such conditions are enumerated in Table 1.1.

EVALUATION OF THE PATIENTS

A detailed history is very important for accurate diagnosis and further treatment. While taking history the character of pain, its location, frequency, duration, radiation, its relation with food and factors aggravating or relieving the pain should all be noted. Intensity of pain is related to underlying tissue pathology. Visceral pain on account of ischemia or inflammation are dull and poorly localized in center of the abdomen. Pain in the flank is related to disease of kidney and ureter. In contrast, the parietal pain is sharper in nature and is better localized to one of the four quadrants of abdomen.

Sudden onset of severe pain suggests bowel perforation or arterial embolization with ischemia of bowel. In cholecystitis and pancreatitis pain is severe and continuous. Spasmodic/colicky pain is found in intestinal obstruction, biliary colic and renal or ureteric stones. Radiation of pain to shoulder and scapula is typical of gallbladder inflammation and biliary colic. In pancreatitis, pain is referred to back, whereas pain due to stone in the kidney or ureter radiates to groin and perineal area.

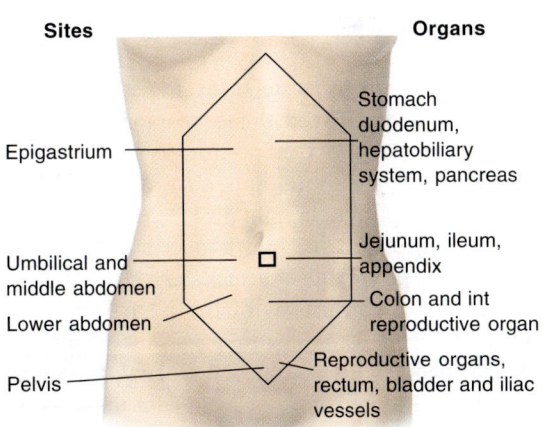

Sites   **Organs**

Epigastrium — Stomach duodenum, hepatobiliary system, pancreas

Umbilical and middle abdomen — Jejunum, ileum, appendix

Colon and int reproductive organ

Lower abdomen —

Pelvis — Reproductive organs, rectum, bladder and iliac vessels

Fig. 1.1: Location of visceral pain

Table 1.1: Common surgical causes of acute abdomen

Inflammatory conditions
- Acute appendicitis
- Acute cholecystitis
- Acute pancreatitis
- Meckel's diverticulum
- Amebic liver abscess

Perforations
- Perforations of GI tract due to disease or trauma

Obstruction or gangrene
- Adhesion
- Stricture
- Growth
- Volvulus
- Intussusceptions

Ischemic
- Acute mesenteric thrombosis or embolism
- Ischemic ulcers
- Strangulated hernia

Hemorrhagic
- After surgery or trauma
- Hemorrhagic pancreatitis
- Spontaneous rupture of spleen

Acute abdomen of gynecological emergencies
- Rupture of uterus
- Endometritis
- Ectopic pregnancy
- Acute salpingitis
- Pyosalpinx
- Torsion of ovarian cyst
- Rupture of ovarian follicles

History of fever, nausea, vomiting, diarrhea, absolute constipation, hematochezia, and hematuria all should be noted. Pain of acute appendicitis is generally associated with nausea and vomiting. Vomiting is also a feature of acute cholecystitis and pancreatitis. Repeated vomiting is generally found in small bowel obstruction, whereas vomiting is a late feature in large bowel obstruction. The nature of vomiting (bilious or non-bilious) depends whether the site of obstruction is distal or proximal to ampulla of Vater. Fecal vomiting is suggestive of late stage of large bowel obstruction. A past history of diarrhea may indicate possibility of chronic inflammatory disease like that of Crohn's disease or ulcerative colitis.

Non passage of flatus and feces is feature of acute bowel obstruction. Past history of any trauma, surgical intervention like ERCP and history of previous operations should be taken. History of intake of any medication should also be noted (intake of NSAID may cause perforation of bowel). Gynecological history like date of last menstrual period, vaginal discharge, dysmenorrhea should always be obtained.

CLINICAL EXAMINATION

A thorough clinical examination is of immense value in reaching the diagnosis of acute abdomen. Laboratory investigations and imaging studies later only help in confirming the suspected diagnosis in majority of the cases. General appearance and posture of the patient should be observed. Vital signs are recorded and presence of pallor, cyanosis or icterus should be looked for. Tachycardia, hypotension, anxious look may indicate the serious intra-abdominal condition and shock. The actual abdominal examination involves close inspection, palpation, percussion and auscultation along with per vaginal and per rectal examination.

On inspection couture of abdomen, whether it is scaphoid, flat or distended (as in intestinal obstruction) and whether it is held still with very little or no movement with respiration (as in perforation peritonitis) is noted. Hernial sites as well as the genitalia should always be inspected in all cases of acute abdomen.

Palpation is a crucial step in examination of acute abdomen. Generalized tenderness and rebound tenderness are signs of peritonitis (perforation peritonitis). In acute appendicitis localized tenderness is present in right iliac fossa. Tenderness on deep palpation in right hypochondrium with positive Murphy's sign indicates acute cholecystitis. Epigastric tenderness with the past history of cholelithiasis or alcoholism suggests the possibility of acute pancreatitis. At times careful palpation may also detect inflammatory or malignant mass in the abdomen. Table 1.2 lists the common abdominal signs of clinical importance.

Table 1.2: Common abdominal signs of clinical importance		
Signs	*Description*	*Diagnosis*
Charcot's sign	Intermittent fever, pain and jaundice	Acute cholangitis
Murphy's sign	Palpation of right upper abdominal quadrant during deep inspiration results in right upper quadrant abdominal pain	Acute cholecystitis
Obturator sign	Flexion of right thigh at right angles to trunk and external rotation of same leg in supine position result in hypogastric pain	Appendicitis (pelvic appendix)
Rovsing's sign	Pain at right iliac fossa on palpation of left iliac fossa	Appendicitis
Turner's sign	Local areas of discoloration around umbilicus and flanks	Acute hemorrhagic pancreatitis
Kehr's sign	Left shoulder pain when patient is supine or in Trendelenburg's position	Hemoperitoneum especially ruptured spleen

Abdomen will be tympanic on percussion in cases of gaseous distension of bowel. Presence of shifting dullness indicates presence of free fluid in the peritoneal cavity. Obliteration of liver dullness because of presence of gas under the right dome of diaphragm suggests bowel perforation.

Auscultation of bowel sound is equally important. Increased and hyperactive bowel sounds are present in intestinal obstruction. Absence of bowel sounds indicates either peritonitis or paralytic ileus. Bruits heard during auscultation are due to the turbulent blood flow in the vascular system and indicates arterial stenosis.

BIOCHEMICAL INVESTIGATIONS

Common laboratory investigations for acute abdomen are as follows:

- Complete hemogram with total and differential count of WBC
- Blood urea, serum creatinine and electrolyte
- Serum amylase and lipase
- Alkaline phosphatase
- Bilirubin with total and direct and amino-transferase
- Serum lactate dehydrogenase
- Urine for routine and microscopic examination.

Routine laboratory tests are of minimum value other than amylase. The white cell count and hematocrit is helpful in supporting the diagnosis.

Elevated TLC denotes inflammation but one should be aware of the fact that acute cholecystitis and acute appendicitis can be present even when the TLC is within normal range. Low hematocrit in emergency only signifies chronic or subacute anemia and it does not reflect the magnitude of acute hemorrhage. Significance of any laboratory investigation should never be judged in isolation but to be considered as a part of whole clinical picture.

IMAGING STUDIES

- Upright chest X-ray including both domes of the diaphragm may show gas under right dome of the diaphragm in 70% of the cases of perforation peritonitis.
- Multiple air fluid levels in erect posture and gas filled loops of small bowel in supine position are seen in intestinal obstruction.
- Plain film may at times show the pancreatic calcinosis in chronic pancreatitis. It also helps in detecting renal stones. Renal stones are radiopaque in 90% of the cases, whereas 10–15% of gall stone are radiopaque.
- Plain X-ray may also show gas in portal and biliary tree suggestive of cholecysto-enteric fistula/gall stone ileus.
- Soap bubble appearance signifies free gas in retroperitoneum, i.e. in epigastrium it is generally associated with infected pancreatic necrosis and

if found in right upper quadrant it may be associated with retroperitoneal perforation of duodenum. Presence of gas in both the gutter indicates the perforation of colon.

- Gaseous distension of small bowel with no gas in the colon signifies complete small bowel obstruction but if gaseous distension seen in both small and large bowel it indicates paralytic ileus.

Although history and physical examination usually provides the essential information required for reaching the diagnosis, the modern imaging techniques like USG and CT scan are helpful in certain cases. The most difficult diagnostic dilemma in emergency was used to be regarding acute appendicitis in young women and ischemic bowel in elderly patients. With the help of CT scan both can be diagnosed with greater certainty. Although the CT scan has got high sensitivity and specificity but it is not available in all the emergency set up. Therefore the role of USG is very useful. It provides rapid, safe and low cost, non-invasive evaluation of patients of acute abdomen having pathology of liver, gallbladder, CBD, pancreas, appendix, kidney, ovaries, or uterus. Transvaginal USG is another helpful procedure in evaluating gynecological conditions. It is useful in demonstrating intra-abdominal fluid-being it ascites, pus or blood, localized or diffused. CT scan becomes superior when USG findings are not very accurate on account of gas-filled bowel. CT scan is very helpful in accurately diagnosing pancreatitis, hemorrhagic pathology and mesenteric vessel thrombosis.

DIAGNOSTIC LAPAROSCOPY

Laparoscopic evaluation of peritoneal cavity is useful in detecting the presence of pus, feces, bile or blood. Laparoscopy offers an organ specific diagnosis and at the same time provides treatment, thereby avoid the need for laparotomy. Its application depends on the surgeon's experience and prompt access to laparoscopic instrumentation. Laparoscopy is found to be useful especially in female to know the source of right lower quadrant pain. Many favor the laparoscopic appendicectomy in emergency although

its benefits are marginal but found to be attractive in very obese patient, where it significantly reduces the wound complication.

ACUTE APPENDICITIS

It has been recognized as one of the most common causes of acute abdominal pain worldwide. It is characterized by inflammation of the appendix. If untreated, mortality is high, mainly because of peritonitis and shock. No single sign, symptom, or diagnostic test accurately confirms the diagnosis of appendicitis in all cases.

PATHOPHYSIOLOGY

Acute appendicitis may result from obstruction of the lumen of the appendix either by fecalith, epithelial debris or worms. Once obstruction occurs in the appendix, it gets filled with mucus secretion and bacterial overgrowth, which results in increase of the pressures within the lumen. This results in thrombosis and occlusion of the small vessels, and stasis of lymphatic flow. Rarely, spontaneous recovery can occur at this point. As the disease progresses, the appendix becomes ischemic and then necrotic. Bacteria begin to leak out through the dying walls and pus forms within and around the appendix. The end result of this cascade is appendiceal rupture causing peritonitis, which may lead to septicemia and eventually death if not treated timely.

In clinical practice acute appendicitis can be simple or complicated. Simple acute appendicitis implies inflammation of appendix and complicated when it associated with gangrene or perforation. Another entity is **appendicular mass** which is an inflammatory phlegmon alongwith omentum and adjacent viscera, which cover the complicated appendix. If the pus develops within the mass it is known as appendicular abscess.

SYMPTOMS

The typical history in a patient with appendicitis includes pain starting in the peri-umbilical region (referred pain) which shifts to the right iliac fossa (due to the involvement of parietal peritoneum). There is usually associated loss of appetite and fever, although fever is not a necessary symptom. Anorexia is present in about 75% of patients and vomiting may occur in 50% of cases. When vomiting occurs, it nearly always follows the onset of pain. The diagnosis of appendicitis is very unlikely if vomiting precedes the abdominal pain. If an inflamed appendix lies in contact with the bladder or ureter, it can cause irritative voiding symptoms, hematuria, or dysuria.

SIGNS

Tenderness and rebound tenderness in right iliac fossa (RIF) is the commonest finding. In case of a retrocecal appendix, however, even deep pressure in the right lower quadrant may fail to elicit tenderness. Similarly, if the appendix lies entirely within the pelvis, there is usually complete absence of the abdominal rigidity. In such cases, a digital rectal examination elicits tenderness in the recto-vesical pouch. The Rovsing's sign (pain in the right lower quadrant on deep palpation of the left lower quadrant), the obturator sign (right lower quadrant pain with internal rotation of the flexed right hip), and the psoas sign (right lower quadrant pain with hyperextension of the right hip) can be present. However, absence of these signs should never be used to rule out appendiceal inflammation.

INVESTIGATIONS

Laboratory Investigation

Total leukocyte count (TLC) is raised in 80 % of all cases of acute appendicitis, usually in the range of 12,000–14,000/cc.

Radiological Investigations

X-ray

It has never been considered as routine or mandatory component of evaluation. Pneumoperitoneum in abdominal radiograph suggest diagnosis other than acute appendicitis. Rarely perforated appendix may present as a pneumoperitoneum.

Ultrasonography

Features which suggest appendicitis on ultrasonography includes:
- Non compressible appendix with anteroposterior dimension of 7 mm or more (Fig. 1.2).
- Echogenic periappendiceal mesenteric/omental fat
- Localized periappendiceal fluid collection.
- Presence of appendicolith with a localized probe tenderness is highly suggestive of acute appendicitis.
- Gaseous distension of right lower quadrant bowel loops may suggest perforation, CT would be preferred in such condition.

In some cases (15% approximately) ultrasonography of the iliac fossa does not reveal any abnormalities despite the presence of appendicitis. Acute appendicitis is mostly a clinical diagnosis and the utility of ultrasound is more to rule out other diseases which may be confused with appendicitis, especially in female patients. It is a non-invasive, rapidly available and avoids any radiation exposure.

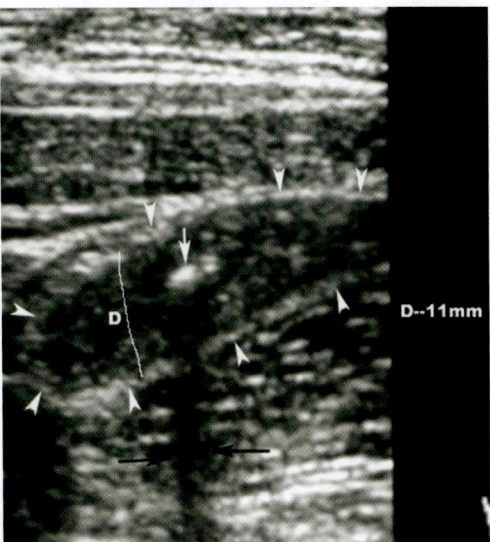

Fig. 1.2: Showing ultrasound finding of acute appendicitis, white arrow points to appendicolith, D is the diameter of the appendix measuring more than 7 mm

CT Scan

CT scan has got 95% sensitivity and specificity to diagnose acute appendicitis. Features of appendicitis on CT scan include.

- Enlarged appendix greater than 6 mm in diameter on cross-section (Fig. 1.3A)
- Lack of oral contrast in the appendix
- Appendiceal wall enhancement with intravenous contrast
- Appendicolith (Fig. 1.3B)

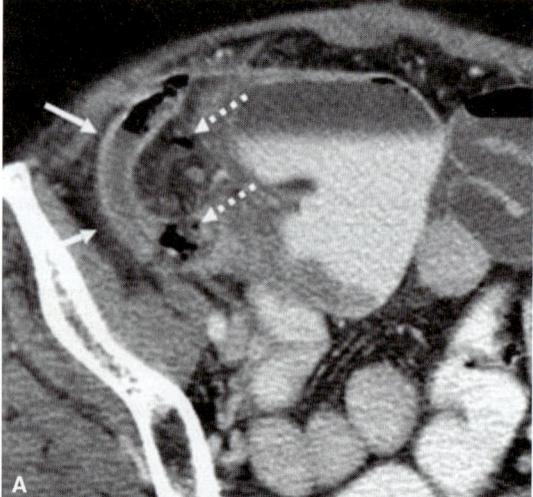

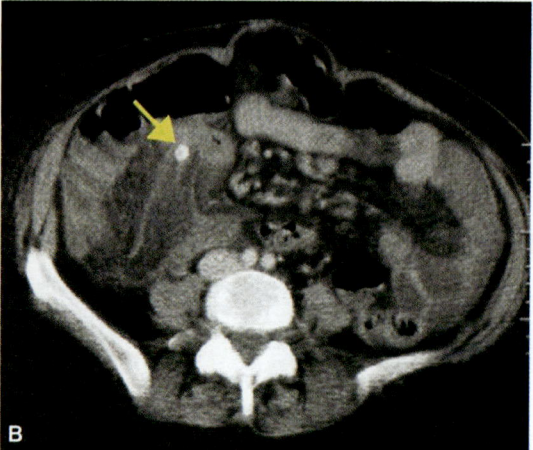

Figs 1.3A and B: CT scan finding of acute appendicitis with appendicolith

- Fat stranding around the appendix
- Cecal wall thicking
- Phlegmon in right lower quadrant
- Abscess or extraluminal gas
- Fluid in right lower quadrant of pelvis.

TREATMENT

Treatment of acute appendicitis is appendicectomy. Prior to the operation, patient is kept nil- per- oral with intravenous fluids for hydration. Intravenous antibiotics like ciprofloxacin and metronidazole are administered to cover against gram-negative bacterias and anerobes.

It is a useful practice to palpate the abdomen once the patient is anesthetized which allows better detection of an appendicular mass.

Appendicectomy

Classically the incision lies over McBurney's point; which is a surface marking at the junction of lateral one-third and medial two-thirds of an imaginary line joining the right anterior superior iliac spine and the umbilicus. An incision is made perpendicular to this line which is known as the gridiron or McBurney's incision (Fig. 1.4A). Another commonly used incision is Lanz incision which is made horizontally over McBurney's point along the skin crease. A lower midline laparotomy incision should be considered in patients where the diagnosis is doubtful.

The skin incision given, the subcutaneous fat is divided down to the external oblique aponeurosis which is cut in the line of the incision (Fig. 1.4B). Internal oblique muscle is then split in direction opposite to the original incision. Peritoneum is then picked by two forceps and opened by scalpel blade in the line of incision. If there is purulent or seropurulent fluid present in the peritoneal cavity, then sample is taken for culture.

Caecum is identified and the taeniae are followed down to base of the appendix. Attempt is then made to deliver the caecum and appendix through the wound. In case of difficulty in delivery the incision is enlarged by dividing the fibers of internal oblique (Rutherford Morrison).

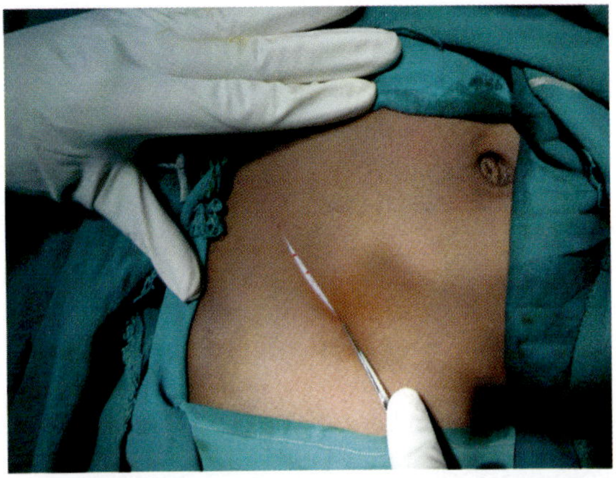

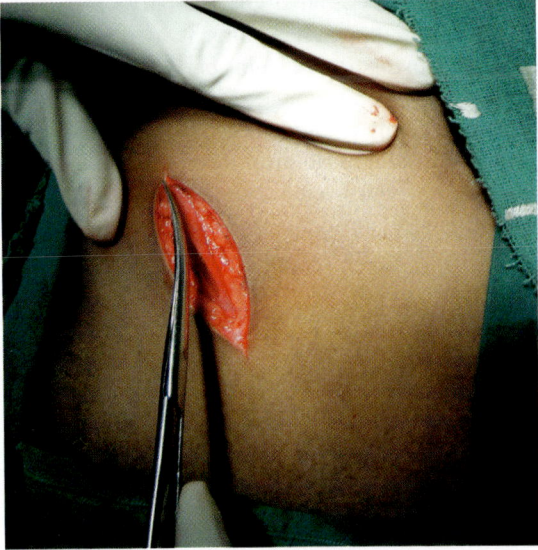

Fig. 1.4A: McBurney's incision for appendicectomy

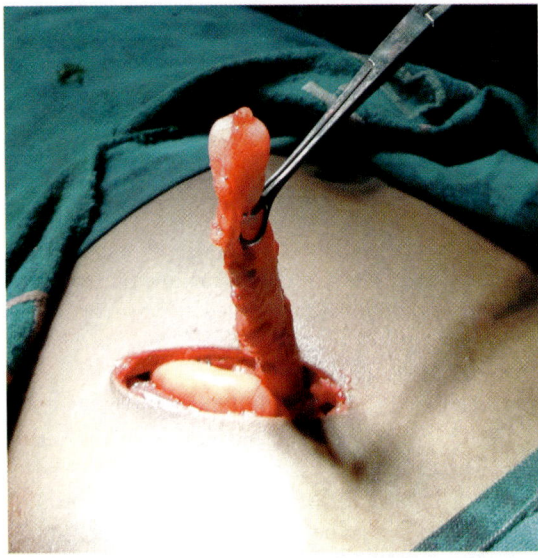

Fig. 1.4C: Appendix is delivered out of the incision and is held with babcock forceps

Fig. 1.4B: External oblique is cut

Once the appendix is delivered it should be held with a babcock forceps (Fig. 1.4C). The meso-appendix containing appendicular artery is then clipped and divided and the pedicles tied with absorbable vicryl suture.

The base of the appendix is crushed and ligated the appendix is then divided with a scalpel blade (Fig. 1.4D). The stump of appendix is buried with

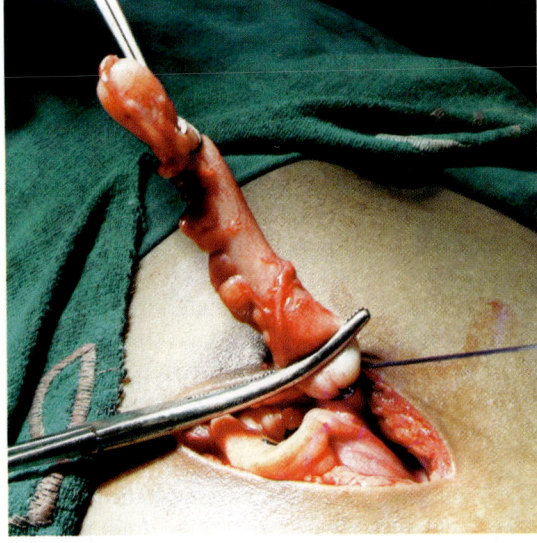

Fig. 1.4D: Base of appendix ligated with vicryl suture

either a purse string or a 'Z' stitch. In case the base is unhealthy it should not be buried. After confirming the hemostasis and cleaning the area the peritoneum is closed using a continuous absorbable suture. The muscle fibers can be loosely approximated with some interrupted stitches. The external oblique defect must be securely repaired with a continuous absorbable suture. Skin is closed with interrupted nylon sutures.

Problems during Appendicectomy

- If there is difficulty in hooking the appendix or exposure is poor or adhesions are present then incision should be extended by converting to Rutherford Morrison incision (muscle cutting incision).
- If there is difficulty in finding appendix (appendix may be retrocecal and buried in the retroperitoneum) trace the taenia coli up to the base. If it is buried, the peritoneal reflection lateral to the colon should be incised and cecum is mobilized to see the posterior aspect.
- If base of the appendix and cecal wall is unhealthy then unhealthy (necrotic/gangrenous) part of the cecum is excised and defect in the cecum is closed with interrupted vicryl suture.
- If appendix is normal, then try to search for other pathology like Meckel's diverticulum, mesenteric lymphadenitis, terminal ileitis, ectopic pregnancy or torsion of ovarian cysts in females. If the appendix looks macroscopically normal and no other pathology is found then also appendicectomy should be done as patients with a right iliac fossa scar will be assumed to have had an appendicectomy by other medical staff. Moreover, 15% of macroscopically normal appendixes prove to be acute appendicitis under microscopy.
- If tip is adherent to cecum retrograde appendicectomy should be tried starting at base and proceeding forward.
- On opening, if an abscess or appendicular mass is found, then abscess need to be drain and if it possible to remove the appendix safely, appendicectomy is carried out. Otherwise, appendicectomy is planned after 4–6 weeks (interval appendicectomy).
- If the base of the appendix and cecum is unhealthy then abdominal drain should be placed.

- In case of caecal malignancy or suspicision of carcinoma tumor more than 2 cm, right hemicolectomy should be done.
- If terminal ileitis found then appendicectomy should not be done.
- At many times during exploration of cecum the purulent fluid tracking down the right paracolic gutter may suggest perforated duodenal ulcer or acute cholecystitis. In such condition a second upper abdominal incision may require to deal the perforated duodenal ulcer, whereas acute cholecystitis if found may be treated conservatively.

Role of Laparoscopic Appendicectomy

In cases of appendicitis, coma laparoscopic appendicectomy is also an alternative approach. Laparoscopic appendicectomy is associated with reduced postoperative pain, early discharge and lower incidence of wound infection. Laparoscopic appendicectomy if performed in complicated cases may lead to complications. Liberal use of diagnostic laparoscopy in suspected appendicitis has led to high incidence of unnecessary removal of normal appendix. The emerging consensus in this regard is to leave the normal appendix and relatives of patient is informed accordingly. But in cases of open surgery appendix should be removed in order not to confuse with appendicitis in future.

No drain should be put unless required, as in conditions like appendicular abscess, perforation or fecal contamination due to cecal perforation.

Appendicitis in Pregnancy and Children

Diagnosis of appendicitis in pregnant patient is confusing because of the location of appendix and the tenderness in abdomen varies with gestational period. Even the raised TLC, nausea, vomiting and anorexia can also be associated pregnancy. Therefore any suspicion of appendicitis in pregnancy, early surgical interference and appendicectomy in all the trimester should be performed. Negative laparotomy results in minimal fetal loss, whereas delay in diagnosis may cause appendicular perforation and gangrene with peritonitis which is responsible for high incidence of fetal death, maternal morbidity, and mortality. Laparoscopic appendicectomy is preferred in first and second trimester of pregnancy.

Acute appendicitis in young children as well as in elderly should be taken for the surgery early due to non development of omentum in children and associated atherosclerosis of the vessel with a possibility of gangrenous change in older people.

Management of Appendicular Mass (Ochsner Sherren Regime)

It includes
- Nil by mouth
- Analgesics for relieve of pain
- Antibiotics to cover most of the organisms
- Measuring the size of right iliac fossa lump
- Recording of pulse rate and temperature charting.
  Indication for abandoning the conservative management are:
  - Rising pulse rate
  - Persistent, sustained fever over 36 hours
  - Persistence of pain despite analgesia
  - Increase in size of the lump or area of tenderness
  - Fluctuation or skin edema and redness.
In all such condition, surgery should be undertaken.

ACUTE CHOLECYSTITIS

Emergency admission for acute cholecystitis is quite common. Acute cholecystitis is most often caused by cholelithiasis (95% of the cases). It occurs due to blockage of the cystic duct by the stones. This leads to inspissation (thickening) of bile, bile stasis, and secondary infection by gut organisms, predominantly *E. coli* and *Bacteroides* species.

SYMPTOMS

Cholecystitis usually presents as pain in the right upper quadrant. The pain is constant, and lasts for hours. The pain may be referred to the right flank or right scapular region (Boas's sign). Typically, an attack subsides in 2 to 3 days and completely resolves in a week. Symptoms of biliary colic are self limiting, disappearing with in few hours, whereas in acute cholecystitis the symptoms and signs persists. Further it is accompanied by local (local peritonitis or tender mass) or systemic (fever and leukocytosis) evidence of inflammation, whereas such features are not found in biliary colic. Presence of high grade fever, shock and jaundice indicates the development of complications such as empyema, perforation or ascending cholangitis.

SIGNS

Low grade fever and tenderness in right upper quadrant are classically seen in cases of acute cholecystitis. **Murphy's sign** is tested by gently placing the hand below the costal margin on the right side at the mid-clavicular line. Patients will experience pain and will catch the breath just before the zenith of inspiration.

Boas's sign is hyperesthesia (increased or altered sensitivity) below the right scapula can be a present in acute cholecystitis.

DIFFERENTIAL DIAGNOSIS

Differential diagnosis includes peptic ulcer disease, liver abscess, and acute pancreatitis, renal colic and acute appendicitis.

INVESTIGATIONS

Blood Investigations

Routine blood investigation with liver function test is essential. TLC is usually elevated. Deranged liver function test with raised direct bilirubin and alkaline phosphatase may indicate choledocholithiasis.

Radiology

Ultrasonography is a sensitive and specific modality for diagnosing acute cholecystitis. The two major diagnostic criteria are cholelithiasis and sonographic

Murphy's sign. Other criterias are gallbladder wall thickening greater than 3 mm, mucosal separation, pericholecystic fluid collection, gallbladder distension, GB hydrops (AP diameter >5 cm) and intramural air.

The reported sensitivity and specificity of CT scan is in the range of 90–95%. CT is more sensitive than ultrasonography in the depiction of pericholecystic inflammatory response and in localizing pericholecystic fluid/abscesses and pericholecystic gas.

Hepatobiliary scintigraphy with technetium-99m DISIDA/HIDA (hydroxyiminodiacetic acid) is also sensitive and accurate for diagnosis of chronic and acute cholecystitis. Non-visualization of gallbladder with visualization of the tracer in common bile duct and small intestine is consistent with cystic duct obstruction. It has a sensitivity of 95%. This can be used if the ultrasound findings are not consistent with clinical diagnosis of cholecystitis.

It is advisable to do MR/MRCP in cases of deranged LFT, dilated CBD and past history of jaundice in conjunction with USG which has got the sensitivity and specificity of more than 80% for detecting CBD stones.

Ultrasound is the most commonly performed investigation to diagnose acute cholecystitis. CT scan is mostly performed to rule out other acute condition like pancreatitis.

TREATMENT

Patients with acute cholecystitis need to be hospitalized. Traditionally patients are managed conservatively with nil per oral, nasogastric aspiration, and intravenous fluids. Intravenous antibiotics (ciprofloxacin and metronidazole) are administered to cover gram-negative bacteria and anerobes. Analgesics are given for pain relieve.

Role of Surgery

All cases are readmitted for elective cholecystectomy at 6–12 weeks after resolution of acute episode.

Recently, there has been change in the policy of interval cholecystectomy and surgeons had been performing open cholecystectomy for acute cholecystitis which is found to be safe and gives rapid recovery. The role of urgent laparoscopic cholecystectomy had also gained importance which is technically easier within 2–4 days of starting of symptoms, but should always be performed by experienced surgeon. At times, conversion to open operation is required if it is not possible to satisfactorily demonstrate the anatomy. Male sex, advancing age, obesity, thickened gallbladder wall gallbladder with surrounding adhesion and complicated cholecystitis are also important factors for conversion to open cholecystectomy.

- In most of the cases of acute cholecystitis, when the risk of surgery is small, either open or laparoscopic cholecystectomy can be done within 2–4 days after the start of symptoms.
- Open cholecystectomy is preferred in cases of gallbladder perforation, empyema, gangrene and acalculous cholecystitis of gallbladder.

In cases of severe sepsis and co-morbid condition where patient is unfit for cholecystectomy, percutaneous cholecystostomy provides an alternative to cholecystectomy. Percutaneous cholecystostomy is performed radiologically under USG or CT guidance. Cholecystectomy is done at a later stage after the patient has been stabilized fully.

Complication of Surgery

Most important complication following gallbladder surgery is damage to bile duct in open as well as laparoscopic surgery. Over all incidence of bile duct injury is approximately 0.3–0.5%.

Basic guidelines for preventing the iatrogenic bile duct injury during laparoscopic/open cholecystectomy are:

- Maximum cephalic fundal traction for visualization of calot's triangle.
- Lateral inferior traction at Hartmann's pouch to open the angel between cystic duct and common hepatic duct.

- Dissection should start at the neck of the gallbladder, and proceed from lateral to medial direction.
- Clips to be placed close to the gallbladder after visualizing both their limbs.
- Avoid electrocautery near the CBD and applied clips.
- Bleeding to be controlled after accurate identification of the source.
- Dissection should be close to gallbladder during removal from liver bed.

While doing open surgery adequate incision, good retraction and able assistance help in proper exposure and safe cholecystectomy. All above precaution should be taken during cholecystectomy. During open surgery if the anatomy is not clear a cholecystostomy or a partial cholecystectomy is the preferred option.

Special Situation

In problematic situation like fibrotic triangle of calot, portal hypertension or in coagulopathy, partial or subtotal cholecystectomy is advocated. Gallbladder is resected starting at fundus, the posterior wall is left attached to hepatic bed and its rim is diathermized or over sewen with the running suture. Aserhirshberg has summarized it aptly, it is better to remove 95% of gallbladder (subtotal cholecystectomy) than 101% (together with a piece of bile duct).

Percutaneous cholecystostomy has been considered as a useful procedure for patients of acute cholecystitis with severe sepsis, co-morbidity and those not fit for surgery. Many surgeons prefer the percutaneous cholecystostomy as treatment of choice for acalculous cholecystitis followed by interval cholecystectomy.

In the recent era, laparoscopic cholecystectomy has emerged as the gold standard treatment for gallbladder disease.

Choledocholithiasis associated with Acute Cholecystitis

Some patients do suffer from acute cholecystitis with stone in bile duct but is rarely combined with acute pancreatitis, acute cholangitis or jaundice. The emphasis should be on treatment of acute cholecystitis. Ductal stone if present is secondary and can be dealt later on.

Acalculous Cholecystitis

Acute cholecystitis can sometimes occur without the presence of stones and is known as acalculous cholecystitis. It is mostly seen in patients with uremia, shock, burns, patients on intravenous feedings for a long-time, severe viral infection or in immunocompromised conditions. The actual pathogenesis of acalculous cholecystitis is believed to be related with bile stasis and gallbladder ischemia. Gallbladder thickness with no gallstone in ultrasound confirms the diagnosis of acalculous cholecystitis. Clinically diagnosis is extremely difficult in cases of acalculous cholecystitis in postoperative cases following major surgery, critically ill and traumatized patients, as the abdominal complains are masked in these cases. Whenever suspected, diagnosis needs to be confirmed by ultrasound. CT scan has been shown to be equally good in diagnosing acalculous cholecystitis. Acalculous cholecystitis rapidly progress to necrosis and perforation. Therefore, early cholecystectomy is indicated. Whenever cholecystectomy is not possible, percutaneous cholecystostomy may be undertaken. It has been observed that subsequent interval cholecystectomy is rarely required.

During investigation of acute abdomen for pain in the right upper quadrant, gallbladder sludge and polyps may accidentally be noted in USG. Biliary sludges are generally the microliths and they settle in majority of time with conservative management. Polyps if demonstrated in patients who are symptomatic should always undergo for interval cholecystectomy. In the absence of symptoms, patients having solitary polyp of size more than 10 mm should also be treated by cholecystectomy as they are associated with increase incidence of malignancy.

ACUTE PANCREATITIS

Acute pancreatitis is defined as acute inflammation of the pancreas. Gallstone and alcohol comprise 80% of all cases of acute pancreatitis. The etiology in males is more often related to alcohol and in females to biliary tract disease (gallstone).

ETIOLOGY

A common mnemonic for the causes of pancreatitis spells "I get smashed", an elusion to heavy drinking (one of the many causes):

- I Idiopathic
- G Gallstone. Gallstones that travel down the common bile duct and subsequently get stuck in the ampulla of Vater causes obstruction in the outflow of pancreatic juices to the duodenum. The backflow of these digestive juices lead to lysis (dissolving) of pancreatic cells and subsequent pancreatitis.
- E Ethanol (alcohol)
- T Trauma
- S Steroids
- M Mumps (paramyxovirus) and other viruses (Epstein-Barr virus, cytomegalovirus)
- A Autoimmune disease (Polyarteritis nodosa, Systemic lupus erythematosus)
- S Scorpion sting (e.g. Tityus trinitatis), and also snake bites
- H Hypercalcemia, hyperlipidemia/hypertrigly-ceridemia, hyperparathyroidism
- E ERCP (Endoscopic retrograde cholangio-pancreatography)
- D Drugs (SAND—steroids and sulfonamides, azathioprine, NSAIDS, diuretics such as furosemide and thiazides, didanosine)

Acute pancreatitis can be mild or severe. Mild pancreatitis has minimal organ dysfunction and usually has uneventful recovery. whereas severe pancreatitis is associated with features of systemic inflammatory response syndrome (SIRS) or multiple organ dysfunction syndrome (MODS) and/or local complication such as necrosis, pseudocyst and abscess. According to Atlanta conference the pancreatic necrosis is defined as diffuse or local area of nonviable pancreatic parenchyma typically associated with peripancreatic fat necrosis.

PATHOPHYSIOLOGY

The association between the etiological factors and pathogenesis remains poorly understood. Early in the course of acute pancreatitis, acinar cells exhibit ultrastructural changes of ischemia. Next follows disruption of cell membrane by lysolecithin from phospholipase activity; near by tissues by proteases lipases; and blood vessel by elastase. Extravascular leukocytes, platelet accumulation and fibrin deposition follows, whilst edema, hemorrhage and necrosis spread along peripancreatic planes. Within the peritoneal cavity, an aseptic exudates forms and fat necrosis produces yellow and white 'studs'. The inflammatory cell mediators, the cytokines, interleukins and oxygen derived free radical amplify the local responses. The circulatory absorption of these will manifest as systemic symptoms.

However, the exact trigger events of pathogenesis is still elusive. The various proposed etiology of pathogenesis includes biliary reflux, pancreatic duct hypertension or obstruction, reflux of activated enzyme, hypoxemia, free radical production and vascular endothelial injury.

SYMPTOMS

The cardinal symptom of acute pancreatitis is upper abdominal pain usually in the epigastric region, which is characteristically dull aching, sudden in onset and gradually intensifies in severity. The pain radiates to the back which is relieved on sitting and aggravated by lying down. In approximately half of the cases nausea and vomiting are often present along with anorexia. In its severe form patient may presents with shock or respiratory distress (pleural effusion or ARDS).

PHYSICAL SIGNS

Fever and tachycardia are common abnormal vital signs. Abdominal tenderness, muscular guarding, and distension are observed in most patients. Bowel sounds are often hypoactive due to paralytic ileus. Guarding tends to be more pronounced in the upper abdomen. A minority of patient exhibit jaundice. Some patients experience dyspnea, which may be caused by irritation of the diaphragm (resulting from inflammation), pleural effusion, or a more serious condition, such as acute respiratory distress syndrome.

Patients with severe acute pancreatitis are often pale, diaphoretic, and listless. Hemodynamic instability may be evident in some cases. The Cullen's sign is a bluish discoloration around the umbilicus resulting from hemoperitoneum. The Grey Turner's sign is a reddish-brown discoloration along the flanks resulting from retroperitoneal blood dissecting along tissue planes. Erythematous skin nodules may result from focal subcutaneous fat necrosis. All these signs may not be observed in all cases of acute pancreatitis.

Rarely, abnormalities on fundoscopic examination may be seen in severe pancreatitis termed Purtscher retinopathy. This ischemic injury to the retina appears to be caused by activation of complement and agglutination of blood cells within retinal vessels. It may cause temporary or permanent blindness.

INVESTIGATIONS

Blood Investigations

Full blood count, blood sugar, renal function test, liver function test, serum calcium, serum amylase and lipase, arterial blood gas, serum LDH all should be done in suspected cases of acute pancreatitis.

a. **Amylase:** Usually the serum amylase level starts rising from 2 to 12 hours after the onset of symptoms and peaks at 12 to 72 hours. It usually returns to normal within one week. Although it lacks sensitivity and specificity, the measurement of the serum amylase level is the most widely used method of diagnosing pancreatitis. However, a variety of non pancreatic conditions also result in increased amylase levels. The urinary amylase strips may provide rapid screening. Hyper-amylasemia should be excluded in every case of acute abdomen.

b. **Lipase:** Lipase levels increase within 4 to 8 hours of the onset of clinical symptoms and peak at about 24 hours. Levels decrease within 8 to 14 days. The specificity (50 to 99%) and sensitivity (86 to 100%) of lipase measurements are better than those of amylase.

c. **C- reactive protein :** Increased level of C- reactive protein >150 mg/dl, indicates more severity of the acute pancreatitis.

Imaging

X-ray

Chest X-ray is helpful in excluding the perforated viscus or presence of plural effusion. Abdominal X-rays may show "sentinel loop" (dilated duodenum and proximal jejunum due to localized ileus) or "colon cut off" sign (gas-filled ascending and transverse colon and failure to visualize descending colon). Plain X-ray at times may also reveal the calcified gallstone and pancreatic calcinosis.

Computed Tomography

The current gold standard for diagnosis of acute pancreatitis and pancreatic necrosis is dynamic contrast enhanced computed tomography which also help in grading its severity. If possible high quality multislice spiral unit is preferable for evaluation.

Indication: CT abdomen should not be performed before the first 48 hours of onset of symptoms as early CT (<48 h) may result in equivocal or normal findings. Baseline CT scan (with oral and intravenous contrast) is indicated in the following situations:

- The diagnosis is in doubt,
- Severe pancreatitis is suspected because of high fever (> 38.8°C), distention, leukocytosis),
- Patient has an elevated severity score as determined by the MODS or APACHE II criteria,
- Patients with persisting organ failure, signs of sepsis, or deterioration in clinical status.

Findings in CT Scan (Fig. 1.5)

Intrapancreatic	Diffuse or segmental enlargement, edema, gas bubbles, pancreatic pseudocysts and phlegmons/abscesses.
Peripancreatic/extrapancreatic	Irregular pancreatic outline, obliterated peripancreatic fat, retroperitoneal edema, fluid in the lessar sac, fluid in the left anterior pararenal space.
Locoregional	Gerota's fascia sign (thickening of inflamed Gerota's fascia, which becomes visible), pancreatic ascites, pleural effusion (seen on basal cuts of the pleural cavity), adynamic ileus.

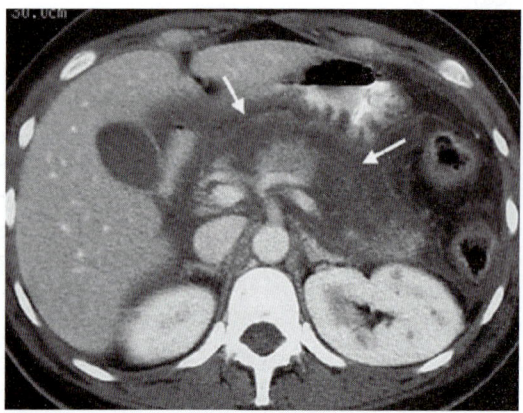

Fig.1.5: CECT showing peripancreatic and retroperitoneal edema (arrow)

Balthazar Scoring for the Grading of Acute Pancreatitis

The CT Severity Score is the sum of the CT Grade and Necrosis Grade Scores.

CT Grade	Appearance on CT	CT Points
Grade A	Normal CT	0 points
Grade B	Focal or diffuse enlargement of the pancreas	1 point
Grade C	Pancreatic gland abnormalities and peripancreatic inflammation	2 points
Grade D	Fluid collection in a single location usually in anterior pararenal space	3 points

Grade E	Two or more fluid collections and/or gas bubbles in or adjacent to pancreas	4 points

Necrosis Percentage	*Points*
No necrosis	0 points
0 to 30% necrosis	2 points
30 to 50% necrosis	4 points
Over 50% necrosis	6 points

CT severity index
= (points for grade of acute pancreatitis) + (points for degree of pancreatic necrosis)

Morality and complications according to the CT severity index is as follows.

Severity index	Mortality	Complications
0–1	0%	0%
2–3	3%	8%
4–6	6%	35%
7–10	17%	92%

PROGNOSTIC INDICES IN ACUTE PANCREATITIS

Ranson's Score

Ranson's score for alcohol and gallstone induced pancreatitis is observed both on admission and after 48 hours.

Ranson's Score (Alcohol induced)

On admission	After 48 hours
1. Age in years > 55 years	1. Calcium (serum calcium < 2.0 mmol/L or < 8.0 mg/dL)
2. White blood cell count > 16000 cells/mm^3	2. Hematocrit fall > 10%
3. Blood glucose > 11 mmol/L (> 200 mg/dL)	3. Oxygen (hypoxemia PO_2 < 60 mmHg)
4. Serum AST > 250 IU/L	4. BUN increased by 1.8 or more mmol/L (5 or more mg/dL) after IV fluid hydration
5. Serum LDH > 350 IU/L	5. Base deficit (negative base excess) > 4 mEq/L
	6. Sequestration of fluids > 6 L

Ranson's Score (Gallstone induced)

On admission	After 48 hours
1. Age in years > 70 years	1. Calcium (serum calcium < 2.0 mmol/L or < 8.0 mg/dL)
2. White blood cell count > 18000 cells/mm^3	2. Hematocrit fall > 10%
3. Blood glucose > 220 mg/dL	3. Oxygen (hypoxemia PO_2 < 60 mmHg)
4. Serum AST > 400 IU/L	4. BUN increased by 2 or more mg/dL after IV fluid hydration
5. Serum LDH > 250 IU/L	5. Base deficit (negative base excess) > 4 mEq/L
	6. Sequestration of fluids > 4 L

Glasgow or Imrie Criteria (Simplified Ranson Criteria for Predicting Severity)

The mnemonics "PANCREAS" makes it easy
- **P** arterial PO_2 < 9 kpa
- **A** albumin < 32 g/l
- **N** Urea nitrogen >10 mmol/l
- **C** calcium<2 mmol/l
- **R** raised white cell count >16 mmol/l
- **E** enzyme LDH > 600 mmol/l
- **A** age> 55 yrs
- **S** sugar: glucose > 10 mmol/l

The presence of three or more criterias reached before or at 48 hr of an attack, predicts a severe attack.

TREATMENT

The patient with acute pancreatitis and necrosis are usually very sick. Most of them have the Ranson's score of more than 3 and APACHE II score of more than 8. Preferably they should be managed in the intensive care unit. Management and monitoring of patient developing necrosis should be more intensive and to be taken care in the following way:
- General management
- Confirmation of diagnosis
- Prevention of infection
- Nutritional support
- Monitoring of complications

Intravenous Fluid and Pain Control

The physiological problem in acute pancreatitis is fluid and electrolyte loss to the third space. That is why accurate and adequate fluid resuscitation is the mainstay in the initial management of acute pancreatitis. Ringer lactate should be the fluid of choice unless contraindicated on account of deranged kidney function. A central venous catheter is necessary when the patient present with shock, fluid correction should be given according to the CVP and it should be maintained at around 8–10 mm Hg. Later on urine output can be taken as guide for fluid requirement.

Pain of acute pancreatitis is severe in nature and in most cases requires administration of narcotics. Meperidine or its analogues are preferred over morphine.

Bowel Rest/Nutritional Support

Patients should be kept nil per oral for at least initial 24 hour to give the bowel rest. Patients should start orally as soon as the nausea decreased or pain subsides or bowel activity returns, normally in mild cases it takes around 24–48 hour.

In patients with mild uncomplicated pancreatitis, no benefit is observed from nutritional support, and the energy (caloric) intake received by the intravenous dextrose 5% is sufficient.

- Oral feedings should be initiated once the patient's pain and anorexia resolve.
- Early initiation of enteral nutritional supplementation and maintenance of a positive nitrogen balance is important in patients with severe pancreatitis in absence of substantial ileus or duodenal obstruction. Thus, in all patients admitted to the ICU, nasojejunal or post pyloric (in which a feeding tube is endoscopically or radiographically introduced to the third portion of the duodenum) feedings should be attempted to maintain a barrier against bacterial translocation.
- TPN should generally be reserved as a second-line therapy behind enteral feeding. Central line feeding is safe and enhances the anabolic response

which prevents the muscle wasting. But the TPN is associated with catheter induced sepsis, electrolyte and metabolic disturbances.

Role of Antibiotics

Studies have not shown benefit of giving antibiotics prophylactically in all cases of acute pancreatitis. However, if the CT scan shows necrosis and there is risk of septic complication, the use of prophylactic antibiotics is appropriate. Many times when secondary infection supervenes it is usually with the resistant bacterias or fungal organism. If antibiotic is used it should only be given for a defined period.

Role of Early ERCP

The role of early ERCP is equally controversial. Urgent ERCP and biliary drainage is indicated in patients with features of ascending cholangitis and presence of CBD stone.

Surgery

Role of emergency surgery is very limited in cases of uncomplicated acute pancreatitis, but in severe episode of acute pancreatitis with following conditions surgery has got definite role.

Indication of Surgery

1. Infected pancreatic or peripancreatic necrosis (Gas bubbles on CT scan or positive bacterial culture on fine needle aspiration, usually CT or US guided) of the pancreas.
2. Irreversible clinical deterioration despite maximum supportive care for two weeks.
3. Pancreatic abscess.

Whenever the patients is subjected to surgery the main objective during surgery should be

- To evaluate the necrotic and infected material
- To drain the toxic product of inflammation
- Prevent reaccumulation of toxic product
- To avoid injury to adjacent visceral and vascular structure.

The current surgical practice in necrotizing pancreatitis involves necrosectomy of the devitalized pancreatic and peripancreatic tissue. Necrosectomy is usually done via a bilateral subcostal incision. Necrosed part of the pancreas is removed by blunt finger dissection technique, taking care of all the viable pancreatic tissue. Whenever necessary, debridement with adequate drainage with facility for irrigation of lesser sac should be done. At times abdomen may be left open (laparostomy) and planed relaparotomy to be done as and when required.

Following necrosectomy local complications are intra-abdominal and retroperitoneal collection, bleeding from pancreatic bed, pancreatic fistula, small bowel and colonic fistula. Forty percent of patients following necrosectomy develops pancreatic fistula, which may often require additional surgery for closure.

Role of Cholecystectomy

It is optimal for patients admitted with gallstone pancreatitis to have a cholecystectomy prior to discharge and not to be postponed for a later date. Patients discharged with gallstone pancreatitis without a cholecystectomy are at high risk for recurrent bouts of pancreatitis.

Complications

Complication of severe acute pancreatitis may be of many fold. ARDS, renal failure, encephalopathy, and GI hemorrhage usually occur in the early phase whereas the bacterial and fungal infection is seen in the intermediate phase and the pancreatic abscess in the late phase.

Life-threatening hemorrhage into the GI tract, retroperitoneum and peritoneal cavity is seen in 1–3%, with mortality of more than 50%. Frequency of vascular necrosis in the form of pseudoaneurysm formation is in the range of 10%. Pancreatic abscess and pseudocyst are the late complications. Percutaneous intervention or surgical drainage is usually successful. Mortality is in the range of 10%. But acute necrotizing pancreatitis with infection may have a very high mortality.

PSEUDOCYST

Pseudocyst is one of the late complications of acute pancreatitis which can be described as fluid-filled cavities arising from the pancreas and surrounded by a wall of fibrous or inflammatory tissue, but lacking an epithelial cover.

According to the Atlanta classification there are four entities of pancreatic pseudocyst:
1. Acute fluid collection, occurring early (< 3 weeks) in the course of acute pancreatitis lacking a wall of granulomatous or fibrous tissue.
2. Acute pseudocyst, a cavity surrounded by fibrous or granulomatous tissue, that is consequence of acute pancreatitis or trauma.
3. Chronic pseudocyst, arising in chronic pancreatitis without preceding episode of acute pancreatitis.
4. Pancreatic abscess, an intra abdominal collection of pus in proximity of pancreas resulting from acute or chronic pancreatitis or trauma.

Diagnosis

A variety of diagnostic tools including CT scan, ultrasonography, ERCP, cyst aspiration, chemistry or cytology are used for diagnosis of pancreatic pseudocyst. USG being inexpensive and non-invasive, should be used as the first line of investigation in the diagnosis of pancreatic pseudocyst, whereas CT scan is mandatory for planning the therapy of pancreatic pseudocyst (Fig. 1.6). CT imaging yields the highest sensitivity of 82–100%. ERCP is less informative regarding the size and surrounding visceral structures than CT and USG. But ERCP renders important information regarding the anatomy of pancreatic and biliary ductal system which becomes helpful in endoscopic therapy.

Treatment

Indication for therapeutic intervention for pancreatic pseudocyst
- Complicated pancreatic pseudocyst
  - Compression of large vessel as seen on CT
  - Gastric duodenal outlet obstruction

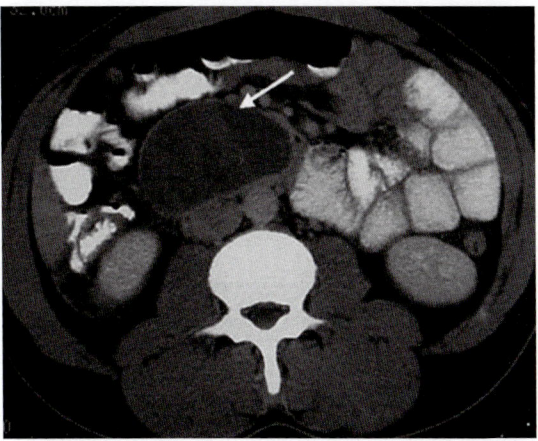

Fig. 1.6: Pseudocyst following acute pancreatitis

-   – Common bile duct obstruction
-   – Hemorrhage into the pancreatic pseudocyst
-   – Infected pancreatic pseudocyst
- Symptomatic pancreatic pseudocyst
  - satiety
  - nausea
  - vomiting
  - pain
  - upper GI bleed
- Pseudocyst more than 5 cm, unchanged in size and morphology for more than 6 weeks.

Pancreatic pseudocyst shows a wide variety of clinical presentations. Cystic pancreatic lesion arising after an episode of acute pancreatitis may resolve without treatment during a period of 4–6 weeks. There are many minimally invasive techniques for the drainage of pseudocyst. The aim of endoscopic drainage treatment is to create a connection between the pseudocyst cavity and gastrointestinal lumen which can be accomplished by either by transpapillary or a transmural approach. The transmural approach requires access through the stomach (cystogastrostomy) or duodenum (cystodudenostomy). Pseudocyst should have a mature capsule (wall >3 mm, <1 cm) impress the stomach wall and have a minimum size of 5–6 cm to become eligible for endoscopic drainage.

Despite recent developments in minimally invasive techniques surgical drainage is still the principal method for the management of pancreatic pseudocyst. It traditionally includes internal drainage.

In case of an infected pseudocyst or in patients with sepsis, percutaneous drainage should be favored.

LIVER ABSCESS

Amoebiasis is a parasitic infestation caused by protozoa *Entamoeba histolytica* (EH). Life cycle of EH has three stages: trophozoite, precyst, and cyst. Infection generally results from ingestion of cyst usually by contaminated water or food.

Ex-cystation takes place in lower ileum and the active trophozoite invades the ileal and colonic mucosa and later get carried away to the liver by the portal venous system. The trophozoites get lodged in the venules of the liver causing thrombosis and then infarction leading to necrosis of liver tissue, usually in upper and posterior portion of the right lobe of liver.

A liver abscess occurs when bacteria or protozoa destroy hepatic tissue, producing a cavity, which fills with infectious organisms, liquefied liver cells, dead RBC and leukocytes. Necrotic tissue then walls off the cavity from the rest of the liver. Therefore, abscess is a collection of liver necrotic tissue, active dead EH, dead RBC and WBC, and all these together form the anchovy sauce because of its characteristic color. 75–90% of abscess gets localized in the right lobe of liver. These protozoa colonize and destroy the liver cells leading to liquefaction and necrosis. Amount of liver destruction depends on the size of the colony of *E.histolytica*, resistance of patients as well as the secondary infection. In 50% of cases the amebic abscess may contain staphylococci and streptococci as well, if gets secondarily infected.

Symptomatology

Common symptoms in acute amebic liver abscess include right hypochondrial pain, weight loss, anorexia, malaise, fever with chills, nausea and vomiting. Referred pain to the right shoulder may be present. Symptoms of right pleural effusion, such as dyspnea and pleural pain can develop if the abscess extends through the diaphragm to pleural cavity. Many patients do have the past history of amebic dysentery with the passage of blood in the stool.

Fever and tender hepatomegaly are the most common signs. Mid-epigastric tenderness is generally seen in cases of left hepatic lobe involvement. Decreased breath sounds in the right basilar lung zones, with signs of atelectasis and effusion may be present. Jaundice may be present in 25% of cases and usually associated with biliary tract disease or with the presence of multiple abscesses.

Course of Amoebic Abscess

- In early stage of infection resolution may occur with proper treatment
- Once abscess forms liver enlarges
- Abscess become encapsulated and remain dormant
- If untreated it may burst into peritoneal cavity or pleural cavity or into right lung.

Investigations

Blood

- Raised WBC (more than 12, 000–30,000/dl)
- Abnormal liver function test with most common abnormality includes elevated prothrombin time
- Positive serology suggest current or previous invasion.

The absence of serum antibodies to *E. histolytica* after 1 week of symptoms is strong evidence against the diagnosis of invasive amoebiasis of the colon or liver. ELISA is very sensitive and easily available method with a sensitivity of more than 90%. The test may be negative in the first week of symptomatology but if found to be positive it is very helpful in differentiating from pyogenic liver abscess. Purified native and recombinant parasitic antigens have been utilized in serological studies with good results. More than 95% of the patients with amoebic liver abscess have serum antibodies to the 170 KD subunit of the galactose inhabitable adherence lectin. This antigen is highly specific for differentiating acute phase serum from convalescent phase serum in areas of high endemicity. Newer diagnostic strategies involve detection of protein antigens in feces or serum by monoclonal antibodies and detection of parasitic DNA by use of nucleotide probes and PCR amplification.

Chest X-Ray

Chest X-ray may show
- Elevated diaphragm
- Pleural effusion.

Ultrasonography

It is inexpensive, easy to perform with a diagnostic accuracy of more than 90%. The classical appearance is a non-homogeneous, hypoechoic, round or oval mass with well defined borders. It is also helpful in defining the site and volume of the abscess. Ultrasound guided percutaneous needle aspiration of the abscess can also be performed with diagnostic as well as therapeutically intention to identify the causative organism.

CECT shows liver abscess as hypoattenuated lesions (Fig. 1.7).

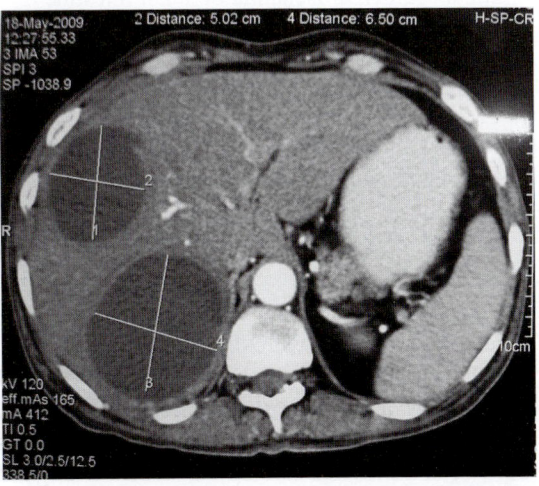

Fig. 1.7: CECT showing liver abscess

Amoebic Liver Abscess

Medical Therapy

Medical therapy should be instituted using either a single agent or a combination of drugs for the extra-luminal parasite. Nitroimidazoles (including metronidazole) are effective in over 90% of cases. Therapy should continue for at least 10 days. The dose of metronidazole is 40 mg/kg/day in divided dosages. Chloroquine, emetine, and dehydroemetine may also be used. Single-agent therapy with metronidazole yields excellent results and the alternative toxic drugs are indicated rarely and used mostly in seriously ill patients when the risk of failure of therapy is unacceptable. The response to anti-amoebic drugs is usually evident within 48–72 hours with the subsidence of signs and symptoms.

Aspiration

The aspirate is anchovy sauce type in half of the patients. The chocolate color is due to admixture of dead RBC and WBC with necrotic liver tissue. Ultrasound and CT guided aspiration is always preferred. The indications are
- Persistence of symptoms despite adequate medical therapy for 48–72 hours
- High chance of rupture because of location and size, rim of liver tissue around the abscess<10 mm
- Suspicion of secondary infection or pyogenic in nature
- Presence of large abscess with previous aspiration more than 250 ml
- Left lobe abscess.

Resolution of the abscess should be followed by repeated ultrasonography or the liver.

Surgery

Indications

- Rupture/impending rupture
- Failure to respond to medical therapy
- Inadequacy in aspiration of left lobe
- Laparotomy is also indicated in patients with multiple liver abscess which are inaccessible for drainage.

Complications

- Pleural effusion (15%), empyema (7%), pneumonitis, lung abscess
- Generalized peritonitis, localized peritonitis and ileus
- Pericardial effusion
- Secondary infection, bacteremia, hepatic failure, hemobilia and brain abscess.

Pyogenic Liver Abscess (PLA)

Pyogenic abscess, which is most often polymicrobial, generally involves both lobes of liver. Cases of liver abscess in infants have been associated with umbilical vein catheterization and sepsis. When abscesses are seen in children and adolescents, underlying immune deficiency, severe malnutrition, or trauma frequently exists.

Biliary tract disease is now the most common source of pyogenic liver abscess. Obstruction of bile flow due to stones, malignancy, stricture or congenital diseases are common predisposing factors. Liver abscess after intra-abdominal sepsis (such as with diverticulitis acute appendicitis) is most likely to be caused by hematogenous spread through the portal bloodstream. Hematogenous spread by hepatic arterial flow may also occur in infectious endocarditis.

Abscesses arising from hematogenous transmission are usually caused by a single pathogen; those arising from biliary obstruction are usually caused by a mixed flora. Pyogenic abscesses usually are multiple. The right hepatic lobe is affected more often than the left hepatic lobe. The predilection for the right hepatic lobe can be attributed to anatomical considerations and vascular supply.

Symptomatology is like that of amebic liver abscess.

Management

Pyogenic liver abscess may become fatal if not diagnosed and treated appropriately. Management of these cases are by USG guided percutaneous drainage with suitable antibiotic coverage according to the sensitivity of pus culture. Most commonly broad spectrum antibiotics should be started, which include a combination of penicillin, aminoglycosides and metronidazole. Usually 4–6 weeks of therapy is required. Initially, antibiotics are given parenterally and then switch over to oral medication depending on response. Surgical drainage becomes mandatory if it does not respond to medical therapy and in presence of sepsis. In multiloculated abscess all efforts should be to break the loculi taking care of hemostasis. Biopsy should always be taken from the wall of the abscess. Drains to be placed before the closure.

ACUTE MESENTERIC ISCHEMIA

INTRODUCTION

Acute mesenteric ischemia (AMI) is not a single entity but refers to a group of disorders with different etiology characterized by reduction of blood supply to the bowel leading to ischemia and eventually to gangrene of bowel wall. It could be arterial or venous in origin. Despite recent advances in diagnosis and treatment, mortality rate continue to remain high. Mesenteric ischemic disorders broadly can be classified into five types:

- Acute mesenteric ischemia
- Chronic mesenteric ischemia
- Mesenteric venous thrombosis
- Focal segmental ischemia of small intestine
- Colonic ischemia.

ETIOLOGY AND CLASSIFICATION

Acute Mesenteric Ischemia

It could be of embolic, thrombotic, or nonocclusive in nature.

Arterial Embolism

Arterial embolism accounts for approximately one-third of acute cases of AMI. The embolizations include mural thrombi after myocardial infarction or arterial thrombi associated with mitral stenosis and atrial fibrillation. Emboli at times may be of malignant origin for example arterial myxoma or renal cell carcinoma. Whatever may be the etiology, the vascular occlusion in acute mesenteric emboli is sudden and patients are unable to develop a collateral flow, therefore leading to worst ischemia in comparison to thrombotic AMI.

Arterial Thrombosis

Arterial thrombosis accounts for another one-third of acute cases of AMI. It is usually due to acute worsening of ischemia in patients who have pre-existing atherosclerosis of the mesenteric arteries. Thrombosis often involves at least two of the major splanchnic vessels. In these conditions patients symptoms do not develop until two or three artery are stenosed or completely blocked. Because of the pre-existing atherosclerotic stenosis they do had the development of collateral circulation. It has been observed that thrombosis tends to occur at the origin of the superior mesenteric artery (SMA). SMA leading to a greater extent of bowel infarction.

Nonocclusive Etiology

This condition is defined as having mesenteric vasoconstriction following hypoperfusion with intestinal necrosis of bowel with a patent arterial tree. It is generally associated with profound illness, sepsis and cardiovascular collapse which in turn lead to marked vasoconstriction to the mesenteric vascular bed. It is supposed to be a lethal form of mesenteric ischemia with a mortality rate more than 70%. The most common setting is severe systemic illness with systemic shock usually secondary to reduced cardiac output, in cocaine ingestion, ergot poisoning, digoxin use, and with alpha-adrenergic agonists or hypercoagulable states.

Mesenteric Venous Thrombosis

This condition is seen in only 5–10% of cases. It occurs in the absence of any identifiable predisposing factor. It usually seen in hematological hypercoagulable state (sickle cell anemia, polycythemia vera, etc.) and inflammatory condition like peritonitis, cholangitis, pancreatitis, etc. It is also observed during the damage control surgery when a portal vein or superior mesenteric vein is ligated in cases of penetrating abdominal injury.

Chronic Mesenteric Ischemia (CMI)

This condition is usually found as an end-stage arthrosclerosis. There is a preponderance among the female. Majority of the patients of chronic mesenteric ischemia do suffer from coronary artery and peripheral vascular disease. This condition is seen mainly affecting the two or more of the vessel supplying the bowel. In cases where there are poorly developed collaterals, even a single vessel occlusion can cause symptom. The characteristic symptomatology is postprandial abdominal pain (abdominal angina), with fear of taking food and weight loss.

Pathophysiology

Mesenteric vessels are known to have rich collateral flow. As a result, gradual occlusion of vessel is well tolerated, if time permits for development of collateral of vessels. Sudden obstruction is poorly tolerated with profound consequences. Compromised bowel mucosa release toxic material to the circulation with systemic consequence. Whenever the serosal surfaces of the bowel get involved, it leads to perforation and peritonitis.

The intestinal mucosa has a high metabolic rate and accordingly, a high blood flow requirement (normally receiving 20 to 25% of cardiac output), making it very sensitive to the effects of decreased perfusion. Ischemia disrupts the mucosal barrier, allowing release of bacteria, toxins, and vasoactive mediators, which in turn leads to myocardial depression, systemic inflammatory response syndrome, multisystem organ failure, and death.

SIGNS AND SYMPTOMS

Usual presentation of AMI includes

- Acute abdominal pain out of proportion to tenderness
- Gut emptying at the onset of pain
- Distension of abdomen
- Blood diarrhea as result of mucosal shading
- Associated oliguria
- Metabolic acidosis

Mesenteric ischemia is generally a disease of the older population, with the typical age of onset being older than 60 years; however, with risk factors and other predisposing factors, it may be seen in younger patients. The clinical presentation is largely dependent on the underlying etiology. The classic picture of a patient with AMI involves severe abdominal pain mostly central, dull aching, poorly localized with minimal response to opioids and paucity of significant abdominal findings. Patient usually gives a similar type of history, often related to meals (intestinal angina). Nausea and vomiting are frequent, and diarrhea may occur in as many as 50% of patients with mesenteric ischemia. The classic triad of SMA embolism includes GI emptying, abdominal pain with underlying cardiac disease. Sudden onset of pain may suggest the possibility of arterial embolism (although not diagnostic), whereas a more gradual onset is typical of venous thrombosis.

The abdomen is usually soft with little or no tenderness. Mild tachycardia may be present. Later, as necrosis develops, signs of peritonitis appear, with marked abdominal tenderness, guarding, rigidity, and absent bowel sounds. Melena or hematochezia occurs in 15% of cases, and occult blood is detected in approximately 50% of patients. Alternative diagnosis like severe acute pancreatitis, perforated viscus, ruptured aneurysm should always be excluded.

INVESTIGATION

Laboratory

- Leukocytosis of more than 15,000 cell/mm^3 is seen in approximately 75% of cases
- Hyperamylasemia – raised serum and peritoneal fluid amylase
- Metabolic acidosis due to raised serum D-lactate level
- Raised serum D-dimer level is present in all cases of AMI irrespective of etiology.

All these features are not usually seen in chronic mesenteric ischemia.

X-ray Abdomen

Plain abdominal X-rays are useful mainly to rule out other causes of pain (e.g. perforated viscus). There is pattern of adynamic ileus with dilatation of small and large intestines with fluid levels and portal venous gas or pneumatosis intestinalis may be seen late in the disease.

Duplex Ultrasound

It is non invasive and useful test for evaluating the mesenteric vasculature and is generally considered as an imaging modality of choice in chronic mesenteric ischemia.

CT Scan

It is not the preferred evaluation technique for detecting the vascular abnormalities in mesenteric ischemia. The catheter angiography is a better choice, however, the CT scan is useful to find the sequels of AMI which include bowel wall thickening and luminal dilatation. Late signs include air in the intestinal wall and mesenteric/ portal venous system which is typical of necrosis of bowel.

Angiography

This is the gold standard test for mesenteric artery ischemia. Patients with clear peritoneal signs should directly undergo exploratory laparotomy for both diagnosis and treatment. For others, selective mesenteric angiography is the diagnostic and therapeutic procedure of choice. Four reliable angiographic criteria for diagnosis of AMI are:

- Narrowing of the multiple branches of SMA
- Alternate dilation and narrowing of intestinal branches
- Spasm of mesenteric arcades
- Impaired filling of intramural vessels.

Early diagnosis is particularly important because mortality increases significantly once intestinal infarction has occurred. Mesenteric ischemia must be considered in any patient > 50 years of age with known risk factors or predisposing conditions who develops sudden, severe abdominal pain.

TREATMENT

The principle of treatment are adequate hydration, broad spectrum antibiotics and early surgical intervention. CVP monitoring and urine output guides the fluid resuscitation. Various studies had showed improved survival following early diagnosis and aggressive management using preoperative aortography and selective injection of intra-arterial papaverine, prostaglandin E1 and tolazoline into the SMA via angiographic catheter. Intra-arterial papaverine during angiography can be used regardless of the etiology of the intestinal ischemia. Papaverine is an opium derivative that functions as a phosphodiesterase inhibitor, which acts to relax vascular smooth muscle. It is usually infused directly into the SMA, thus improving intestinal blood flow.

Definitive treatment options depend on the etiology of intestinal ischemia as well as the hemodynamic stability of the patient.

The use of papaverine is for the relief of vasoconstriction and to prevent progressive ischemia and thus avoid laparotomy. Papaverine has resulted significant reduction in mortality of these patients. Papaverine given as 60 mg bolus over 2 min, followed by an infusion of 30 to 60 mg/h is useful even when surgical intervention is planned and is sometimes given during and after surgical intervention as well. Use of papaverine helps in reducing the length of intestinal resection.

Surgical embolectomy by exposing the SMA or retrogradely via ileocolic arteries are the preferred option. If there is any doubt regarding the embolectomy then anastomosis of ileocolic artery to the common iliac artery should be performed. Intra-arterial thrombolysis is another option.

Papaverine infusion and arterial reconstruction either through aorto-superior mesenteric arterial bypass grafting or reimplantation of the SMA to the aorta are the preferred option.

For nonocclusive mesenteric ischemia, papaverine infusion is the mainstay of treatment. For mesenteric venous thrombosis, anticoagulation with heparin/warfarin either alone or in combination with surgery is the preferred treatment. For chronic mesenteric ischemia (MI), management options include angioplasty with or without stent placement or surgical revascularization. Several studies have found, a high rate of success with percutaneous stent revascularization for CMI, although repeated interventions may be necessary.

All cases of mesenteric ischemia with signs of peritonitis, regardless of the etiology, require immediate surgical intervention for the resection of ischemic or necrotic intestines.

If there is generalized patchy ischemia of bowel which appears to be reversible, then proximal superior mesenteric artery is exposed at base and pulsation and flow is assessed by Doppler ultrasonography. In case of thrombus, thrombectomy is done and arteriotomy is closed by patch angioplasty.

The main difficulty at laparotomy is to predict intestinal recovery and thus accurately assess the length of bowel that need to be resected. Clinical assessment depends on the color, contractility and capillary bleeding. Although 70% of small bowel can be resected without any nutritional consequences, however, it is essential to document accurately how much bowel is removed and the length and type of bowel which remains. This will enable the probable consequences for nutrition to be assessed, if further resection is required at later date. The decision to perform a second look surgery 24 hour, later is made at the time of first surgery. The bowel ends are exteriorized or cross stapled if a second look surgery is planed. Primary anastomosis should not be performed. All patients should be anticoagulated with heparin.

Mortality/Morbidity

Mortality rates are high and range from 60 to 100% depending on the source of obstruction. Early and aggressive diagnosis and treatment has been shown to significantly decrease the mortality rate if the diagnosis is made prior to the development of peritonitis.

For Perforation Peritonitis and Intestinal Obstruction—Please see the respective chapters.

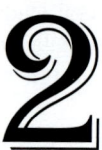

Perforation Peritonitis

Inflammation of the peritoneum (peritonitis) can be caused by a number of agents like bacteria, fungus, viruses, chemical irritants, blood and foreign bodies.

TYPES OF PERITONITIS

Peritonitis is of three types based on the source and nature of the microbial contamination.

Primary Peritonitis

It is defined as the inflammation of the peritoneal cavity without any associated visceral perforation. Mostly infection is monomicrobial. Spontaneous bacterial peritonitis of ascitic fluid in a liver failure patient and peritonitis caused by ascending infection via the female genital tract are examples of primary peritonitis.

Secondary Peritonitis

It refers to the peritoneal contamination arising from an intra-abdominal source usually from visceral perforation.

Tertiary Peritonitis

It develops following the treatment of secondary peritonitis either due to failure of host inflammatory response to contain the infection or a superinfection.

ROUTES OF PERITONEAL INFECTION

Infection can reach the peritoneal cavity by the following routes

- Gastrointestinal perforation
- Exogenous contamination (penetrating injury, surgical drains, surgical intervention)
- Bacterial translocation from the gut without perforation (intestinal obstruction, appendicitis, bowel ischemia)
- Female genital tract infection (pelvic inflammatory disease)
- Hematogenous spread (septicemia).

Peritonitis: Localized or Diffuse

Localized Peritonitis

Peritoneal cavity is divided into greater sac and lesser sac (Fig. 2.1). Greater sac is further divided into subphrenic spaces, pelvis and peritoneal cavity proper. Peritoneal cavity proper is divided by transverse colon into supracolic and infracolic compartment. Peritonitis can be localized around a compartment by formation of adhesions in-between surrounding structures, omentum, and intestines. This usually occurs if the course of the pathological process is slow and there is no massive leakage of gastrointestinal contents. In cholecystitis and appendicitis peritonitis is usually localized.

Symptoms and signs in localized peritonitis are those of underlying pathological condition. Abdominal pain is the prominent symptom. Tachycardia is present and there is localized guarding and rebound tenderness.

With appropriate treatment localized peritonitis gets resolved, however in some cases there may be formation of pus or progression to diffuse peritonitis.

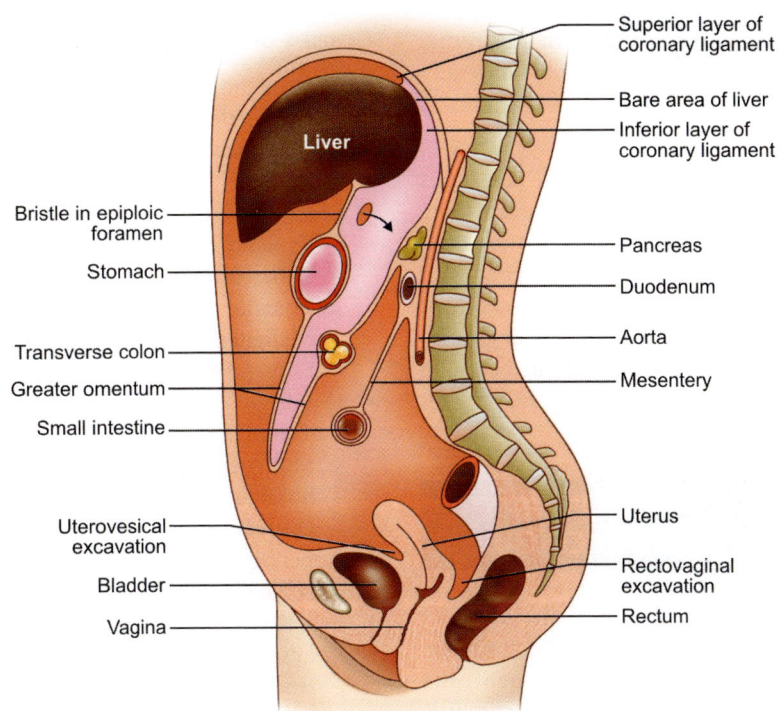

Superior layer of
coronary ligament

Bare area of liver

Inferior layer of
coronary ligament

Liver

Bristle in epiploic
foramen

Stomach

Pancreas

Duodenum

Aorta

Transverse colon

Mesentery

Greater omentum

Small intestine

Uterovesical
excavation

Bladder

Vagina

Uterus

Rectovaginal
excavation

Rectum

Fig. 2.1: Blue area is the lesser sac. Red area is greater sac

Diffuse Peritonitis

Factors which facilitates the development of diffuse peritonitis are:

- Sudden leakage of gastrointestinal contents: In bowel perforation gastrointestinal contents come out from the bowel to the peritoneal cavity very rapidly and spread to whole of the peritoneal cavity without any chance of getting localized.
- Disruption of localized collection due to rough handling can lead to diffuse peritonitis as in appendicular abscess/mass.
- Young children are more prone to diffuse peritonitis as infection is less likely to be contained because of under developed small omentum.
- Virulent organism and immunodeficient host (due to steroids, AIDS) are other factors which causes development of diffuse peritonitis.

CLINICAL PRESENTATION

Clinical presentation of diffuse peritonitis may be different depending upon the duration of the illness.

Early

There is severe generalized abdominal pain that gets worse by movement or breathing. Pain is first noted at the area of the pathology, e.g. in epigastrium in gastric perforation and then the pain becomes generalized. Fever and vomiting may be present. Characteristically the patient lies still to avoid any movement which causes aggravation of the pain. Tachycardia, generalized rigidity, guarding and rebound tenderness is present all over the abdomen. Abdominal tenderness and guarding may be absent if the anterior abdominal wall is unaffected as in pelvic peritonitis. Pelvic peritonitis is associated with urinary frequency and is tender on per-rectal examination. Bowel sounds are generally absent.

Late

If the resolution or localization of diffuse peritonitis does not occur then patient gradually becomes more sick and toxic. Abdomen gets distended progressively. If remains untreated patients goes into circulatory failure and shock. Limbs become cold and clammy, eyes are sunken, tongue is dry, pulse become feeble and thready and patient bears an anxious look (Hippocratic facies).

SECONDARY PERITONITIS DUE TO PERFORATION OF GUT

It is commonly seen condition in the surgical emergency. Despite the advances in the antibiotic treatment and intensive care management, the mortality and morbidity associated with perforation peritonitis continues to be high because of late presentation of the patient to the hospital. Early detection of the condition and prompt operative treatment is of paramount importance to reduce the morbidity and mortality.

Common Sources of Perforation Peritonitis

- Duodenum
- Stomach
- Ileum
- Jejunum
- Appendix
- Colon
- Esophagus.

In our country, duodenum and ileum are the most common sites seen in perforation peritonitis followed by appendix and stomach. Colonic perforations are uncommon in contrast to the western patients because of rarity of diverticular diseases in Indian population.

Causes of Perforation Peritonitis

- Gastroduodenal
  - Peptic ulcer disease
  - Malignancy
  - Trauma
- Small intestine
  - Typhoid
  - Tuberculosis
  - Trauma
  - Malignancy
  - Strangulation
- Colon
  - Trauma
  - Malignancy
  - Strangulation
  - Diverticulitis
- Appendix
  - Appendicitis
- Esophagus
  - Iatrogenic
  - Boerhaave syndrome.

Bacteriology

Bacterial load in the proximal bowel is very less; while in the distal ileum and colon bacterial load is high. For this reason gastric and duodenal perforation are sterile to begin with, while ileal and colonic perforation are usually infected right from the beginning. Gram negative bacilli (*E.coli*, *Klebsiella*) and *Bacteroides* (anerobic) are the chief bacterial organisms in perforation peritonitis. Gram-negative bacteria contain endotoxins (Lipopolysaccharides) in the cell wall. These lipopolysaccharides causes the release of tumor necrosis factor (TNF) from the leukocytes which is the main cause of the inflammatory response associated with the perforation peritonitis. Systemic absorption of endotoxins causes development of septic shock. The proportion of anerobic to aerobic organism increases with the passage of time.

Evaluation of Perforation Peritonitis

Diagnosis of perforation peritonitis is essentially clinical. Abdominal pain is the prominent feature.

Pain associated with peritonitis is sudden, severe, continuous and generalized. In cases of perforated peptic ulcer there is history of sudden onset of pain abdomen in the epigastrium which soon becomes generalized. In cases of appendicular perforation pain starts at the periumbilical area and then shifts to the right iliac fossa and then may become generalized. Any movement aggravates the pain and hence the patient lies absolutely still to avoid movements.

Fever can be present as a feature of systemic inflammation. Peritonitis is associated with intestinal ileus and there can be obstipation and abdominal distention.

In history, patient should be asked about previous episodes of epigastric pain and dyspepsia which will suggest peptic ulcer disease. History of ingestion of NSAIDs should be obtained which suggests peptic ulcer perforation. In typhoid (enteric fever) there is a preceding history of high-grade fever prior to the onset of acute abdominal pain. Intestinal perforation usually occurs in 2nd or 3rd week of enteric fever. In tuberculosis patient will give history of evening rise of fever, weight loss, and loss of appetite. Contact history with a tubercular patient or previous treatment with antitubercular drugs may suggest tuberculosis as a cause of perforation. In rare cases of malignant perforation there may be history of gastrointestinal bleeding, weight loss, and anorexia.

Examination

Patient looks sick and anxious. Tachycardia is present and there may be hypotension because of fluid deficit (third space loss of fluid) or sepsis. Patient may be febrile and tachypneic as a result of systemic inflammatory response. Signs of dehydration like dry tongue, shrunken eyes and oliguria should be looked for. In case of shock limbs are cold and clammy.

Abdominal Examination

Abdomen is standstill with very little movement with respiration. Tenderness, board like rigidity and rebound tenderness is found on palpation. Liver dullness will be obliterated due to presence of free air under diaphragm. Bowel sounds are absent. Bogginess may be present in the pouch of Douglas indicating presence of pelvic collection.

MANAGEMENT OF PATIENTS

Resuscitation of the patient is carried out first. Patient is kept nil per oral, nasogastric tube is inserted and intravenous crystalloids (ringer lactate) is started. Fluid resuscitation is very important as peritonitis is associated with tremendous amount of third space loss. Foley catheter is placed to measure the urine output which should be at least 0.5 ml/kg/hour. Antibiotics (third generation cephalosporin-ceftriaxone and metronidazole) are administered to cover against gram-negative bacilli and anerobes. Any metabolic and electrolyte disorder is corrected. Central venous line should be inserted in hypotensive patients not responding to fluid resuscitation to measure the CVP and guide further fluid administration. Inotropes (dopamine, dobutamine) are started in hypotensive patient after the CVP is brought to 8 cm of water with intravenous fluids.

INVESTIGATIONS

Radiological Investigations

As stated earlier, diagnosis of perforation peritonitis is principally clinical. Erect chest X-ray with both domes of the diaphragm may show free gas (Fig. 2.2). Though absence of free gas does not exclude the diagnosis of perforation peritonitis. Frequently X-ray does not show free gas in many cases especially in cases of appendicular perforations. CECT scan has greater sensitivity to detect free gas and it may also show contrast extravasations from bowel.

Findings associated with free gas on X-ray
- Free air beneath diaphragm-crescent sign
- Visualization of both sides of the bowel wall—Rigler's sign
- Triangular area of free air trapped below central tendon of diaphragm (Fig. 2.3)

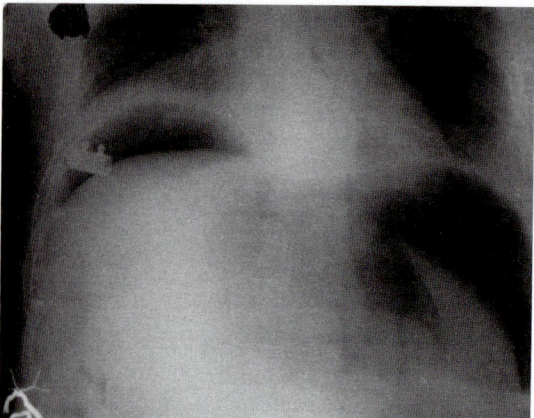

Fig. 2.2: Free gas under the dome of diaphragm indicating hollow viscus perforation

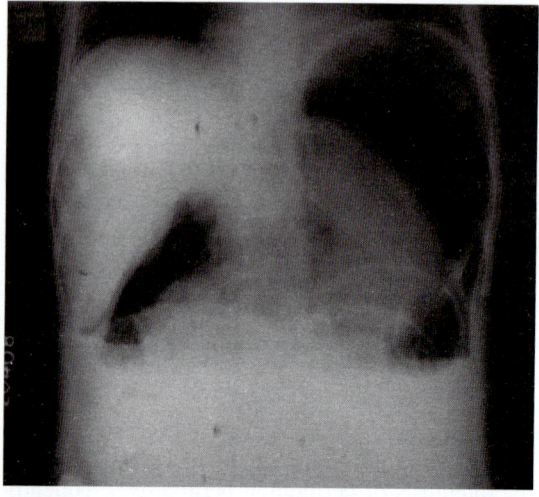

Fig. 2.3: Triangular area of free air trapped below central tendon of diaphragm (*Courtesy* Dr Seema, Lecturer, UCMS, Delhi)

- Large pneumoperitoneum outlining entire abdominal cavity with "laces" representing falciform ligament—Football sign

Blood Investigations

Hemogram, serum electrolytes, renal function test and arterial blood gases (ABG) should be done.

OPERATIVE MANAGEMENT

All cases of frank peritonitis should be taken up for exploratory laparotomy after adequate resuscitation.

OPERATIVE MANAGEMENT OF SPECIFIC CONDITION

DUODENAL PERFORATION

Surgical operative procedures for duodenal perforation can be divided into simple closure (Graham's patch repair) or definitive procedure. In Graham's patch repair of duodenal perforation, acid reduction surgery is not carried out. Using 2-O Vicryl, three sutures are taken at the duodenal perforation site (Fig. 2.4A) and a tongue of omentum is placed into the suture. The sutures are then tied over the omentum (Fig. 2.4B). The basic principle in Graham's patch repair is that perforated site is usually friable and hence primary closure will lead to cut through of the sutures. For this reason omentum is used to patch the perforated site in the duodenum. Another less frequent procedure which used to be practiced earlier is the omentum plug repair. In this, ryles tube is brought through the perforated site of the duodenum and end of which is tied to the omentum. The ryles tube is gently withdrawn from the nasal end causing the omentum to plug the perforated site.

Sometimes the perforation is big and not suitable for omental patch repair. In this scenario loop of jejunum is brought at perforation site and serosa of the jejunum is sutured at the edges of the perforation (jejuna serosal patch repair).

Definitive surgery for duodenal perforation with acid reduction procedure can be done in early cases (less than 6 hours) with minimal contamination. Truncal vagotomy and pyloroplasty including the perforation site or truncal vagotomy, repair of perforation and gastrojejunostomy are the operative options. Acid reduction procedure is done because of the associated recurrence of peptic ulcer and need for long-term acid suppression medicines. However, with the anti-*H. pylori* treatment incidence of

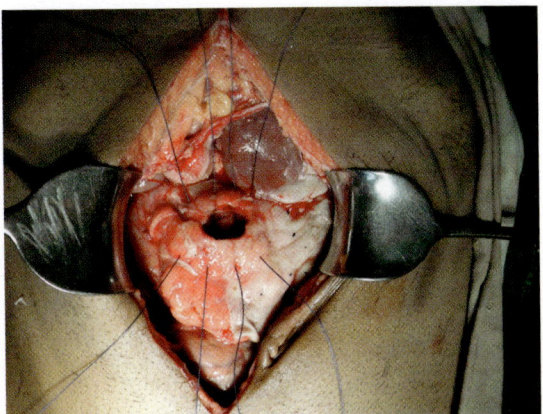

Fig. 2.4A: Vicryl sutures taken around the perforation

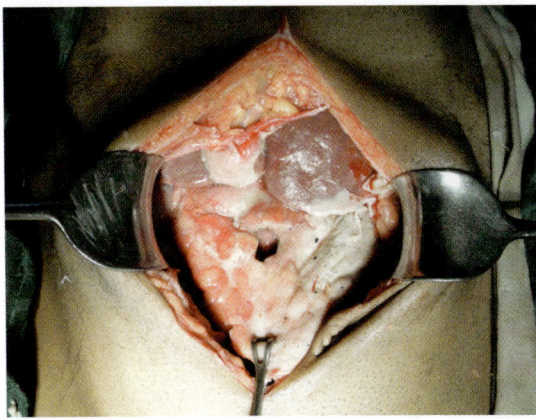

Fig. 2.5: Perforated gastric ulcer

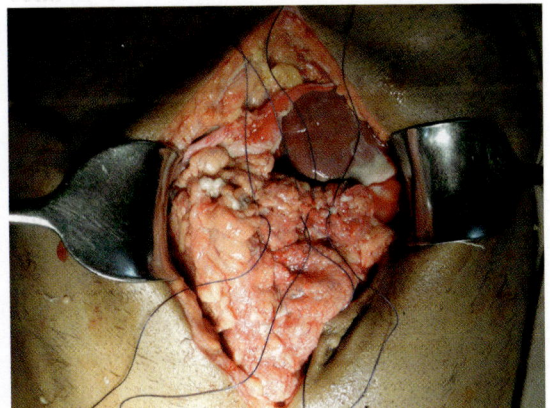

Fig. 2.4B: Omentum placed in between the sutures and sutures are tied over the omentum

recurrence has decreased. In our opinion and also the literature from our country supports that the simple closure of duodenal perforation should be done in the emergency setting. As mentioned earlier all the patients of perforated duodenal ulcer should receive anti-*H. pylori* treatment postoperatively.

GASTRIC ULCER PERFORATION (Fig. 2.5)

Ulcer is excised and closed primarily with interrupted 2-O Vicryl suture in two layers. Acid reduction surgery like truncal vagotomy and drainage procedure or antrectomy should generally be avoided in emergency setting. Ulcer edge should always be sent for histopathological diagnosis to rule out any underlying malignancy.

Perforated gastric carcinoma—If present in the lower half of the stomach then the subtotal gastrectomy should be the choice of surgery.

Ileal Perforation

Whole of the gut is evaluated to rule out multiple perforations or associated strictures.

Solitary Perforation

For single perforation (Fig. 2.6) options include primary repair or exteriorization of the perforation as ileostomy. Primary repair is appropriate if general condition and nutritional status of patient is good and peritoneal contamination is limited.

Exteriorization of perforation as loop ileostomy is done if general condition of patient is bad, nutritional status is poor, there is hypotension or respiratory compromise or the perforation is old with purulent contamination. Primary repair in these scenario are associated with high leak rates and subsequent mortality and remember a living problem (ileostomy) is better than a dead patient. Ileostomy thus made, is closed after one and half-months in elective setting.

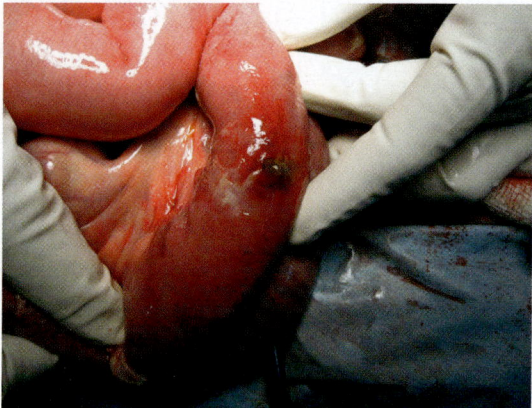

Fig. 2.6: Ileal perforation

Multiple Perforations (Fig. 2.7)

If the perforations are limited to a small segment of bowel then that segment is resected. If conditions are favorable, end-to-end anastomosis is done, otherwise the ends taken out as ileostomy and mucous fistula.

If the perforations are far from each other then most proximal perforation is exteriorized and all other distal perforations are repaired. If conditions are favorable then primary repair of perforations can be done.

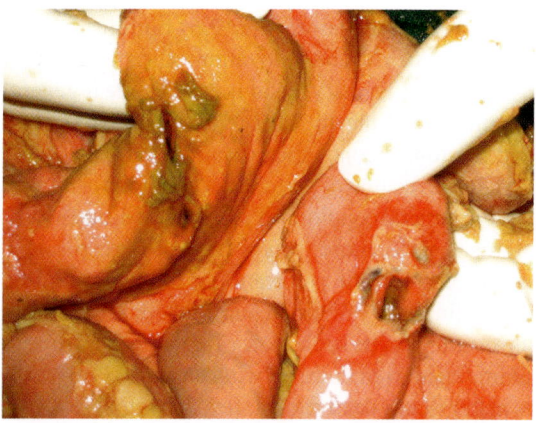

Fig. 2.7: Multiple ileal perforations

Perforation associated with Stricture

Not uncommonly ileal perforations are associated with tubercular stricture. In these scenario all non passable strictures are managed with either stricturoplasty (short segment stricture) or resection anastomosis (long segment stricture).

Colonic Perforation

Causes of colonic perforation are
- Colonic obstruction secondarily to malignancy
- Inflammatory bowel disease
- Complication of colonoscopy
- Volvulus
- Diverticulitis
- Pseudo-obstruction
- Fecal impaction (stercoral perforation).

Caecum is the commonest site of colonic perforation reason of which can be explained by Laplace's law. Laplace's law states that the intraluminal pressure needed to stretch the wall of a hollow tube is inversely proportional to its radius. The caecum has the largest diameter of the colon and requires the least amount of pressure to distend. During a closed loop large bowel obstruction, the wall tension in the caecum increases, causing ischemia to the bowel wall. Threshold for risk of cecal perforation is a diameter of twelve centimeters as seen on X-ray.

Perforation associated with Malignancy

For right sided malignancy extended right hemi-colectomy is done. Another option in sick patient is to do a caeccostomy (at site of perforation) and defi-nitive procedure is carried a later date. For left sided lesion it is appropriate to exteriorize the perforated site of the colon and carrying out definitive operation electively at later date. If the patients general condition is good then the definitive surgery can be carried out in emergency as well.

Perforation associated with Ulcerative Colitis

Subtotal colectomy with Hartmann's procedure is to be done. This included removal of the diseased ascending, transverse, descending and the sigmoid colon with closure of the rectal stump at or above the level of sacral promontory without any pelvic mobilization of the rectum and making an end ileostomy.

Diverticular Perforation

Affected segment of the colon is resected and ends are brought out as colostomy and mucous fistula.

Stercoral Perforation

It is the perforation of the large bowel due to pressure necrosis from a fecal mass. Severe chronic constipation is considered to be the main causative factor in the development of stercoral perforation of the colon. Involved segment of the colon is resected and both the ends are exteriorized.

Appendicular Perforation

Appendicular perforation is suspected when there is a history of parumbilical pain which shifts to the right iliac fossa before becoming generalized. On examination there will be features of peritonitis i.e. guarding, rigidity and rebound tenderness. Appendicular perforations are not usually associated presence of free intraperitoneal gas. If there is suspicion of appendicular perforation then it is better to open the abdomen via a lower right paramedian incision, as this incision can be extended upwards to explore the abdomen if the appendix is found to be normal. Appendectomy is done in cases of appendicular perforation after thorough peritoneal lavage. If the appendicular base and adjoining caecum is friable or necrotic then affected part of the caecum is excised and opening in the caecum thus created is closed with interrupted vicryl sutures. Tube caecostomy is another option in this scenario where a malecot catheter is placed in the caecum and brought through the right iliac fossa. Tube is removed at around 2 weeks after the tract has matured.

3 Acute Intestinal Obstruction

Intestinal obstruction is a common disorder and is frequently seen in the surgical emergency. If not recognized and managed properly it may lead to significant morbidity and mortality. Knowledge of pathophysiology of bowel obstruction is essential for understanding the management.

TYPES OF INTESTINAL OBSTRUCTION

Dynamic Obstruction

Dynamic obstruction is caused by mechanical compromise of the intestinal lumen and is characterized by increased peristalsis against the obstruction.

Adynamic Obstruction

Adynamic obstruction results from absence of peristaltic activity of the bowel as in paralytic ileus and mesenteric vascular occlusion.

VARIOUS TERMINOLOGIES USED IN INTESTINAL OBSTRUCTION

Acute Obstruction

It is characterized by sudden onset of complete occlusion of intestinal lumen.

Subacute Obstruction

It implies incomplete obstruction of the intestinal lumen.

Strangulated Obstruction

When the blood supply of the obstructed bowel is hampered and the bowel turns ischemic, it is called strangulated obstruction.

Closed Loop Obstruction

In this condition bowel is obstructed at both the proximal and distal point. In these, the pressure inside the obstructed loop increases very rapidly and bowel is more susceptible to strangulation and perforation. Mostly this is seen when distally colon is occluded by neoplasm and the ileocecal valve prevents the regurgitation of colonic contents into ileum, thereby part of the colon proximal to the neoplasm gets closed at both the ends.

CAUSES OF INTESTINAL OBSTRUCTION

Dynamic Obstruction

- Adhesive obstruction
- Tuberculosis
- Malignancy
- Intussusception
- Hernia
- Volvulus
- Gallstone ileus
- Ascariasis
- Faecalith impaction
- Inflammatory bowel disease.

Adynamic Obstruction

- Paralytic ileus
- Mesenteric vascular ischemia
- Pseudo-obstruction

PATHOPHYSIOLOGY OF INTESTINAL OBSTRUCTION

Mechanical obstruction of the bowel leads to proximal dilatation of the intestine due to accumulation of gastrointestinal secretions and swallowed air. This leads to increased peristalsis both above and below the obstruction. This may lead to loose stools in early course of obstruction in a few cases. Vomiting occurs early if the level of obstruction is in the proximal bowel. In distal small bowel and colonic obstruction vomiting is a delayed feature.

Increasing bowel distention leads to increased intraluminal pressures. This can cause compression of mucosal lymphatics leading to bowel wall lymphedema. Higher intraluminal pressures and increased hydrostatic pressure in the capillary beds results in massive third space shift of fluid, electrolytes, and proteins into the intestinal lumen. The fluid loss and dehydration that ensue may be severe and contribute to increased morbidity and mortality. If the obstruction is not corrected then venous return is compromised leading to marked edema which further causes compromise of arterial supply due to pressure resulting in intestinal ischemia, necrosis and gangrene (strangulated intestinal obstruction). If left untreated, it further progresses to perforation and peritonitis.

In intestinal obstruction there is always a proliferation of bacteria in the gut proximal to the obstruction. Microvascular changes of the bowel wall leads to the translocation of bacteria and bacterial toxin in to the peritoneal cavity as well as to the mesenteric lymph nodes. Systemic absorption of toxins leads to bacteremia. Most common pathogen involved is *Escherichia coli*.

CLINICAL FEATURES OF OBSTRUCTION

Abdominal Pain

Pain associated with intestinal obstruction is characteristically colicky in nature (waxing and waning type of pain). Changes in the character of the pain may indicate the development of a more serious complication, i.e. constant pain indicates ischemia or strangulation of bowel. It is important to remember that colicky pain is absent in paralytic ileus.

Vomiting

Vomiting is more pronounced in proximal small bowel obstructions. However, in distal intestinal obstruction it is a late feature. Character of the vomitus alters with the progression of obstruction. Initially it is digested and mucoid fluid thereafter it becomes yellowish and bilious finally the vomitus becomes feculent.

Abdominal Distention

Abdominal distention is a classical feature of distal small bowel and colonic obstruction. In proximal small bowel obstruction distention is not a prominent feature.

In case of proximal bowel obstruction (jejunum) vomiting will be the predominant and abdominal distention will be minimal. Whereas, in distal bowel obstruction (ileum or colon) vomiting is a late feature and abdominal distention is more prominent.

Obstipation

Inability to pass flatus and feces (obstipation) is characteristic of complete intestinal obstruction. One must remember the fact that diarrhea may be present initially in intestinal obstruction as the peristaltic activity of the bowel distal to the obstruction results in evacuation of the distal bowel contents.

Fever and Tachycardia

Occur late and may indicate development of strangulation.

Abdominal Tenderness

Localized tenderness in the abdomen indicates the development of ischemic changes in the bowel. Presence of guarding, rigidity and rebound tenderness indicates the possibility of perforation of the bowel.

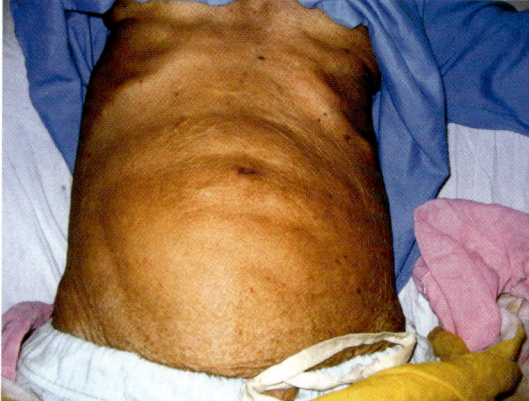

Fig. 3.1: Visible bowel loops in a patient with intestinal obstruction

Peristalsis of the bowel may at times be visible on abdominal inspection (Fig. 3.1).

Bowel Sound

Increased bowel sounds indicates mechanical obstruction. In case of strangulation or ischemia, bowel sounds are absent. In paralytic ileus bowel sounds are characteristically absent. High pitched tinkling bell like sounds can be heard in cases of paralytic ileus because of overflow of fluids from one distended loop to other and not because of peristalsis.

Signs of dehydration should be looked for which are dry skin, sunken eyes and decreased urine output.

Always examine the hernial sites as obstructed hernia is an important cause of intestinal obstruction. PR examination should be done to look for rectal mass, faecalith and any deposits in pouch of Douglas. Ballooning of rectum is consistent with paralytic ileus.

Features Indicating Strangulated Obstruction

- Presence of continuous pain
- Localized or generalized tenderness
- Rigidity, rebound tenderness

- Fever
- Tachycardia
- Leukocytosis.

INVESTIGATIONS

X-ray of Abdomen Erect and Supine

Distended bowel loops in supine abdominal X-ray is indicative of intestinal obstruction. Site of obstruction is determined based on the characteristic appearance of jejunum, ileum, and colon. Jejunum is characterized by valvulae conniventes that completely pass across the width of the bowel and present at equal distance to each other giving a concertina or ladder effect (Fig. 3.2).

Ileum appears as distended loops with no other features (Fig. 3.3).

Caecum appears as a rounded gas shadow in the right iliac fossa. Distended caecum indicates that site of obstruction is in the large bowel.

Colonic loops are present at the periphery in contrast to the small intestinal loops which are seen

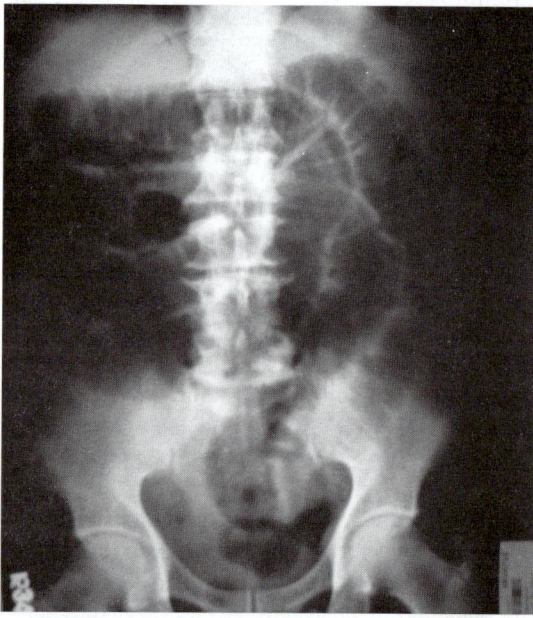

Fig. 3.2: Dilated jejunal loops with valvulae conniventes

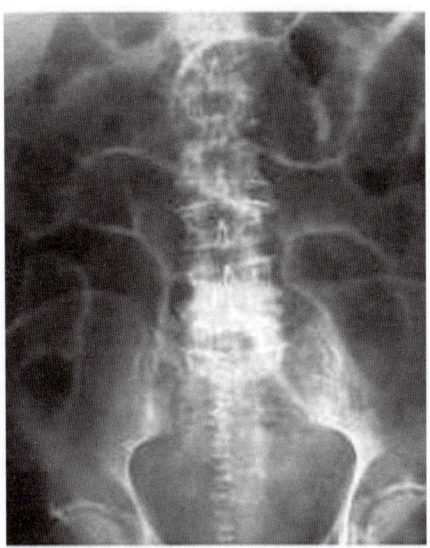

Fig. 3.3: Dilated ileal loops

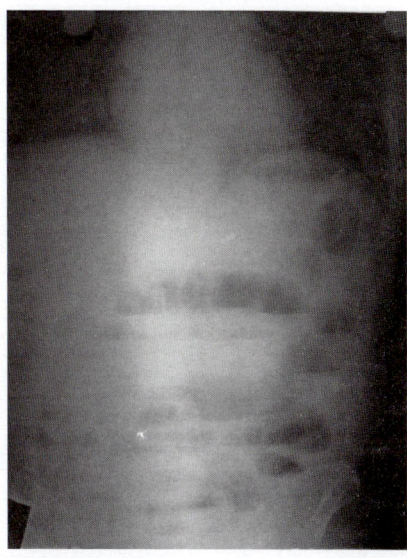

Fig. 3.5: Multiple air fluid levels in intestinal obstruction

in the center. Colon except for caecum shows haustral folds (Fig. 3.4). Haustral folds in the contrast to the valvulae conniventes of the jejunum does not completely transverse the wall and are not equidistant to each other.

Erect abdominal X-ray shows multiple air fluid levels which indicate intestinal obstruction (Fig. 3.5). In children less than two years of age few fluid levels are physiological and in adults two inconstant air

fluid levels – one at the duodenal cap and other at the terminal ileum are considered normal. In small bowel the number of air fluid levels is directly proportional to the degree of obstruction and distal small bowel obstruction is associated with more numbers of air fluid levels compared to proximal obstruction. Obstruction low in the colon usually does not give rise to fluid levels in small bowel because of competent ileocecal valve.

Other Specific Findings

Gallstone Ileus

The classic Rigler's triad includes mechanical bowel obstruction, pneumobilia (evidence of gas in the biliary tree) and an ectopic gallstone within bowel lumen. Only 10% of gallstones are sufficiently calcified to be visualized radiographically (Fig. 3.6).

Specific Laboratory Investigations in Cases of Obstruction

* TLC
* Blood urea
* Electrolytes (Na and K).

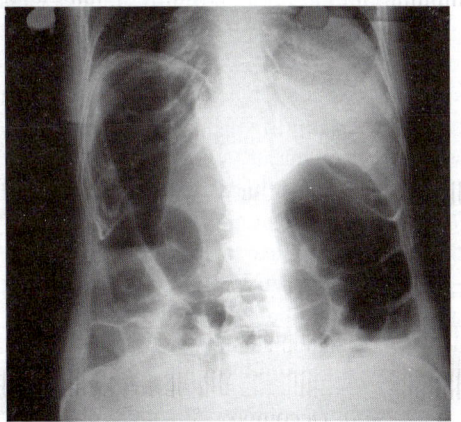

Fig. 3.4: Dilated colonic loops with haustral folds

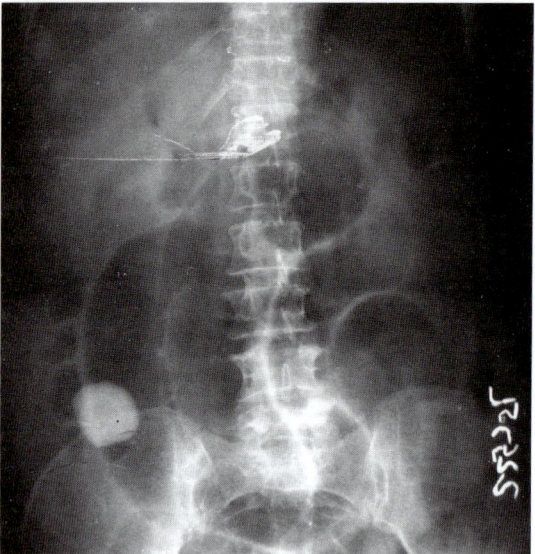

Fig. 3.6: Gallstone ileus—Dilated ileal loops with radiopaque gallstone

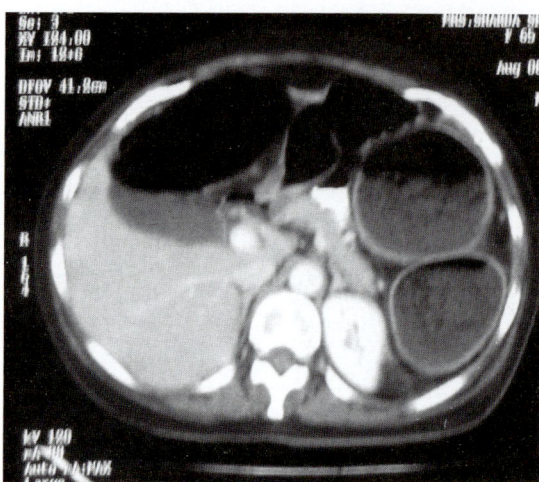

Fig. 3.7: CECT abdomen showing dilated colonic loops

ULTRASONOGRAPHY AND CECT OF THE ABDOMEN

USG and CECT of abdomen are done in some cases of intestinal obstruction. Though the presence of dilated gas filled bowel loops hampers the proper evaluation, ultrasound may detect intestinal mass, liver metastasis and enlarged lymph nodes. CECT of the abdomen is a much more sensitive investigation for these. CECT is a highly accurate method in determining the level and cause of obstruction and it is the investigation of choice when findings of clinical examination or plain X-ray are equivocal (Fig. 3.7).

MANAGEMENT OF INTESTINAL OBSTRUCTION

Principles of Treatment of Intestinal Obstruction

- Provide adequate resuscitation and correct fluid and electrolyte imbalance.
- Establish a diagnosis (mechanical vs paralytic ileus, presence of intestinal ischemia, site of obstruction and specific cause of obstruction).
- Remove the cause of obstruction.

Initial Management

Fluid Resuscitation

As intestinal obstruction is associated with fluid loss, fluid replacement is of paramount importance. Intravenous crystalloids, normal (0.9%) saline or lactated Ringer's solution, is used for intravascular volume repletion.

Adequacy of fluid replacement is judged by urine output which should be at least 0.5 ml/kg/hr. Measurement of central venous pressure (CVP) is helpful to evaluate the fluid resuscitation, particularly in elderly patients, patients with other comorbid conditions and patients in shock. CVP should be 5–8 cm H_2O at the midaxillary level. Electrolyte replacement should be guided by test results.

Nasogastric Aspiration

Decompression: Decompression of the stomach with a nasogastric tube will decompress the bowel and reduces the risk of airway contamination from aspiration.

Acute mechanical obstruction should be operated after initial resuscitation.

NON-OPERATIVE CONSERVATIVE MANAGEMENT

Conservative management of intestinal obstruction is by "drip and suck" regimen, i.e. administration of intravenous fluid and providing intestinal rest by nasogastric aspiration. Partial subacute obstruction especially adhesive obstruction due to previous operation should be treated conservatively. Majority of these obstructions resolves spontaneously by conservative method. Careful monitoring of patient should be done regarding adequate fluid replacement (NG aspirate should be replaced be normal saline and potassium) and keeping urine output above 0.5 ml/kg/ml. Serial abdominal examination is done to detect any features of strangulation.

Conservative management should be abandoned at first suggestion of strangulation. Although non-operative management can be continued for several days in the absence of any suggestion of strangulation, surgical exploration is generally indicated if the obstruction fails to resolve after 24 to 48 hours.

Non-operative Management for Specific Disorders

Sigmoid volvulus Detorsion of the sigmoid volvulus should be attempted using a sigmoidoscope or colonoscope and concomitant rectal tube placement. If successful, patient should be undertaken for elective operation during the same hospitalization. Inability to detort the sigmoid volvulus via endoscope requires immediate surgical intervention. If signs of ischemia or peritonitis are present then patient should be straight away taken for exploratory laparotomy.

Fecalith impaction Fecalith should be removed by manual evacuation and soap water enemas.

OPERATIVE MANAGEMENT

If features of strangulation or perforation are present, then exploratory laparotomy is done soon after patient is resuscitated. Acute complete intestinal obstruction is also a clear indication for exploration. The patients who fails to respond to 24 to 48 hours of conservative management as suggested by abdominal girth, failure to pass flatus, high nasogastric output, and increased bowel sounds, should also be subjected for exploration. It is of utmost important that patients is fully resuscitated before being taken up for surgery.

Exploratory Laparotomy for Obstruction

Abdomen is opened by midline laparotomy. If patient has previous midline incision then there is a high possibility of bowel being adherent to the anterior abdominal wall at the site of the scar. In this situation the incision is extended cranially or caudally to the previous scar and abdomen is entered through a fresh virgin area taking care not to injure underlying bowel.

After entering the abdomen first the caecum is evaluated at the right iliac fossa. Dilatation of the caecum indicates that the site of obstruction is in the colon, distal to the caecum. Collapsed caecum indicates that the site of obstruction is at the small intestine. The exact site of obstruction is then determined by identifying the point where there is dilatation of the bowel proximally and bowel is collapsed distalled. Whole of the small and large intestine is to be carefully evaluated as there can be more than one lesion.

Principles of Surgical Intervention

- Removal of obstructing lesion
- Decompress the bowel—Small bowel are best decompressed by retrograde stripping of bowel and forcing the intestinal contents and gases into the stomach where it aspirated by applying suction on large bore nasogastric tube. In friable intestine, decompression can be done by inserting a 14 G needle mounted on a syringe in the

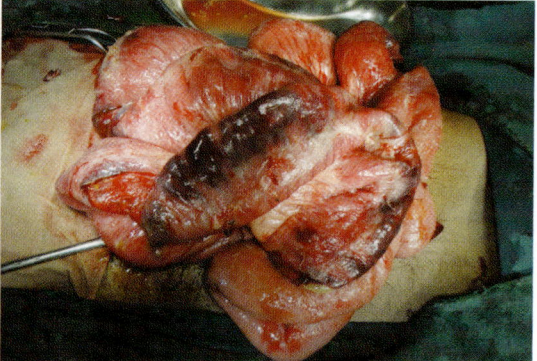

Fig. 3.8: Ischemic segment of bowel

intestinal lumen and applying suction on the end of the syringe which sucks out the gas contained in the intestines making it easier to handle.

- Assessment of bowel viability and resection of irreversibly ischemic areas of bowel—If the bowel appears dusky and cyanotic indicating ischemia then that segment is wrapped in warm moist abdominal pads for at least 10 minutes and patient is administered 100% oxygen and then bowel is reassessed for viability (Fig. 3.8). Signs of viable bowel are
  - Pink color of the bowel
  - Presence of peristalsis
  - Presence of mesenteric pulsation

Bowel viability is sometimes difficult to judge and generally short segment of intestine with doubtful viability should be resected as leaving behind ischemic bowel will result in perforation and peritonitis. Doubtful long segments of intestine poses a difficult problem as resection of large segment may result in short bowel syndrome. If segment of bowel with doubtful viability is left behind then planned relook laparotomy should be done. Alternatively, if bowel is resected but viability at the resected ends is doubtful then ends of the bowel should be brought out as stomas.

- Restore the continuity of intestine—If bowel is resected then continuity of bowel is restored by anastomosing the cut ends. However, if there is doubt that the anastomosis may not heal then it is

best to take the cut ends of the bowel as stomas. These conditions are—poor nutritional status of patient, hypotension, poor respiratory condition and oxygen saturation, presence of feco-purulent contamination and doubtful viability of the resected ends.

Definitive Management of Specific Causes of Intestinal Obstruction

Adhesions and Band

Adhesions are the commonest cause of intestinal obstruction. Approximately 90% of adhesive intestinal obstructions are result of previous operation and most of these obstructions are relieved with conservative management and patients can be kept on conservative management for longer duration compared to other causes of obstruction. If patient is not responsive to conservative management or there is development of ischemia then explorative laparotomy should be done. If patient has got previous midline incision then abdomen is opened from the same incision but initial entry into the peritoneum should be done few centimeters beyond the previous incision at a virgin area to avoid the bowel loops adhered to the scar. Adhesions causing obstruction should be taken down by doing adhesionolysis by sharp dissection (Fig. 3.9).

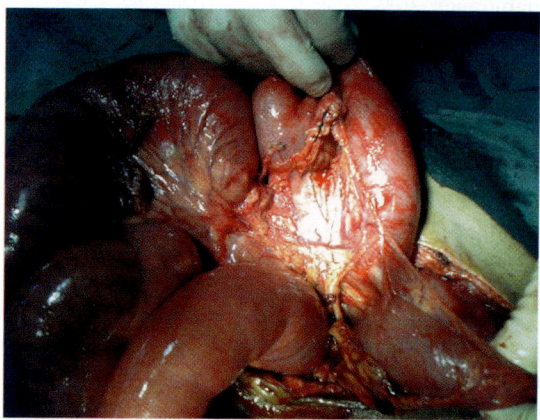

Fig. 3.9: Adhesive intestinal obstruction

Sometimes intestines are very densely plastered to each other as in tuberculosis and it is not always possible to do complete adhesinolysis. In this scenario, adhesinolysis is done till the point where it can be done safely without perforating the bowel and making a stoma. Patient is administered antitubercular treatment afterwards.

Hernia

Though femoral hernias are more prone to get obstructed but most commonly obstruction is seen in inguinal hernias especially indirect inguinal hernia. Intestinal obstructions due to hernia are dangerous as they quickly progresses to strangulated obstruction as these are closed loop obstruction. Tense and tender hernial sac indicates strangulated obstruction.

After initial resuscitation and stabilization patient is taken up for operation at the earliest. For inguinal hernias exploration is done by a standard incision over the inguinal canal which can be extended to the root of scrotum. It important that hernial sac is first opened at the fundus so that any contaminated fluid in the sac can be aspirated and thus avoiding it to enter the peritoneal cavity. Also it is important to evaluate the viability of the bowel contained in the sac. Generally the neck of the hernia sac forms the constricting ring. The neck of the sac is carefully divided to release the constriction. If the bowel is viable then it is returned to the peritoneal cavity. If there is doubt about the viability of the bowel it should be checked and reassessed as described earlier.

Hernia sac is ligated at the deep ring and posterior wall is reinforced with prolene mesh (hernioplasty). However, in cases of strangulated hernia mesh should not be placed as there is a high chance that mesh can get infected. In these cases herniorrhaphy (Bassini's repair) should be done.

Ascariasis Ball

Worm bolus is distangled and then pushed into the large bowel by milking, from where worms get expelled out of the rectum spontaneously. Thereafter

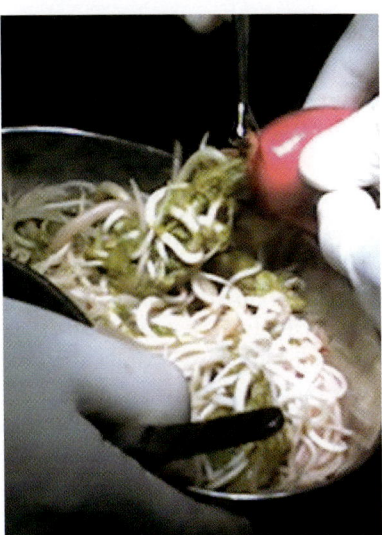

Fig. 3.10: Ascariasis ball being removed via an enterotomy (*Courtesy* Dr Abdul Hai, UCMS, Delhi)

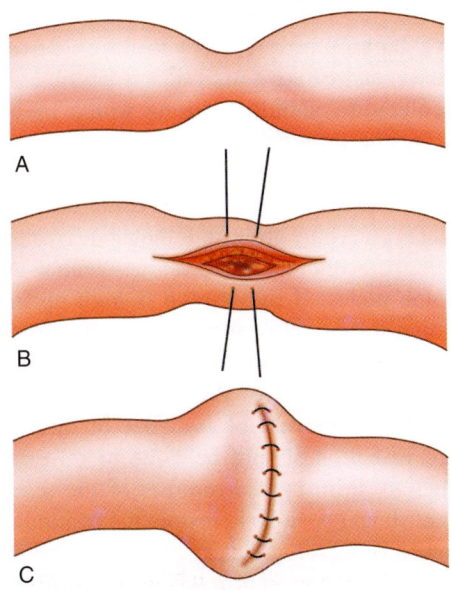

A

B

C

Figs 3.11A to C: Stricturoplasty (A) Stricture in the intestine (B) Stricture segment opened longitudinally (C) Opened segment closed horizontally

postoperatively patient should be given antihelminthic drugs. If it is not possible to push the ascariasis ball to caecum then they are removed by an enterotomy which is closed subsequently (Fig. 3.10).

Stricture

For short segment strictures of benign etiology stricturoplasty is done (strictured portion is opened longitudinally and closed horizontally Fig. 3.11). For long segment strictures resection of the strictured portion and anastomosis is done. Biopsy should always be taken from the strictured area as sometimes it can be malignant. Formal appropriate resection should be done for malignant stricture.

Malignancy

Colonic and rectal malignancies are frequently encountered as cause of intestinal obstruction during surgical emergency operation. Operative options for obstructing colonic malignancy includes:

Right Sided Colonic Malignancy

During laparotomy, if there is no evidence of metastasis and curative resection is possible, right hemicolectomy should be done which involves resecting the terminal 20 cm of ileum, caecum, appendix, ascending colon, hepatic flexure and proximal one-third of transverse colon along with mesentery and entire group of lymphnodes including epicolic, paracolic, intermediate and central group of lymph nodes. If the growth is high up in the ascending colon or close to the hepatic flexure, then extended right hemicolectomy is done where proximal two-thirds of the transverse colon is removed. In the event of evidence of metastasis limited resection should be done to relieve the obstruction. Primary anastomosis of the resected segment should be done to restore the continuity of the bowel. However, if the general condition is poor or there is hypotension or respiratory insufficiency it is advisable to exteriorize the cut ends of the bowel and restoration of the continuity is done after one and half months electively.

Left Sided Malignant Obstruction

Common sites of malignancy in the left side are sigmoid colon and rectum. In case the general condition of the patient is not good, immediate relief of the obstruction can be done by performing a proximal diversion colostomy either in transverse colon or in the sigmoid colon. However, if the general condition of the patient is good and there is no evidence of any metastasis a curative resection of left hemicolectomy can be done for growth involving descending colon or sigmoid colon. Resection should include distal one-third of transverse colon, splenic flexure, entire descending colon and sigmoid colon. End-to-end anastomosis can be done in case conditions are favorable, otherwise both the ends should be exteriorized and taken for closure at a later date.

Obstructing Anorectal Malignancy

Curative resection in anorectal malignancy is not done in emergency set up. Obstruction is relieved by performing a sigmoid colostomy and at laparotomy presence of metastasis should be looked for. All such patients are subjected to definite management afterwards.

On imaging investigation if the tumor is extending beyond the rectal wall or lymph nodes are enlarged, then chemo-radiation should be given and then definitive surgery anterior resection or abdomino-perineal resection is done depending upon the location of the tumor.

Ileocecal Tuberculosis

Obstructing ileocecal tuberculosis are hyperplastic. Ulcerative form of intestinal tuberculosis does result in obstruction. In such obstructing conditions ileocecal junction is thickened, leading to marked narrowing of the lumen causing obstruction. Features which suggest the etiology to be tuberculosis are presence of mesenteric abscesses, enlarged and caseating mesenteric lymph nodes (Fig. 3.12), and tubercles over the bowel serosa (Fig. 3.13). Fistulae and abscess are not common in

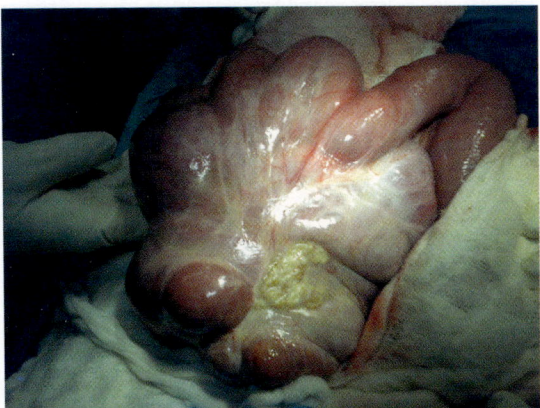

Fig. 3.12: Caseating mesenteric lymph nodes of tuberculosis

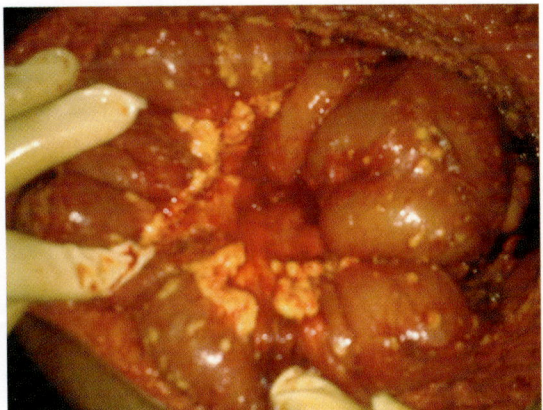

Fig. 3.13: Tubercles over bowel serosa and mesentery

tuberculosis compared to Crohn's disease. Right hemicolectomy is done with ileotransverse anastomosis either end to end or end to side. However, limited hemicolectomy is also a suitable procedure where 10 to 15 cm of terminal ileum, caecum, appendix and part of ascending colon is resected and ileoascending colon anastomosis is done. In case there is difficulty in resection, obstruction can be bypassed by side-to-side ileotransverse anastomosis. All such patient should receive full course of antitubercular treatment.

Gallstone Ileus

It refers to the mechanical intestinal obstruction due to impaction of one or more large gallstones within the GI tract. Biliary-enteric fistula is the major pathologic mechanism of gallstone ileus. The most common locations of impaction of gallstone are the terminal ileum and the ileocaecal valve because of their anatomical small diameter and less active peristalsis. Preoperative diagnosis is difficult in many cases; however, history of repeated attacks of cholecystitis and air in biliary tree on abdominal X-ray may suggest the diagnosis of gallstone ileus. Many times the diagnosis is only realized during laparotomy on palpating intraluminal hard structure at the site of obstruction. Incision is made just proximal to the site of impaction in the healthy bowel and the stone is extracted. Proximal bowel is carefully palpated to look for any other stones and enterotomy is closed. Cholecystectomy and repair of biliary-enteric fistula is done after 4 to 6 weeks electively.

Sigmoid Volvulus

In sigmoid volvulus on abdominal X-ray, sigmoid colon appears as a bent tyre (Fig. 3.14). Patients with sigmoid volvulus should preferably be operated in lithotomy position for assess to the anus. After opening the abdomen, colon is untwisted (Fig. 3.15). The bowel is then decompressed by introducing a flatus tube through the anus, which the abdominal surgeon manipulates into the distended loop. Sigmoid colectomy and primary anastomosis is the ideal procedure. If the bowel is loaded with faeces on table irrigation of the colon should be done. If there a doubt about viability of the colon or there is intra-abdominal sepsis, then primary anastomosis should not be done and both the ends are taken out as stoma. Sigmoidopexy where sigmoid colon is fixed to the parietal peritoneum is associated with high rates of recurrence and is an obsolete procedure.

Caecal Volvulus

There is axial rotation of the caecum and ascending colon in this condition. Manual derotation of the

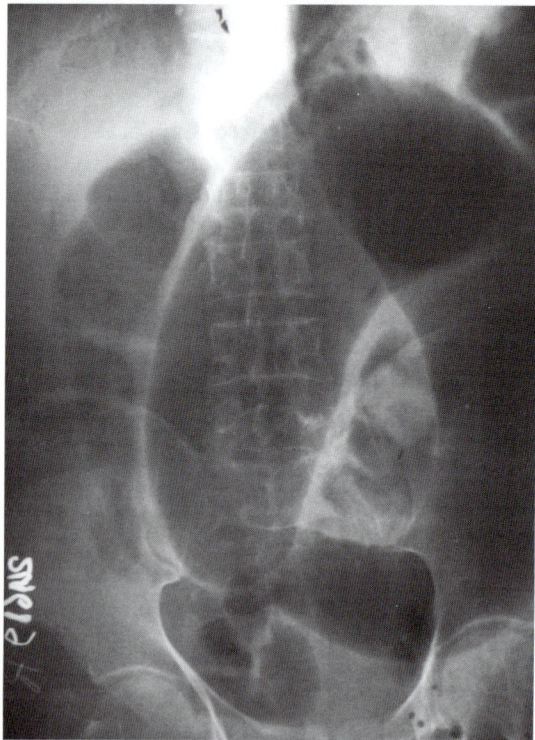

Fig. 3.14: Abdominal X-ray showing bent tyre appearance of sigmoid colon indicating sigmoid volvulus

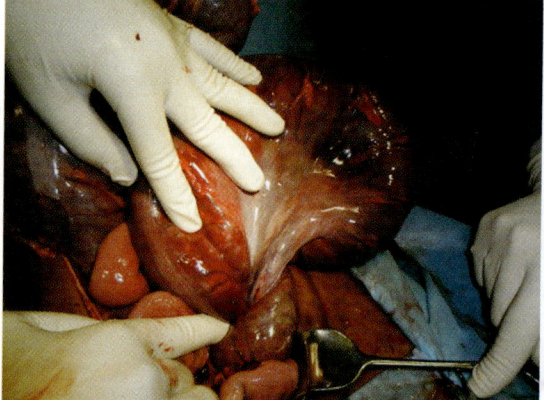

Fig. 3.15: Intra-operative photograph of a sigmoid volvulus

caecum is done and then the viability of the caecum is assessed. If the caecum is nonviable and gangrenous despite giving 100% oxygen and putting warm wet towel for 5 minutes, then limited right hemicolectomy is done.

Acute Colonic Pseudo-obstruction (Ogilvie's Syndrome)

It is a syndrome which is characterized with features of large bowel obstruction but without any mechanical obstruction. It is postulated to occur because of increased sympathetic tone compared to the parasympathetic tone. It is associated with severe illness, malignancy, severe metabolic disorders and opiate medication. The diagnosis of colonic pseudo-

obstruction is one of exclusion. Water soluble contrast enema or colonoscopy should be done to exclude mechanical obstruction. Treatment includes nasogastric decompression and rectal tube placement, correction of metabolic disorder and discontinuing medicines that decreases colonic motility, e.g. opiates and anticholinergic drugs. Colonoscopic decompression is successful in majority of the patients. Persistent colonic distention despite colonoscopic decompression or presence of peritonitis requires laparotomy. Caecostomy or loop colostomy is effective in relieving the distention.

Paralytic Ileus

In paralytic ileus there is actually no compromise of intestinal lumen; instead there is loss of peristalsis of bowel. It is associated with abdominal distention, vomiting, and obstipation, however, there is no colicky pain and bowel sounds are absent. Per-rectal examination shows ballooning of the rectum and X-ray will reveal distention of both small and large intestines. Paralytic ileus is seen after general anesthesia, hypokalemia, metabolic disorders, spinal cord injury and retroperitoneal hematoma. Management is conservative with nasogastric aspiration and intravenous fluids and correction of underlying disorder.

Gastrointestinal Hemorrhage

ACUTE UPPER GASTROINTESTINAL BLEEDING

Acute upper GI (gastrointestinal) bleed is a potentially life-threatening emergency. The bleeding is said to be from the upper gastrointestinal tract if the source of bleeding is present proximal to the ligament of treitz (duodenojejunal junction).

Patients with upper GI bleed (UGIB) present with hematemesis and melena. Melena is passage of black, liquid and tarry stools and it occurs because of the degradation of heme into hematin by gastric acid. Hematochezia (passage of bright red blood from rectum) usually indicates lower GI bleed but it is important to remember that massive upper GI bleed (bleeding more than 1000 ml) can sometimes also lead to hematochezia because of rapid transit of blood without degradation by gastric acid.

All patients who develop acute gastrointestinal bleed need urgent assessment and all patients should be admitted for careful monitoring and management.

Cause of acute upper gastrointestinal bleeding can be non-variceal (80%) or portal hypertensive variceal bleeding (20%). Peptic ulcer disease still represents the most frequent cause of upper GI bleeding, accounting for 40% of all the cases. Other common causes of non-variceal bleeding are Mallory-Weiss tear, gastroduodenitis, esophagitis and gastric tumors. Among the portal hypertensive bleeding, the gastroesophageal variceal bleeding accounts for more than 90% of the cases.

COMMON CAUSES OF UPPER GI BLEED

- Peptic ulcer disease
- Esophageal and/or gastric varices (portal hypertension)
- Mallory-Weiss tear
- Gastritis and duodenitis
- Gastric tumors
- Erosive esophagitis
- Dieulafoy's lesion.

APPROACH TO A PATIENT WITH UPPER GASTROINTESTINAL BLEEDING

Short History

- The amount of blood loss, number of episodes of bleeding and occurrence of melena is to be asked from the patient or relatives. It is important to distinguish hemetemesis (blood in the vomitus) from hemoptysis (blood in the sputum).
- Whether the patient had previous episodes of upper GI bleed, was he evaluated for it and whether the diagnosis was established.
- History of ingestion of NSAIDs (non-steroidal anti-inflammatory drugs) like aspirin, diclofenac.

Resuscitation

After these short enquiries resuscitation of the patient is done. Resuscitation of a hemodynamically unstable patient begins with assessing and addressing the ABCs (i.e. airway, breathing, circulation). Patients with severe blood loss and hemorrhagic shock may have altered sensorium or unconsciousness. In such circumstances, patients cannot protect their airway, especially when hematemesis is present and are at increased risk for aspiration. This situation must be recognized early and patients must be electively intubated as aspiration can be potentially lethal.

Once the airway is secured, the next step in evaluation is assessing the patient's circulation. Pulse rate and blood pressure of the patient is noted. Systolic BP of less than 100 mm Hg or tachycardia >100 beats/min suggests significant blood loss (20% of the circulating volume). Intravenous access is then established with two wide bore cannulas (16 Gz), blood sample is taken for cross matching and crystalloid intravenous fluid (Ringer lactate) is started. A rough guideline for the total amount of crystalloid fluid volume needed to correct the hypovolemia is the 3-for-1 rule, i.e. replace each milliliter of blood loss with 3 ml of crystalloid fluid. This restores the lost plasma volume. Nasogastric tube is then inserted and lavage with saline is done to see if there is continued bleeding. Urinary catheter is inserted to assess the urine output. Blood transfusion is started if there is evidence of significant hemorrhage (class 2 and above, *see* Table 4.1). Central venous line is inserted and fluid resuscitation is guided by the measurement of central venous pressure which is kept at 5–8 cm of water. The role of gastric lavage in the management of patient with upper GI bleed is controversial. Although there is no evidence that lavage helps to stop bleeding, it may be helpful in cleaning stomach before urgent endoscopy. Hemostasis is not improved with the use of iced saline solution.

The early administration of prophylactic antibiotics is beneficial in all patients of variceal bleeding as it improve the survival by reducing infection which is likely to occur in the patients having cirrhosis.

Detailed History and Examination

After this initial resuscitation when the patient is hemodynamically stable, a detailed history is taken and examination is done to evaluate the cause of the bleeding.

In patients with peptic ulcer disease there will be previous history of epigastric pain. History of NSAID intake may indicate gastric erosions. In cases of portal hypertension because of cirrhosis, history of jaundice and abdominal distention due to ascites may be present. In alcoholic cirrhosis there will history of chronic alcohol intake. Signs of liver disease like icterus, palmar erythema, spider angioma, asterixis should be looked for. Presence of splenomegaly and caput medusae indicates portal hypertension. Splenomegaly without the symptoms and signs of liver disease indicates EHPVO (extrahepatic portal vein obstruction) or NCPF (noncirrhotic periportal fibrosis) as the cause of portal hypertension. Mallory-Weiss tear will have history of vomiting and retching followed by bleeding.

Investigations

- Hemoglobin/Hematocrit—Hematocrit estimation is better than hemoglobin level as hemoglobin levels may be falsely high because of dehydration.
- Coagulation profile [prothrombin time (PT), activated partial thromboplastin time (APTT), and International Normalized Ratio (INR)]. Prolonged PT is indicative of deranged liver function.

Table 4.1: Estimated blood loss in shock				
Classification of shock				
	Class 1	*Class 2*	*Class 3*	*Class 4*
Blood loss, mL	Up to 750	750–1500	1500–2000	>2000
Blood loss,% blood volume	Up to 15%	15–30%	30–40%	>40%
Pulse rate, bpm	<100	>100	>120	>140
Blood pressure	Normal	Normal	Decreased	Decreased
Respiratory rate	Normal or Increased	Decreased	Decreased	Decreased

- Liver function tests are needed to calculate the Child-Pugh score in patients of portal hypertension (Table 4.2). Elevated aminotransferase, alkaline phosphatase and gamma-glutamyltranspeptidase levels are indicative of liver disease.
- Serum electrolytes.

Upper GI Endoscopy

It should be carried out after the patient is stabilized. In most cases this is done electively on the next available routine list but certainly within 24 hours of admission. Only a minority of profusely bleeding patients needs "out of hours" emergency endoscopy. Endoscopy will establish the cause of the bleeding and the therapeutic intervention can be done at the same time to stop the bleeding. Early endoscopic hemostatic therapy significantly reduces rate of recurrent bleeding, need for emergent surgery, and mortality in patients with upper GI bleed.

SPECIFIC MANAGEMENT IN UPPER GI BLEED AS PER THE CAUSE

Portal Hypertension Related Variceal Bleeding

Some important facts regarding variceal bleeding are as follows

- 90% of patients with portal hypertension have varices.
- 30% of patients with varices will have an upper gastrointestinal bleed.
- 80% of GI bleed in patients with portal hypertension comes from varices.

- 70% of patients who once had upper GI bleed will have a rebleed.
- Survival is dependent on the degree of hepatic impairment.
  Risk factors for variceal hemorrhage are:
  - Portal pressure more than 12 mmHg
  - Advanced liver disorder (child—C category)
  - Large size varices
  - Endoscopically "Red sign" on varices.
  Variceal bleeding is a medical emergency associated with recurrene and death as well. Management is based on pharmacological, endoscopical and surgical therapy.

Pharmacological Therapy

Variceal bleeding may initially be treated with intravenous vasopressin with nitroglycerine, somatostatin, or one of its analogues, (e.g. octreotide). These agents cause splanchnic and systemic vasoconstriction and thereby control bleeding. Pharmacological therapy has evolved into an effective first line treatment in patients with probable variceal bleeding. Dose of vasopressin is 20 IU in 200 ml saline, IV over 20 minutes and then 0.4 unit/min for up to 24 hours. Side effects include abdominal griping, and coronary and renal artery vasoconstriction. For this reason, it is used in combination with nitroglycerin (50 µg/min).

The newer drug terlipressin has been found to have less systemic vasoconstriction in comparison to vasopressin and glyopressin. Terlipressin has also been found to decrease renal vasoconstrictor system actively and improve renal function in patient with hepatorenal syndrome as well. But this drug is

Table 4.2: Child-Pugh score (Class A–5 to 6, class B–7 to 9, class C–10 to 15)			
	Child-Pugh score		
Measure	*1 point*	*2 points*	*3 points*
Bilirubin (total)	<2 mg/dl	2–3 mg/dl	>3 mg/dl
Serum albumin	>3.5 mg/dl	2.8–3.5 mg/dl	<2.8 mg/dl
INR	<1.7	1.71–2.20	> 2.20
Ascites	None	Suppressed with medication	Refractory
Hepatic encephalopathy	None	Grade I–II (or suppressed with medication)	Grade III-IV (or refractory)

contraindicated in patients with cardiovascular diseases. The dose of terlipressin is 1–2 mg every 4 hours.

Somatostatin and its analogue (octreotide) have proven to be superior, have fewer side effects and stop variceal bleeding in 80% of patients. Somatostatin is administered as a continuous infusion of 250 mcg/ hr, after an initial bolus of 250 mcg. Octreotide is given as an intravenous infusion of 50 mcg/hr after the initial bolus of 50–100 mcg. A combination of continuous infusion of octreotide for 5 days along with either sclerotherapy or band ligation has been shown to be superior to either sclerotherapy or band ligation alone in reducing early rebleeding and mortality. No major side effects and practically no complication are associated with the use of somatostatin or its analogue octreotide or vapreotide. The dose of vapreotide is bolus of 50 microgram followed by 50 microgram/hr.

Administration of lactulose and neomycin orally help in reducing the severity of hepatic encephalopathy in cirrhotic patients.

Emergency Endoscopy

Band Ligation: Varices appear as prominent venous channels in the esophagus or gastric fundus (Fig. 4.1). Varices are graded according to their size, tortuosity and extent (Table 4.3). Endoscopic therapy is successful in controlling acute variceal bleeding

Table 4.3: Grading of esophageal varices	
Grade-I	Diameter <5 mm, straight, limited to the distal esophagus
Grade- II	Diameter 5–10 mm, tortous, denser, extending above the midesophagus
Grade- III	Diameter >10 mm, filling the esophageal lumen with little or no normal mucosa between the columns, a thin wall and red color sign

in over 90% of patients after one or two treatment sessions. Band ligation is now regarded as the endoscopic treatment of choice in the management of esophageal varices. Banding eradicates varices with fewer endoscopic treatment sessions and less complications compared to injection sclerotherapy. Band is applied by endoscope at the bleeding varix or the most distal part of the target variceal column. Full contact is made between the end of the ligating device and the varix. Endoscopic suction is applied which results in the aspiration of the varix into the suction device. The draw string is pulled displacing the stretched elastic band which is released and encircles the neck of the varix, resulting in strangulation and subsequent thrombosis (Fig. 4.2).

Maximum of 5–6 elastic bands can be used per session and can be repeated at the interval of 2–3 weeks until the varices have been collapsed.

Sclerotherapy: Endoscopic sclerotherapy has been found to be equally good for controlling the acute episode of bleeding varices. A variety of sclerosants are used for this purpose. Sclerosants are injected either directly into the varices (intravariceal injection) or into the submucosa around the bleeding varix column (paravariceal injection). The intravericeal injection leads to thrombosis of the bleeding varix, whereas the paravariceal causes submucosal edema and stops bleeding by pressure. Later it causes mucosal thickening and prevents rebleeding.

Sclerosant should not be injected into the deeper layers of the esophageal wall as it may cause perforation, periesophageal inflammation and esophageal stricture (Fig 4.3). Commonly used sclerosants are

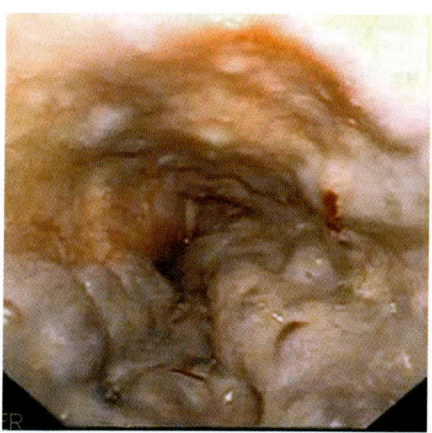

Fig. 4.1: Esophageal varices

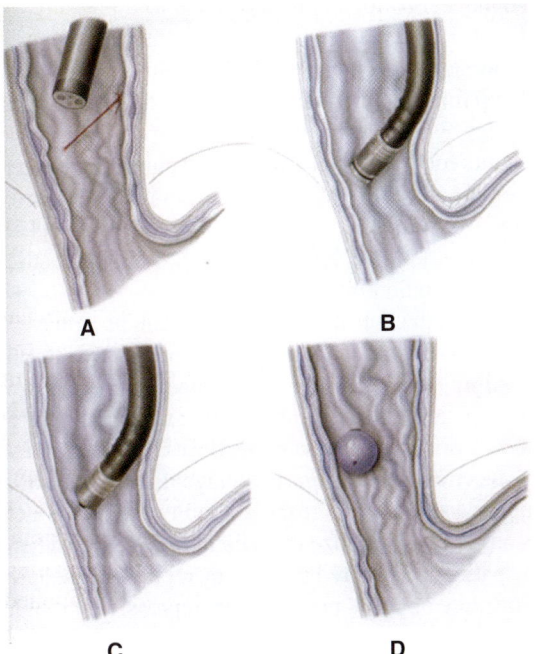

Figs 4.2A to D: Band ligation for bleeding esophageal varices: (A) Upper GI endoscopy is performed to locate the site of bleeding, (B) The endoscope is loaded with the banding device and reinserted into the esophagus. The bleeding varix is suctioned into the cylinder, (C) Rubber band is ejected on the varix, (D) Band ligated on the varix

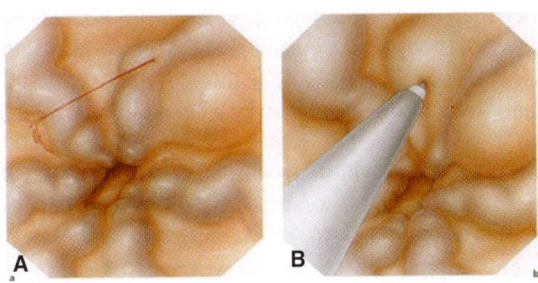

Figs 4.3A and B: Sclerotherapy for bleeding esophageal varices: **(A)** The site of bleeding is identified, (B) Sclerosant is injected immediately adjacent and slightly distal to the bleeding point into the submucosa until a significant prominent bleb appears

absolute alcohol, 5% ethanolamine oleate, sodium teradecyl sulphate and 1% polidocanol. Total of 10–30 ml of sclerosant per session can be given and can be repeated at the interval of 2–3 weeks till the varices have been obliterated. As the varices do recur in more than 50% of the cases the surveillance endoscopy at every 3–6 month interval should ideally be done.

Tissue adhesives such as n-butyl-2 cyanoacrylate are particularly helpful to obliterate fundal varices that respond unreliably to intravariceal injection of sclerosant or band ligation. One ml of adhesive is injected at a time with a maximum of three injections per session.

Re-bleeding after Emergency Endoscopic Therapy

Patients who re-bleed after two emergency endoscopic treatments during a single hospital admission have higher mortality if further endoscopic therapy is pursued. In such patients balloon tube is first inserted, resuscitation is done and then managed with an alternative method like transjugular intrahepatic portosystemic shunt (TIPS), surgically created portosystemic shunt or esophageal transection operation.

Balloon Tamponade

The vessels that feed the esophageal varices originate from the abdomen and enter the chest through the diaphragm around the gastro-esophageal junction. By inflating the balloon in the stomach and pulling it tight against the diaphragm, the balloon acts as a tourniquet, stopping the blood flow from the veins around the stomach to the varices in the esophagus. By inflating the esophageal balloon the pressure is exerted against the esophageal varices in view to achieve the hemostasis.

The Sengstaken–Blakemore tube (Fig. 4.4) is a triple-lumen rubber tube with two balloons: one that is inflated in the lumen of the stomach and pressed against the esophagogastric junction and one that is inflated in the lumen of the esophagus to press

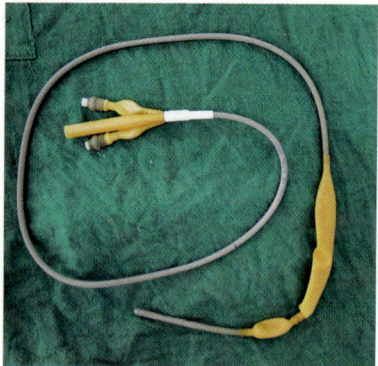

Fig. 4.4: Sengstaken–Blakemore tube

esophageal balloon is then inflated to a pressure of 40 mm Hg with a help of connecting to a sphygmomanometer and the pressure is maintained with a clamp for achieving the compression to the bleeding varices. Esophageal balloon should be deflated every 4 hours for 15 minutes to avoid esophageal pressure necrosis and entire tube is not left in place for more than 24–48 hours. After 12 hours the esophageal balloon is deflated, if there is no bleeding, the gastric balloon should also be deflated.

Although control of the bleeding can be achieved by balloon tamponade in 85% of cases, recurrent bleeding with release of the tamponade occurs in most patients. These tubes are associated with a 20% complication rate that includes airway obstruction, aspiration, esophageal necrosis with rupture, and alar necrosis. Balloon tamponade act as a bridge to stabilize the patient until a time when the patient is prepared for either a repeat endoscopic procedure or portal pressure decompression through a radiological or surgical method.

directly against the varices. Two of the lumens are used to inflate the balloons; the third opens into a port on the distal tip of the tube, and is used to irrigate and drain the stomach and administration of lactulose. Minnesota tube has esophageal and gastric balloons as well as esophageal and gastric drainage ports (Fig. 4.5)

Tube is well lubricated and passed to the back of pharynx, then down to esophagus and stomach and a small amount of air is injected to confirm the placement of tube in the stomach. Once proper placement is confirmed, the gastric balloon is inflated with 300–350 mL of air and is pulled up into the gastric fundus, compressing the gastroesophageal junction. The tube is secured to the facemask of a football helmet placed on the patient's head. The

Transjugular Intrahepatic Portosystemic Shunt

A transjugular intrahepatic portosystemic shunt (TIPS) is a percutaneously created connection within the liver between the portal and systemic circulations. It is the emergency procedure of choice for patients where endoscopic therapy has failed to control the bleeding. A catheter is inserted into a hepatic vein via the jugular vein. A rigid needle is passed through the catheter and advanced from the right or middle hepatic vein, through the liver tissue into right or left portal vein branch. After placement of a guide wire, the tract within the liver tissue is dilated using a balloon catheter (Fig. 4.6). The communication between the hepatic vein and the portal vein is then bridged with an expandable metal stent. Immediate control of variceal bleeding is achieved in over 90% of patients.

Absolute contraindications for TIPS are right-sided heart failure with increased central venous pressure, polycystic liver disease and severe hepatic failure. Relative contraindication are severe hepatic

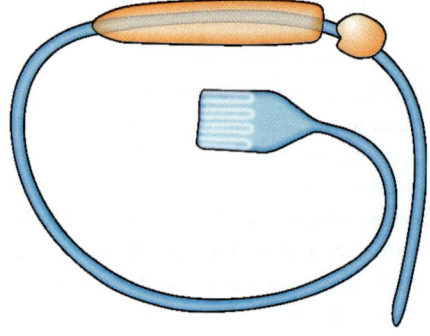

Fig. 4.5: Minnesota tube

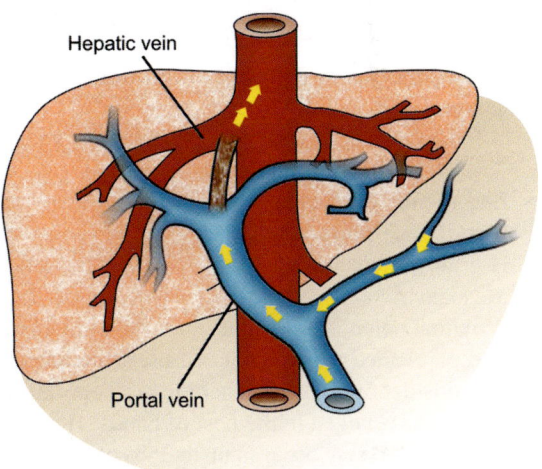

Fig. 4.6: Transjugular intrahepatic portosystemic shunt

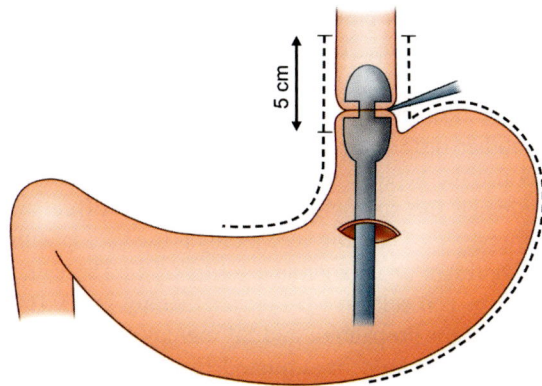

Fig. 4.7: Gastro-esophageal devascularization and stapling of lower esophagus (dotted line indicates the extent of devascularization)

encephalopathy poorly controlled with medical therapy, hypervascular hepatic tumors and portal vein thrombosis. Disadvantages of TIPS include high cost, hepatic encephalopathy (30% increased risk), and only 50% patency rate at one year.

Surgical Options

There are two non shunt procedures including esophageal transection and gastro-esophageal devascularization which is performed during emergency, but the role of surgery has now markedly decreased at present with improved efficacy of endoscopic treatment. Role of emergency procedure to control variceal bleeding is now restricted to patients where endoscopic treatment has failed and TIPS is not possible because of technical reasons.

Esophageal transection and reanastomosis using a staple gun and devascularization of lower 5 cm of esophagus and upper two-thirds of the stomach (Fig. 4.7), is the preferred emergency procedure. But the esophageal stapled transection is now seldom used with the advent of TIPS. It is also not recommended if the patient is a candidate for liver transplantation because of the resulting increased risk of operative morbidity at the time of transplantation.

Sugiura operation which includes esophageal transection with extensive esophageal and gastric devascularization, splenectomy and preservation of coronary and paraesophageal vein is not justified in the emergency setting.

The widespread use of endoscopic techniques and the introduction of the TIPS procedure have made shunt surgery a less attractive choice for acute variceal bleeding.

Emergency shunt surgery has an operative mortality greater than 25%, largely determined by the degree of liver decompensation. Non-selective portacaval shunt (Fig. 4.8) is the most common surgical shunt performed for the control of acute variceal bleeding in the emergency setting.

Secondary Prevention

About 70% of patients who have had one episode of variceal bleeding rebleed. As mortality of acute variceal hemorrhage is high, measures should be taken to prevent further episodes of bleeding (secondary prevention). Non-selective β-blockers like propranolol are the first line for the prevention of re-bleeding. β-blocker lowers the portal pressure by reducing the portal blood flow. Non-selective β-blocker such as propranolol and nadolol are more effective than selective β_1–blockers in reducing the hepatic venous pressure gradient. Propranolol has been found to prevent increases in portal pressure related to physical exercise in patient with cirrhosis and to decrease the rate of bacterial translocation. Another drug used is nitrates which are found to reduce the hepatic venous pressure gradient and to enhance the splanchnic hemodynamic effect of propranolol. This drug is generally is used along with vasopressin or its analogue terlipressin. The usual dose of non selective β-blocker therapy is 80–160 mg/day for propanolol and 80 mg/day for nadolol. The dose should be adjusted to obtain 20–25% reduction in the heart rate.

Non-selective β-blockers is also effective in reducing the risk of first variceal bleeding episode in patients with medium to large size varices (Primary prevention). Endoscopic ligation to eradicate the varices is done if

- The patient is non-compliant to β-blockers
- The patient is intolerant to β-blockers
- β- blockers are contraindicated as in bronchial asthma and congestive heart failure
- The patient is high risk (Child-Pugh type C, large varices)

Surgery for Gastro-esophageal Varices

Surgical procedures aimed at controlling gastro-esophageal varices fall into two groups:

Non-selective Shunts (Fig. 4.8)

- End-to-side portacaval
- Side-to-side portacaval
- H-graft portacaval
- Mesocaval
- Proximal splenorenal shunt
  These are called non-selective because entire splanchnic bed is decompressed. There is high operative mortality (15%) even in the best of hands. Hepatic encephalopathy may occur in up to 35% of patients.

Selective Shunts

Warren distal splenorenal shunt (Fig. 4.9) is the most popular selective shunt. It is called selective shunt because this selective decompresses the gastro-esophageal varices. Hepatic perfusion is maintained and thus, it prevents the development of hepatic encephalopathy. This is a technically difficult operation with increased blood loss, operating time and morbidity. This surgery is considered for patients

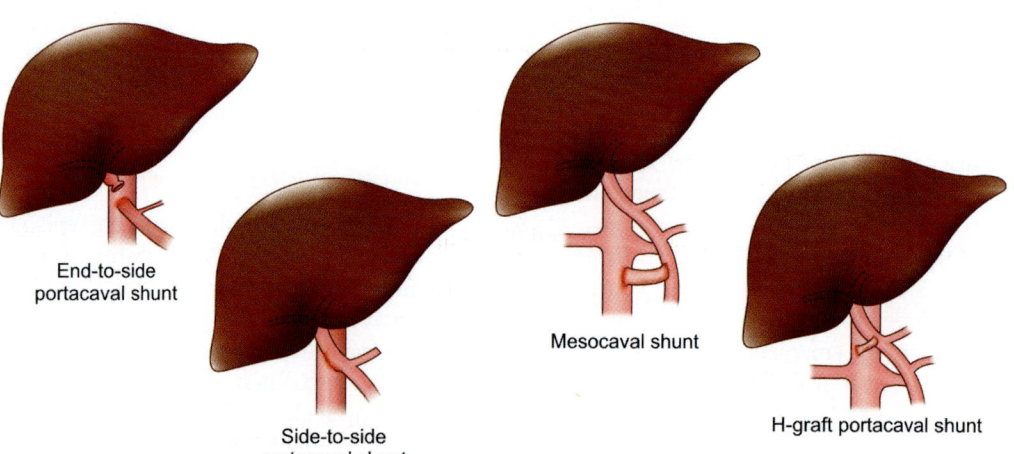

Fig. 4.8: Common non-selective shunt

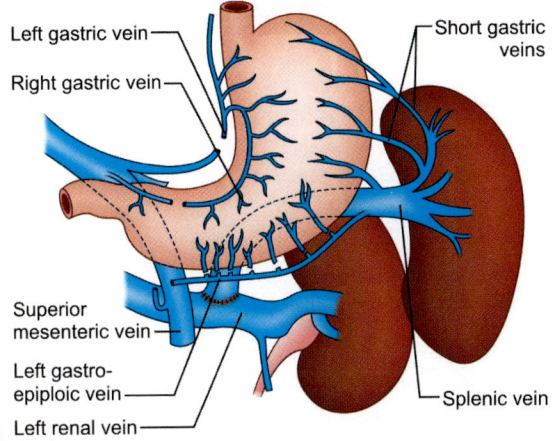

Fig. 4.9: Warren distal splenorenal shunt

Left gastric vein

Right gastric vein

Short gastric veins

Superior mesenteric vein

Left gastro-epiploic vein

Left renal vein

Splenic vein

who have well preserved liver function, who do not have readily available tertiary care including endoscopic therapy and who are unlikely to be compliant for follow up.

Partially decompression shunt like small diameter prosthetic mesocaval or H-graft portacaval shunt

maintaining a good portal perfusion and reducing portal pressure are found to be effective alternative to distal splenorenal shunt.

Role of shunt surgery has greatly diminished for the management of varices. However in India, extrahepatic portal vein obstruction (EHPVO) and non-cirrhotic periportal fibrosis (NCPF) are the cause in majority of the patients of varices. This is in contrast to the western patients where cirrhosis is the most common cause. In EHPVO and NCPF liver is not cirrhotic and hence surgical shunt do no result in development of encephalopathy and prevents rebleeding. Due to this reason shunt surgery is a good option in the management of EHPVO and NCPF who had history of massive GI bleed, especially if the patient is staying in an area where access to endoscopy and blood transfusion is not readily available.

Liver Transplant

Liver transplant is the only definitive treatment that cures the underlying liver disease and eradicates the portal hypertension (Fig. 4.10).

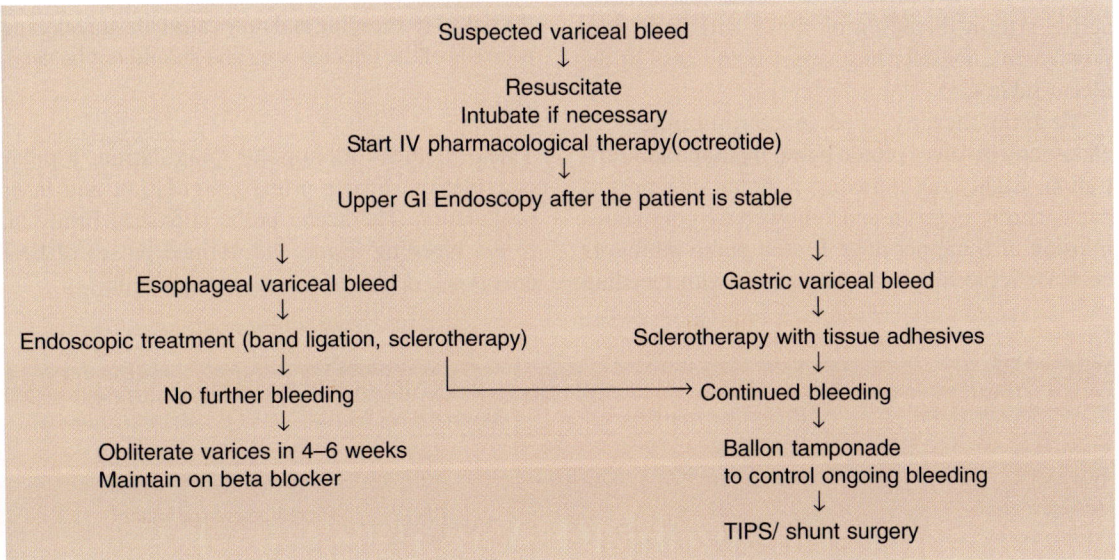

Fig. 4.10: Flowchart for management of acute variceal bleed

PEPTIC ULCER BLEED

Peptic ulcer disease (PUD) is a common cause of UGIB. Duodenal ulcers are more common than gastric ulcers, but the incidence of bleeding is identical for both. In most cases, the bleeding is caused by the erosion of an artery in the base of the ulcer. In approximately 80% of patients, bleeding from a peptic ulcer stops spontaneously. A minority of patients experience recurrent bleeding, and these cases are usually associated with risk factors for rebleeding. These factors include age older than 60 years, the presence of shock upon admission, coagulopathy, active pulsatile bleeding, and the presence of cardiovascular disease. These circumstances are associated with a poorer prognosis and a higher mortality rate.

Upper GI endoscopy is the most effective diagnostic tool for PUD and has become the method of choice for controlling active ulcer hemorrhage. The appearance of the ulcer at the time of endoscopy provides important information regarding the risk of rebleeding. Forrest et al have classified the stigmata of hemorrhage from peptic ulcers based on the endoscopic findings (Box 4.1). The ulcers at highest risk for rebleeding are those that involve active arterial bleeding or those with a visible, protuberant, non-bleeding vessel in the base of the ulcer (Table 4.4).

Medical therapy used in conjunction with endoscopy involves proton pump inhibitor administration. Eighty mg intravenous bolus injection of pantaprozole is given and followed by continuous infusion of 8 mg per hour. Proton pump inhibitors decrease rebleeding rates in patients with bleeding

Box 4.1: Forrest classification
Acute hemorrhage
• Forrest Ia (Spurting hemorrhage)
• Forrest Ib (Oozing hemorrhage)
Signs of recent hemorrhage
• Forrest IIa (Visible vessel)
• Forrest IIb (Adherent clot)
• Forrest IIc (Hematin on ulcer base)
Lesions without active bleeding
• Forrest III (Lesions without signs of recent hemorrhage)

ulcers associated with an overlying clot or visible non-bleeding vessel in the base of the ulcer.

Endoscopic Therapy

Endoscopic modalities available to treat bleeding ulcers are

Injection

The most widely used injection fluid is 1:10 000 adrenaline. This stops active bleeding in more than 90% of cases, but 15–20% of cases will re-bleed. The addition of sclerosants (polidocanol, STD, or ethanolamine) or absolute alcohol does not reduce the risk of re-bleeding and may cause life-threatening necrosis of the injected area and should not be used.

Thermal Energy

These includes monopolar coagulation, bipolar coagulation, heater probe coagulation and laser coagulation. The heater probe is pushed firmly on to the bleeding lesion and defined pulses of heat energy are delivered to cause coagulation.

Table 4.4: Chances of rebleeding, operation and mortality rate according to ulcer characteristic			
Ulcer characteristics	*Rebleeding rate (%)*	*Surgery rate (%)*	*Mortality rate (%)*
Clean base	5	0.5	2
Flat spot	10	6	3
Adherent clot	22	10	7
Visible vessel	43	34	11
Active bleeding	55	35	11

Mechanical Devices

"Endoclips" can be applied to visible vessel.

Role of Surgery

Ten to twelve percent of patients with acute ulcerous hemorrhage require operative procedure to control the bleeding ulcer. In most circumstances, the operation is performed emergently, and the associated mortality rate is as high as 15–25%. If two attempts at endoscopic control of the bleeding vessel are unsuccessful, avoid further attempts (i.e. because of increased rebleeding and mortality rates) and pursue surgical intervention. The indications for surgery in patients with bleeding peptic ulcers are as follows:
- Severe life-threatening hemorrhage not responsive to resuscitative efforts
- Failure of medical therapy and endoscopic hemostasis with persistent or recurrent bleeding
- A coexisting reason for surgery such as perforation, obstruction, or malignancy
- Ongoing transfusion requirement of more than 6 units of packed red cells transfusion in 24 hours
- A second hospitalization for peptic ulcer hemorrhage.

Choice of operation

Bleeding Duodenal Ulcer

Ulcer is exposed by a duodenotomy at the first part of duodenum or by a pyloroduodenotomy. Bleeding duodenal ulcers are characteristically located posteriorly. Direct suture ligation generally controls the bleeding. If direct suture ligation fails then four-quadrant suture ligation at the perimeter of ulcer is done. If that also fails then 3-point ligation of gastroduodenal artery is done. The gastroduodenal artery is ligated both proximally and distally to the arterial bleeding site. The third suture is a horizontal mattress placed to control hemorrhage from the transverse pancreatic branch of the gastroduodenal artery. Failure to place this third stitch may result in recurrent bleeding.

If the patient is stable and there is no preoperative comorbid condition then antisecretory procedure that is truncal vagotomy (Fig. 4.11) along with pyloroplasty/gastrojejunostomy (Fig. 4.12) is done. Anterectomy and vagotomy as acid reduction procedure is also an alternative procedure but generally to be avoided in the emergency set up for the management of bleeding duodenal ulcer.

Bleeding Gastric Ulcer

Gastric ulcers are different than duodenal ulcers as there is 10% chance that gastric ulcer may be malignant and simple ligation of the bleeding gastric ulcer has 30% chance of rebleed. Hence gastric ulcers should be completely excised. The common operations for the management of a bleeding gastric ulcer include
- Truncal vagotomy and drainage procedure with a wedge resection of the ulcer
- Antrectomy with wedge excision of the proximal ulcer
- Distal gastrectomy to include the ulcer with or without truncal vagotomy with Billroth I or Billroth II reconstruction.
- Wedge resection of the ulcer only.

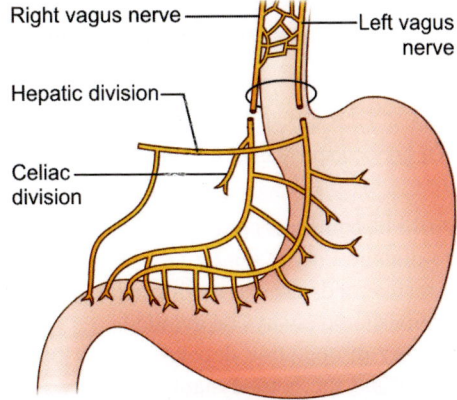

Fig. 4.11: Truncal vagotomy—Right and left vagus nerve trunks are cut

Pyloroplasty

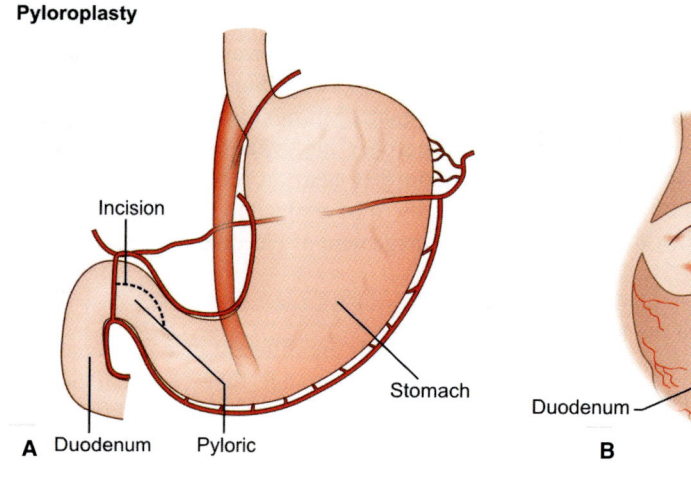

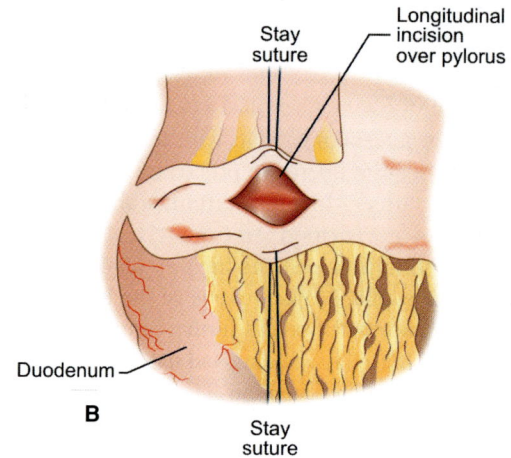

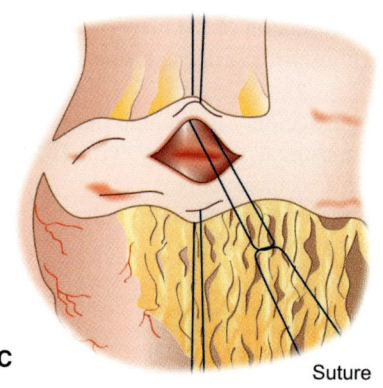

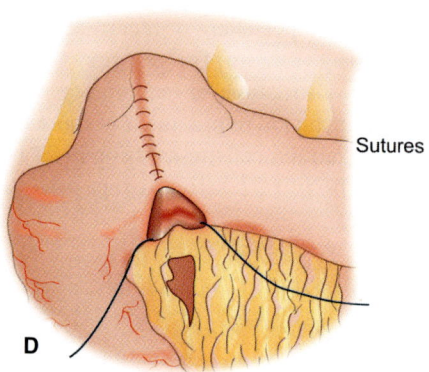

Figs 4.12A to D: Pyloroplasty **(A)** Dotted line showing the site of incision over the pylorus **(B)** Pylorus opened up **(C and D)** Longitudinally opened pylorus is being closed transversely

When the bleeding ulcer is not found in gastrotomy, a pyloro-dudenotomy is done to expose the occult ulcers, erosions and vascular malformations. A blind gastrectomy should always be avoided.

The choice of operation depends on the location of the ulcer and the hemodynamic stability of the patient to withstand an operation. Five types of gastric ulcers occur, based on their location and acid-secretory status.

- Type 1 gastric ulcers are located on the lesser curvature of the stomach at or near the incisura angularis. These ulcers are not associated with a hyper-secretory acid state.
- Type 2 ulcers represent a combination of two ulcers that are associated with a hyper-secretory acid state. The ulcer locations occur in the body of the stomach in the region of the incisura. The second ulcer occurs in the duodenum.

- Type 3 ulcers are prepyloric ulcers. They are associated with high acid output and are usually within 3 cm of the pylorus.
- Type 4 ulcers are located high on the lesser curvature of the stomach and are not associated with high acid output.
- Type 5 ulcers are related to the ingestion of NSAIDs or aspirin. These ulcers can occur anywhere in the stomach.

A vagotomy is added to manage type 2 or type 3 gastric ulcers. These ulcers arise in the pyloric channel or the prepyloric area and are associated with acid hypersecretion physiology. Patients who are hemodynamically stable should undergo a distal gastric resection to include the ulcer for type 1,2, and 3 ulcers, with Billroth I or II reconstruction (Fig. 4.13)

In patients who present with life-threatening hemorrhage and a type 1, 2, or 3 ulcers, biopsy and oversew or excision of the ulcer in combination with a truncal vagotomy and a drainage procedure should be considered. In patients with type 4 ulcers, left gastric artery should be ligated and a biopsy should be performed on the ulcer. Then, the ulcer should be oversewn through a high gastrotomy.

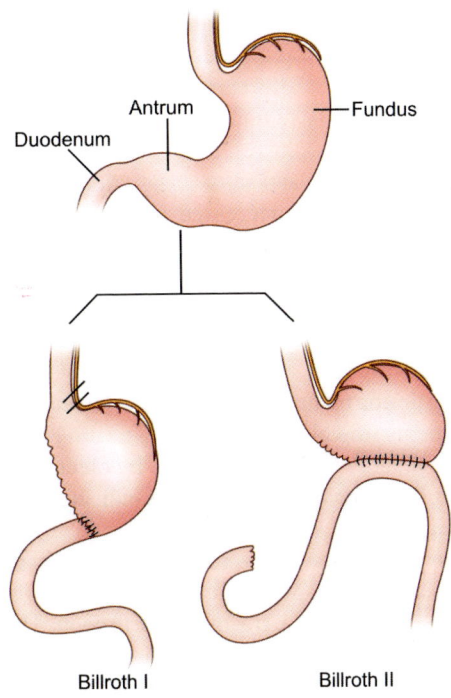

Fig. 4.13: Billroth I and II reconstruction

Eradication of *H pylori*

Helicobacter pylori is present in 90–100% of patients with duodenal ulcers and 70–90% of patients with gastric ulceration. Eradication of the *H. pylori* can reduce the incidence of rebleeding in *H. pylori* related ulcer disease presenting with bleeding. All duodenal ulcers patients and all gastric ulcer patients where there is evidence of *H. pylori* infection on investigation (histopathology, rapid urease test, carbon breath test or serology) should be given anti *H. pylori* treatment in the postoperative period. Triple therapy comprising two antibiotics and an antisecretory drug is the current gold standard for treatment. Anti-*H. pylori* treatment includes proton pump inhibitor (PPI) (20 mg omeprazole) plus amoxicillin 1 gm and clarithromycin 500 mg, all three given twice a day or PPI (20 mg omeprazole) plus metronidazole 400 mg and clarithromycin 250 mg, all three given twice a day for one week.

Stress/Erosive Gastritis

Acute stress gastritis is a disease process characterized by diffuse superficial mucosal erosions that appear as discrete areas of erythema. The bleeding is usually mild, self-limiting and rarely progresses to life-threatening hemorrhage. Stress gastritis and mucosal ulceration are historically associated with head injuries with associated elevations in intracranial pressure and burn injuries. These stress ulcers are called Cushing's ulcer and Curling's ulcer, respectively.

Predisposing clinical conditions have the potential to alter local mucosal protective barriers such as mucus, bicarbonate, blood flow, and prostaglandin synthesis. Any disease process that disrupts the balance of these factors results in diffuse gastric mucosal erosions. This is most commonly observed in patients who have undergone episodes of shock, multiple trauma, acute respiratory distress syndrome, acute renal failure and sepsis. The principal mechanisms involved are decreased splanchnic mucosal blood flow and altered gastric luminal acidity.

Treatment is best accomplished by treating the underlying cause. Aggressive support of hemodynamic parameters ensures adequate mucosal blood flow. Gastric acid suppression is done by administrating proton pump inhibitors (PPIs). Ninety percent of patients stop bleeding with conservative medical therapy. Endoscopic hemostasis by electrocoagulation, laser, or injection therapy is indicated in some points.

Surgical intervention becomes necessary if nonoperative therapy fails and blood loss continues. The goals of operative treatment are to control bleeding and to reduce recurrent bleeding and mortality. These patients are at extremely high risk, and the most expeditious procedure is the best option. Simply oversewing an actively bleeding erosion is sometimes effective enough to control the bleeding. In the setting of life-threatening hemorrhage not amenable to endoscopic control, gastric resection with or without vagotomy with reconstruction may be necessary.

MALLORY–WEISS SYNDROME

Mallory–Weiss syndrome consists of tear in the mucosa of the gastric cardia and occurs because of forceful vomiting, retching, coughing, or straining. These actions create a rapid increase in the gradient between intragastric and intrathoracic pressures, leading to a gastric mucosal tear from the forceful distention of the gastroesophageal junction. The bleeding from a Mallory–Weiss tear spontaneously ceases in 50–80% of patients. For other patients in whom bleeding is visualized at endoscopy, the endoscopic treatment options are electrocoagulation, heater-probe application, or sclerotherapy. Surgical intervention is indicated in patients with continued bleeding after failed attempts at endoscopic

therapies. Bleeding from the gastroesophageal junction is visualized through an anterior gastrotomy and bleeding is controlled by oversewing the lesion.

DIEULAFOY'S LESION

These are submucosal vascular malformation of the proximal stomach, usually within 6 cm of the gastroesophageal junction along the lesser curvature of the stomach. However, it can occur anywhere along the GI tract. This lesion accounts for 2–5% of acute upper GI bleeding episodes. Endoscopically, the lesion appears as a large submucosal vessel that has become ulcerated. Endoscopic treatment modalities can be successful in the management. Although surgical intervention may be required after failed endoscopic therapy, endoscopy is still an important adjunct for management because a nonbleeding Dieulafoy's lesion may be undetectable through a gastrotomy. Hence, the lesion should be marked with India ink at the time of endoscopy. Limited resection of the lesion is all that is needed for Dieulafoy's lesion.

ACUTE LOWER GASTROINTESTINAL BLEEDING

Bleeding in the gastrointestinal tract distal to ligament of Treitz is defined as the lower gastrointestinal bleeding. Acute massive gastrointestinal bleeding presents as hematochezia (fresh bleeding per rectum). However, massive upper gastrointestinal bleeding may also sometimes present as hematochezia. The common causes of lower gastrointestinal bleeding are hemorrhoids, fissure and colonic malignancies. The causes of massive lower GI bleeding are—angiodysplasia, diverticulosis, malignancy, and inflammatory bowel disease. Causes of large bowel and small bowel hemorrhage are given in the Tables 4.5 and 4.6.

EVALUATION AND MANAGEMENT

Initial management is the resuscitation taking care of airway, breathing, and circulation. Vascular access

Table 4.5: Causes of large bowel hemorrhage
• Colonic angiodysplasia
• Colonic carcinoma
• Colonic polyps
• Colitis-ulcerative colitis, Crohn's colitis, infectious colitis
• Post-polypectomy hemorrhage
• Diverticulosis

Table 4.6: Causes of small bowel hemorrhage
• **Vascular lesions**
Angiodysplasia
Telangiectasia
Hemangioma
Arteriovenous malformation
• **Ulceration**
Crohn's disease
NSAID
Meckel's diverticulum
Zollinger–Ellison syndrome
Vasculitis
• **Small intestinal tumors**
Gastrointestinal stromal tumor
Lymphoma
Carcinoid
Small bowel carcinoma
• **Aorto-enteric fistula**
• **Meckel's diverticulum**

is established by two wide bore intravenous cannulas (16 G) and blood is sent for cross matching. Intravenous crystalloids (Ringer lactate) are infused till the blood is arranged. Foley catheter is inserted and fluid resuscitation is governed by monitoring central venous pressure and urine output.

After initial stabilization detailed history is taken and examination is done to detect the cause of the bleeding. Patients with inflammatory bowel disease will have history of frequency of stools with passage of blood and mucus. Patients with rectal malignancy will have tenesmus. There may be associated weight loss with malignancies. Patients with diverticulosis will have pain in the left lower abdomen, constipation and recurrent episodes of diverticulitis. However, many times bleeding due to vascular malformation will have no symptoms prior to the onset of bleeding. Per-rectal examination and procto-scopy will identify the lower rectal and anal canal pathology of malignancy, hemorrhoids, polyps, or fissure.

Investigations for Lower GI Hemorrhage

Upper Gastrointestinal Endoscopy

Upper gastrointestinal endoscopy is the first investigation in a patient with massive and ongoing lower GI bleed, as massive upper gastrointestinal hemorrhage may present as hematochezia.

Further investigations will depend upon whether the bleeding is continuing or it has stopped. If the bleeding is stopped then colonoscopy is done after bowel preparation. The chances of finding the cause of bleeding are more likely when the colonoscopy is done after the episode of bleeding. If the bleeding is continuing but it is slow, then also colonoscopy is the preferred investigation. However, colonoscopy is not helpful if the bleeding is rapid, as the vision will be obscured by the blood. Angiodysplasia (Fig. 4.14) can be treated by bipolar probe coagu-lation or by laser. Malignancy of colon rarely presents with severe bleeding and coagulation of the focal bleeding point can control it, however, appropriate operation according to the pathology should be done in a planned way. In ulcerative colitis mucosa is friable and erythematous with superficial ulcerations and pseudopolyps (Fig. 4.15). Ulcerative colitis is usually continuous from the rectum, with the rectum almost universally being involved.

Push Enteroscopy

Push enteroscopy, where the endoscope is pushed into the jejunum and small intestine, is helpful in diagnosing lesions in the small intestine. In cases of vascular lesion bleeding can be controlled by bipolar coagulation. The site of the lesion can be marked with India ink which helps to identify the site at the time of exploratory laparotomy.

Push enteroscopy is helpful in identifying the bleeding site in 20–40% of bleeding of obscure origin.

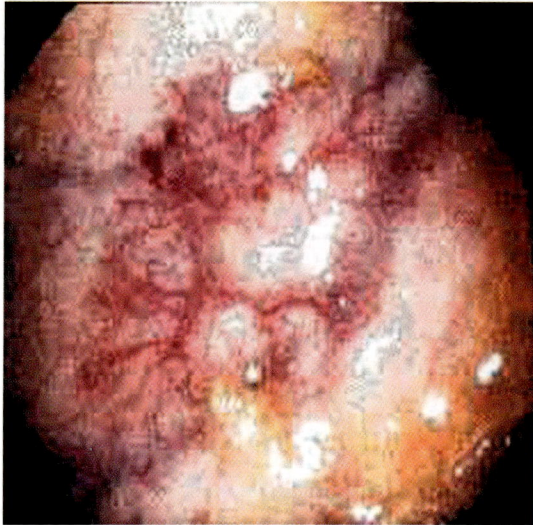

Fig. 4.14: Colonoscopic appearance of angiodysplasia

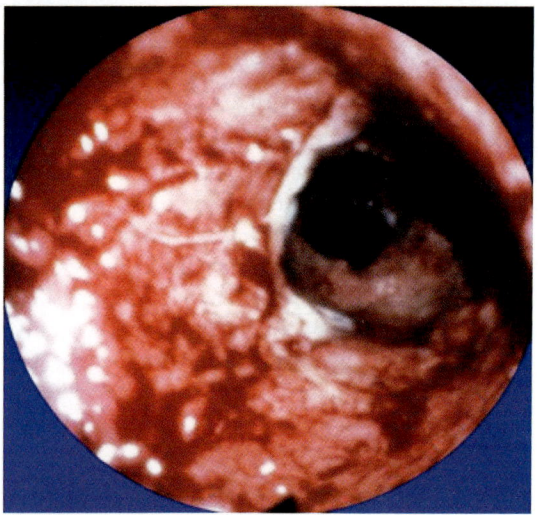

Fig. 4.15: Colonoscopic appearance of ulcerative colitis

Video capsule endoscopy, which allows endoscopic examination of entire small intestine, increases the diagnostic yield in obscure GI bleeding.

Mesenteric Angiography

If the bleeding is ongoing and severe or the source of bleeding is not identifiable by colonoscopy or push enteroscopy, then mesenteric angiography is the next investigation. If the rate of bleeding is more than 0.5 ml/min, then the site of bleeding will be detected by angiography in 50–70% of cases. Angiographic embolization can also be carried out by Gelfoam or metal microcoils embolization, however, there is a risk of bowel ischemia with embolization. Intra-arterial injection of vasopressin has high hemostatic rate but the rate of rebleeding is high. When a small vascular abnormality has been identified in preoperative angiography, identification of that particular lesion at laparotomy may still be very difficult. In such situation Intraoperative angiography is helpful in the management of the case.

Radioisotope Scan

Radioisotope scan using ^{99m}Tc tagged RBC cell is another option to detect the site of the bleeding. If rate of bleeding is more than 0.1 ml/min, then it will be picked up by the isotope scan. However, it only gives a rough idea about the site like proximal or distal small intestine and the exact site cannot be detected. Moreover, therapeutic procedure cannot be done with this investigation (Fig. 4.16).

INDICATIONS FOR SURGERY

- Ongoing and recurrent bleeding
- Transfusion of more than 6 units of packed cells in 24 hours
- Ongoing transfusion requirement
- Persistent hemodynamic instability.

Prior to operation attempt should be made to localize the source of bleeding by colonoscopy, push enteroscopy, angiography or isotope scan. Blind total colectomy carries significantly higher mortality and morbidity, and blind segmental colectomy has a high re-bleeding rate. For these reasons blind resection of bowel should not be done.

If site of bleeding is identified in the colon then limited resection or hemicolectomy should be done. In small intestine segmental resection at the identified site should be done. If site of bleeding was not apparent or was not evaluated preoperatively then intraoperative endoscopy is carried out.

At the time of operation first it is seen whether the blood is in colon or is in both colon and small intestine. If bleeding is present only in colon then colon is to be evaluated first via intraoperative colonoscopy. If blood is in the small intestine then small intestine is evaluated first by push enteroscopy, which is assisted by the intraoperative manipulation. However, in case of incompetent ileocecal junction the blood from the colon may go to the small intestine.

If facilities of angiography, isotope scan or intraoperative endoscopy is not available and patient is explored for lower GI bleed then segment of the intestine can be sequentially clamped to see which segment is getting filled and that segment is resected. This is not an ideal procedure and is done when other investigative modalities are not available.

If the site of bleeding is not localized but it is apparent that it is from colon (no blood in the small intestine) then subtotal/total colectomy (resection of ascending, transverse, descending and sigmoid colon) is done as the last resort to save the life of patient.

There are several conditions of gastrointestinal bleeding of obscure origin. Angiodysplastic and Dieulafoy's lesion are the common gastric lesions that may easily be missed at gastroscopy. Hemobilia, which presents as a characteristic triad of malena, biliary pain and jaundice are generally seen after number of interventions like transhepatic puncture for cholangiography or stenting or after surgery on biliary tree and pancreas. Congenital anomaly like Meckel's diverticulum may at time be a cause of obscure gastrointestinal bleeding. Small bowel tumors, inflammatory and angiodysplastic lesions of colon are also important causes of obscure gastrointestinal bleeding. A diagnostic laparotomy should be performed to assess the actual source of bleeding and treated accordingly.

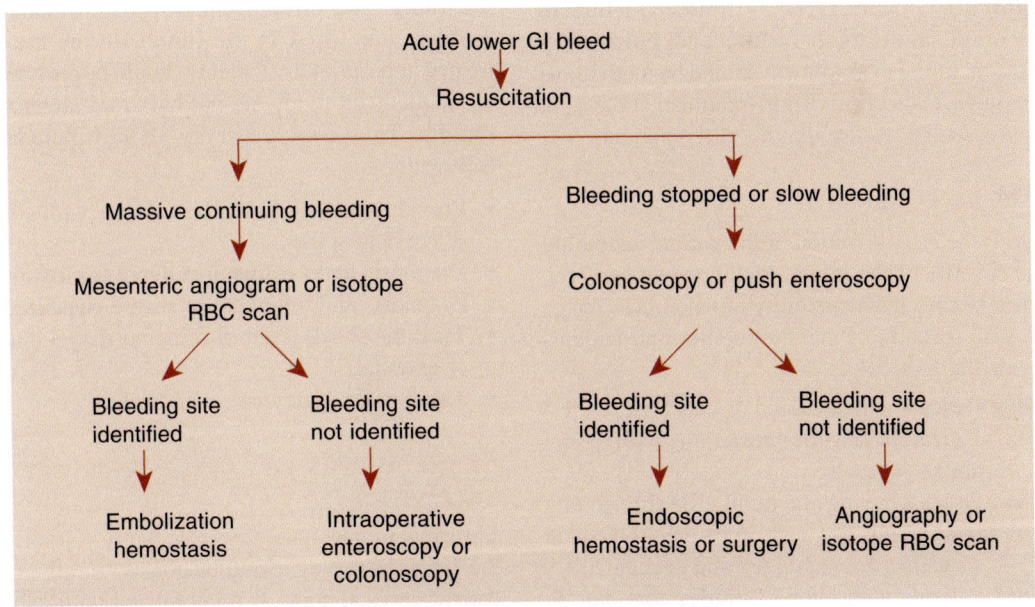

Fig. 4.16: Management of lower GI bleed

5 Initial Resuscitation of Trauma Patients

Road side accidents are a global problem and it spares none. In the present era such trauma is a major cause of morbidity and mortality. Mortality following trauma shows trimodal distribution. Half of the patients die within minutes of injury and these deaths are due to injury to the vital structures like brain stem, heart, and aorta. These mortalities can not be prevented medically. Second peak of mortality occurs within first hour of injury, also known as the golden hour and are because of hemothorax, pneumothorax, hemorrhage and intracranial injuries. These mortalities are mostly preventable. Third peak of mortality occurs after 24 hours are due to septicemia, multiorgan failure and pulmonary embolism. Initial management should be methodical and requires team effort. Right treatment at the right time is essential to save the life of the patient.

TRIAGE

Triage is the categorization of the patient according to the severity of the injury, likelihood of survival, urgency of care and availability of resources. Triage is done in scenario of mass casualties and patients are coded in four colors (Fig. 5.1)

Black Patients who are dead or expected to die
Red Patients having life-threatening injuries and are salvageable.
Yellow Patients having potentially life-threatening injuries but can wait until the immediate casualties are stabilized and evacuated.
Green Patients with simple injuries that can be discharged after initial treatment

INITIAL EVALUATION AND RESUSCITATION OF THE INJURED PATIENT

Initial treatment of injured patient consists of primary survey, resuscitation, secondary survey, diagnostic evaluation and definitive care.

Primary Survey

The primary survey is a structured assessment that aims to identify and treat immediate and life-threatening problems. Primary survey consists of ABC—airway, with cervical spine protection, breathing, and circulation. Any life-threatening problem identified in the initial survey must be treated appropriately. Patients should be reevaluated at frequent intervals, as patients may deteriorate rapidly. The primary survey should include the following:

- Provide and secure the clear airway with control of cervical spine
- Diagnosis and treatment of hypoventilation
- Diagnosis and treatment of severe chest injury
- Treat the shock (control of hemorrhage, internal or external)
- Assessment of neurological disability.

Airway Management with Cervical Spine Control

Ensuring an adequate airway is the first priority in the primary survey. Simultaneously, in all trauma patient cervical spine is immobilized until cervical injury is ruled out. This can be done by a hard

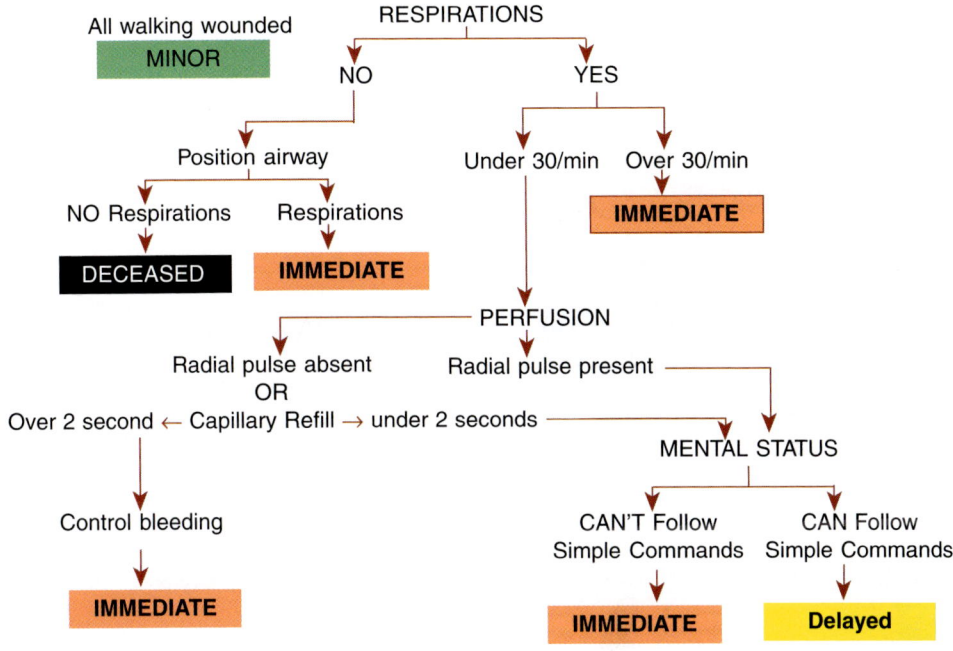

RESPIRATIONS

All walking wounded
MINOR

NO — YES

Position airway — Under 30/min — Over 30/min

NO Respirations — Respirations — **IMMEDIATE**

DECEASED — **IMMEDIATE**

PERFUSION

Radial pulse absent
OR
Over 2 second ← Capillary Refill → under 2 seconds — Radial pulse present

MENTAL STATUS

Control bleeding

CAN'T Follow
Simple Commands — CAN Follow
Simple Commands

IMMEDIATE — **IMMEDIATE** — **Delayed**

Fig. 5.1: Triage of patients in a scenario of mass casualty

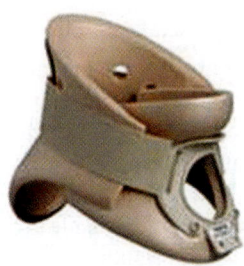

Fig. 5.2: Philadelphia collar

Philadelphia collar (Fig. 5.2) or placing sand bags on both sides of head. Soft collars do not immobilize the cervical spine.

Patients who are conscious and have normal voice do not require further evaluation or early attention to their airway. Patients who have abnormal voice or altered mental status require further airway evaluation. Suctioning of the mouth to remove blood/

vomitus and removal of foreign objects present in the oral cavity can result in immediate relief in many patients.

Jaw thrust or chin lift maneuver with cervical spine control can open the airway in simple cases (Figs 5.3A to C), alternatively one may need to use an oropharyngeal or a nasopharyngeal airway (Fig. 5.4). Options for airway access include nasotracheal intubation, orotracheal intubation, or operative intervention (cricothyroidotomy or tracheostomy).

Patients in whom attempts at intubation have failed or is not possible because of extensive facial injuries require surgical procedure like crico-thyroidotomy or tracheostomy. Cricothyroidotomy and percutaneous transtracheal ventilation is preferred over tracheostomy because of their simplicity and safety. Percutaneous transtracheal ventilation is accomplished by inserting a large bore intravenous catheter through the cricothyroid

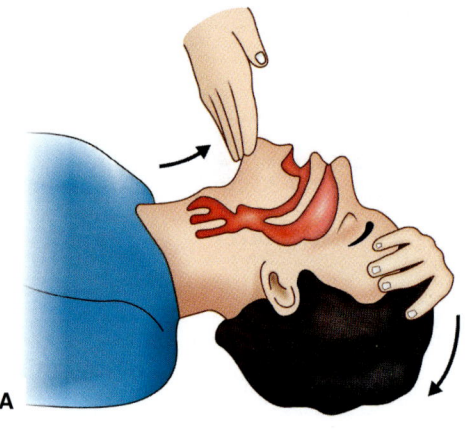

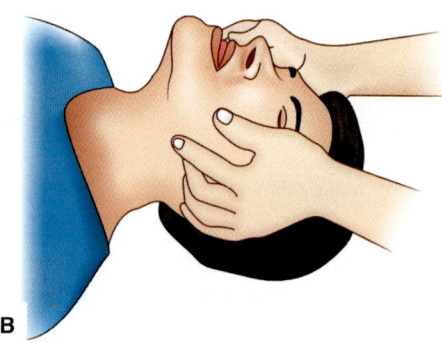

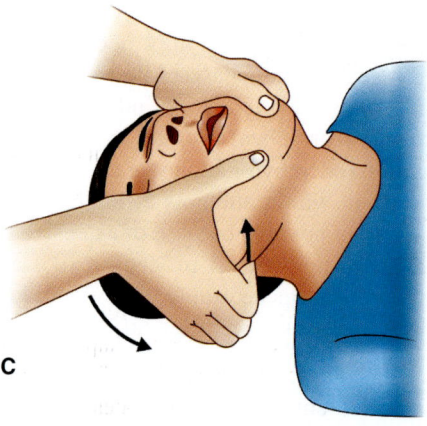

Figs 5.3A to C: (A) Head tilt/ chin lift, (B) Jaw trust, (C) Triple airway maneuver

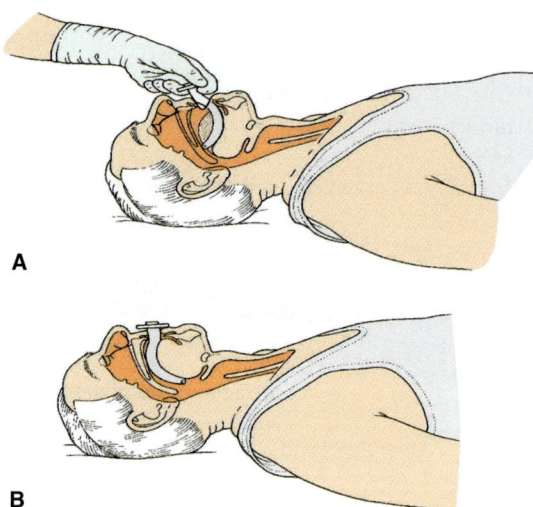

Figs 5.4A and B: Nasopharyngeal airway is inserted upside down into the patients mouth then rotated 180° as it slides into the pharynx

membrane into the trachea and attaching it to an oxygen source.

Procedure of Orotracheal Intubation

- Assure adequate ventilation and oxygenation. Make sure suctioning equipment is immediately available in the event the patient vomits.
- Inflate the cuff of the endotracheal tube to ascertain that the balloon does not leak, then deflate the cuff.
- Connect the laryngoscope blade to the handle, and check the bulb for brightness.
- Have an assistant to manually immobilize the head and neck. The patient's neck must not be hyperextended or hyperflexed during the procedure.
- Hold the laryngoscope in the left hand.
- Insert the laryngoscope into the right side of the patient's mouth, displacing the tongue to the left.
- Visually examine the epiglottis and then the vocal cords.
- Gently insert the endotracheal tube into the trachea without applying pressure on the teeth or oral tissues.

- Inflate the cuff with enough air to provide an adequate seal. Do not overinflate the cuff.
- Check the placement of the tube by auscultating the chest and abdomen with a stethoscope to ascertain tube position.
- Visually observe lung expansion with ventilation.
- Secure the tube. If the patient is moved, the tube placement should be reassessed.
- If endotracheal intubation is not accomplished within seconds, discontinue attempts, ventilate the patient with a bag-valve mask device, and try again later.

Procedure of Cricothyroidotomy

The cricothyroid membrane is the soft avascular membrane just below the Adam's apple (thyroid cartilage) and just above the cricoid cartilage (Fig. 5.5A). In men, this is easily identified by running the finger down the center of the neck. Cricothyroid membrane is felt just beyond the Adam's apple as a small, soft indentation about the width of a finger. The thyroid cartilage (Adam's apple) in women is not usually as prominent as it is in men. It is easier to find their cricothyroid membrane by sliding ones finger up the midline of the neck. The first hard bump felt is the cricoid cartilage. Above it is the cricothyroid membrane.

1. Identify the cricothyroid membrane.
2. Make an incision directly over the cricothyroid membrane. The incision should be about an inch long (Fig. 5.5B).
3. Once through the skin, feel for the soft, compressible cricothyroid membrane.
4. Cricothyroid membrane is then incised and hollow tube is inserted.

An emergency cricothyroidotomy can be left in place for up to 72 hours, but after that, it should be replaced by a tracheostomy. Tracheostomy is indicated in patients with suspected laryngeal injury.

Breathing

Once the airway is secured, adequate oxygenation and ventilation is provided. A patent airway does

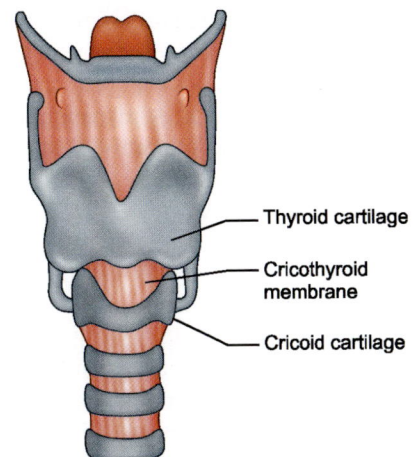

Fig. 5.5A: Anatomy of cricothyroid membrane

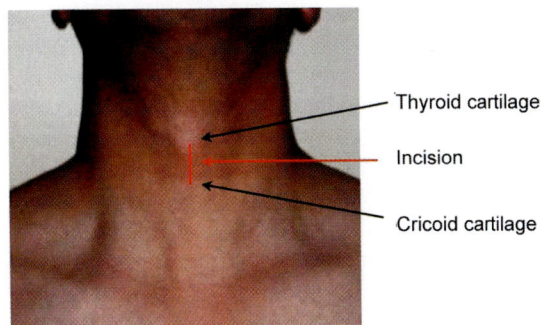

Fig. 5.5B: Incision for cricothyroidotomy

little for a patient who is not breathing, and no ventilation is provided. Expose the chest wall and look for its characteristic rise and fall. Respiratory rate, effort, and symmetry of movement of chest wall are recorded, all of which provide a sensitive indication of underlying pathology. Breathing rate less than 12/min or greater than 28/min indicate significant abnormality. Depth of respiration is seen, trachea is felt to detect any deviation, neck veins are examined whether it is full or collapsed and chest is auscultated for any abnormality of sound and for equality of air entry on both the sides.

Patients who are breathing spontaneously should be given high flow (80%) oxygen, via a face mask and a reservoir bag. Those requiring help to maintain breathing should be given 100% oxygen through a bag valve mask and intubation should be considered. It is essential to rule out life-threatening injuries listed below which may compromise ventilation.

- Tension pneumothorax
- Massive hemothorax
- Open chest wound
- Flail segment (a segment of unstable rib cage after multiple fractures of the ribs and sternum).

Tension Pneumothorax: Tension pneumothorax is the accumulation of air under pressure in the pleural space. This condition develops when injured tissue forms a one-way valve, allowing air to enter the pleural space and preventing the air from escaping naturally (Figs 5.6 and 5.7). Arising from numerous causes, this condition rapidly progresses to respiratory insufficiency, cardiovascular collapse and ultimately death if unrecognized and untreated.

Tension pneumothorax is suspected if the patient has got respiratory distress with any of the following signs-tracheal deviation to the opposite side, distended neck veins, absent or decreased breath sound on affected side of the chest.

Tension pneumothorax is treated by insertion of a large bore needle (16 G) in the 2nd intercostal space in the midclavicular line of the affected thorax (Fig. 5.8). After this a chest tube is inserted in the usual way. Treatment of the suspected tension pneumothorax should not be delayed for the want of a chest X-ray.

Open Chest Wound: An open chest wound can be caused by the chest wall being penetrated by a bullet, knife blade, shrapnel, or other object and there is pleural breach. When a patient with an open chest wound breathes, because of the negative intrapleural pressure, air goes in and out of the wound. This air sometimes causes a "sucking" sound. Because of this distinct sound, an open chest wound is often called a "sucking" chest wound. The area around the open chest wound is exposed by removing the clothing covering the wound. Occlusion of the injury

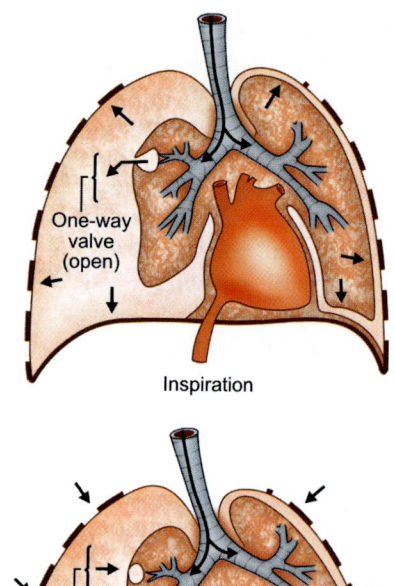

Inspiration

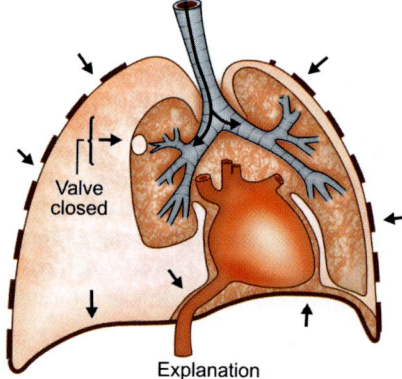

Explanation

Fig. 5.6: One-way valve leading to development of tension pneumothorax

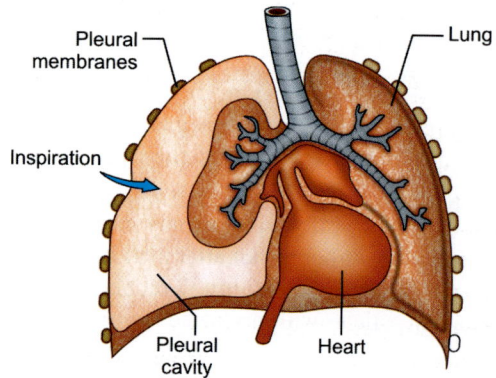

Fig. 5.7: One-way valve leading to development of tension pneumothorax

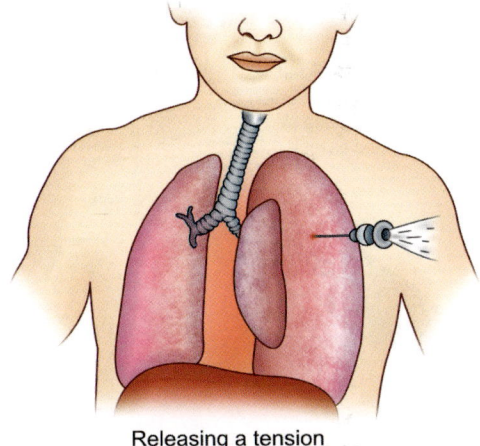

Releasing a tension
pneumothorax

Fig. 5.8: Wide bore needle is inserted in the 2nd intercostal space in the midclavicular line to relieve the tension in tension pneumothorax

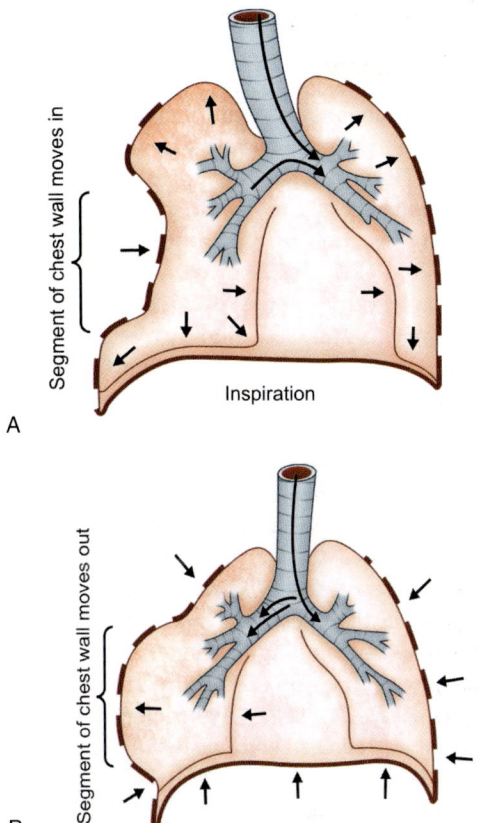

A

Inspiration

B

Explanation

Figs 5.9A and B: Paradoxical movement of flail segment

may result in converting an open pneumothorax into a tension pneumothorax. Proper treatment is to place an occlusive dressing over the wound which is taped on three sides and open on one side. This prevents entry of air into the pleural space during inhalation and the untapped side allows the accumulated air to escape during expiration. Definitive treatment is to place a chest tube and closure of the wound.

Flail chest: A flail chest occurs when a segment of the thoracic cage is separated from the rest of the chest wall. This is usually defined as at least two fractures per rib, in at least two ribs. There is paradoxical movement of the flail segment of the chest wall during respiration and this flail segment does not contribute to lung expansion and ventilation. The flail chest is identified as paradoxical movement of the segment of the chest wall-inward movement on inspiration and outward movement on expiration (Figs 5.9A and B). The main significance of a flail chest, however is that it indicates the presence of an underlying pulmonary contusion. Providing adequate analgesia is mainstay of the treatment. In case of respiratory distress patient

requires endotracheal intubation and mechanical ventilation.

Massive hemothorax: Accumulation of large amount of blood in the pleural cavity (massive hemothorax) may compress the underlying lung and compromise the ventilation. Massive hemothorax is suspected if the patient has got respiratory distress, breath sounds are decreased on the affected side, trachea is shifted to the opposite site and affected side is dull on percussion. Hemothorax should always be suspected if there is rib fracture. The treatment is to immediately insert a chest tube on the affected side.

INSERTION OF CHEST TUBE

Triangle of Safety

Before inserting the chest tube reconfirm the side of insertion of the chest tube based on clinical findings and chest X-ray if it has been done. It is preferable to obtain the chest X-ray but in case of emergency situations insertion of the chest tube should not delayed for the want of X-ray.

The preferred position for drain insertion is patient lying supine on the bed, slightly rotated, with the arm on the side of the lesion behind the patient's head to expose the axillary area. The tube is inserted in the triangle of safety which is bordered by the anterior border of the latissimus dorsi, the lateral border of the pectoralis major muscle, a line superior to the horizontal level of the nipple in a man or the fourth intercostal space in a woman (Fig. 5.10A). The triangle of safety contains no important structures in the chest wall and also chances of inadvertently perforating the diaphragm, even it is raised, are very low. After cleaning and draping, local anesthesia (15–20 ml of 1% lignocaine) is infiltrated into the skin, intercostal muscle down to the parietal pleura. The tract of the injection should be just above the rib to avoid the neurovascular bundle which runs at the lower border of the rib (Fig. 5.10B).

A skin incision of about 2 cm is then made at the anesthetized area and deepened into the subcutaneous fat (Fig. 5.10B). Intercostal muscle is then split using a Kelly's clamp. It is important that

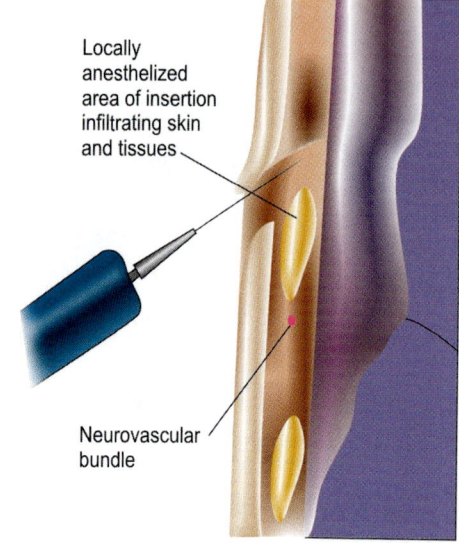

Fig. 5.10B: Infiltration of local anesthesia at the upper border of the lower rib

incision and the tract should be at the upper border of the rib to avoid injury to the neurovascular bundle. Pleura are then punctured with the Kelly's clamp and the jaws of the clamp are opened widely parallel to the direction of the ribs. Finger is then inserted through the incision into the thoracic cavity. It is ensured that an empty space is felt and the lung is not adhered to the bony cage. End of chest tube is grasped with the Kelly's forcep (convex angle towards ribs) and the tube is inserted through the hole made in the pleura (Fig. 5.10C). After the tube has entered thoracic cavity, the Kelly is removed, and the tube is manually advanced and the other end is connected to an underwater seal bag. Chest tube is then fixed to the skin by taking a purse string suture and dressing is applied. Underwater seal bag prevents the entry of air into the pleural cavity.

After the insertion of the chest tube, it is important to note the content which has come out of the tube (air, blood, pus). Air bubbling in the water column of the bag indicates the presence of air leak. Under water seal bag should be always kept at a level below the site of insertion of chest tube. Chest X-ray should

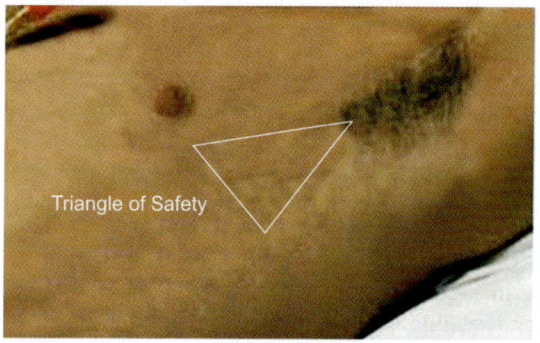

Triangle of Safety

Fig. 5.10A: Triangle of safety for insertion of chest tube

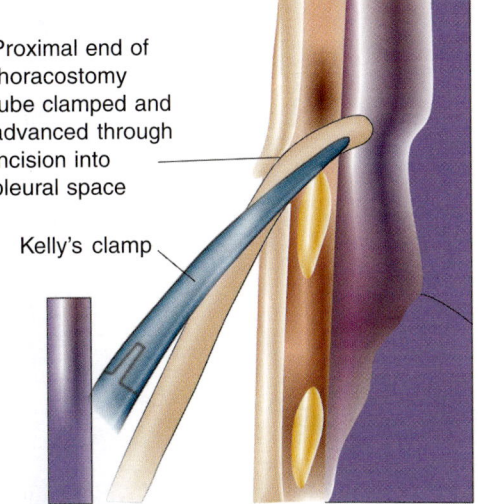

Proximal end of thoracostomy tube clamped and advanced through incision into pleural space

Kelly's clamp

Fig. 5.10C: Insertion of chest tube with the help of Kelly's clamp

must have been decreased by 30–40% before hypotension occurs. Severe external hemorrhage should be controlled by direct manual pressure on the wound. Splinting of extremity decreases the bleeding from the fracture site. Internal hemorrhage may require immediate surgery. Look for source of bleeding in the thoracic cavity, peritoneal cavity or fracture of pelvis or long bones, if patient has got hypotension.

Box 5.1: Signs of hypotensive shock
• Increased respiratory rate
• Decreased blood pressure
• Increased heart rate
• Decreased pulse pressure
• Clammy skin
• Decreased urine output
• Increased capillary refill time
• Decreased level of consciousness

be done after the chest tube insertion to evaluate the position of the chest tube.

Chest tube is removed when the output of the drain has decreased, there is no air leak and the lung has expanded as seen in chest X-ray.

Circulation

After the airway is secured and adequate ventilation is established, circulatory status is evaluated. Blood volume and cardiac output are key concerns in the acute setting; prolonged impairment of the cerebral circulation will ultimately cause death of brain cells. Therefore, it is important to correct the hypovolemia; taking care of both internal and external injuries. Any injured patient who is cold, clammy, sweating, restless and anxious is really in hypovolemic shock. A number of clinical signs are typical of hypotensive shock (Box 5.1). However, no single factor should be used to rule out hypovolemia. At this point hypotension if present is assumed to be caused by hemorrhage.

The commonest mistake is to miss an internal hemorrhage in a young patient because of normal blood pressure. Hypotension is a relatively late sign of hypovolemia in young patients and blood volume

Intravenous access is obtained by inserting two large bore (16 G) cannulas in the peripheral veins. Blood sample is sent simultaneously for cross matching at this point. If veins are collapsed and peripheral venous access is not possible then saphenous vein cut down is performed. Long saphenous vein is reliably found one cm anterior and one cm superior to the medial malleolus (Figs 5.11A to D). At times in shock patients the intense venous spasm of long saphenous vein at ankle may prevent the infusion. In such situation the cut down of the long saphenous vein in the groin allows insertion of large bore cannula for a faster infusion.

Initial fluid for resuscitation is 1 litre of either normal saline or lactated Ringer's solution in an adult or 20 ml/kg in a child. This can be repeated once in case of no response. Plain dextrose should not be given. If patient does not respond even after second bolus of fluid challenge then blood transfusion is indicated. The goal of fluid resuscitation is to establish adequate tissue perfusion. Monitoring of urine output by inserting a Foley catheter is a good and reliable indicator of organ perfusion. Adequate urine output is 0.5 ml/kg/hr in an adult and 1 ml/kg/hr in a child.

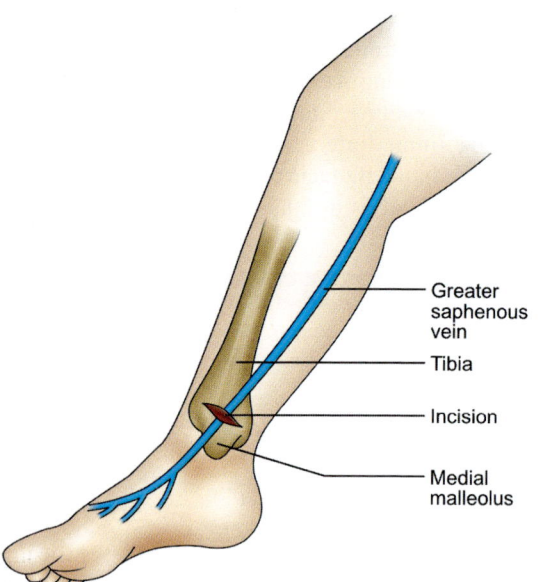

Fig. 5.11A: Site of incision for saphenous cut down (one cm anterior and one cm superior to the medial malleolus)

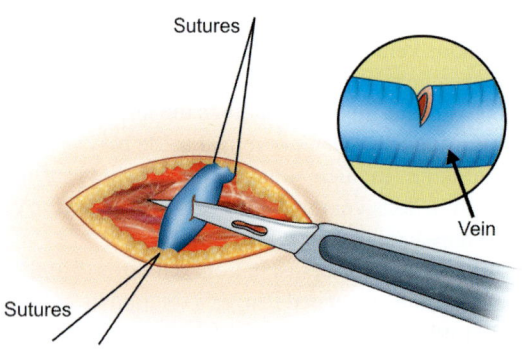

Fig. 5.11B: After dissecting out the saphenous vein two sutures are passed around it. The distal suture is tied and a nick is given on the vein

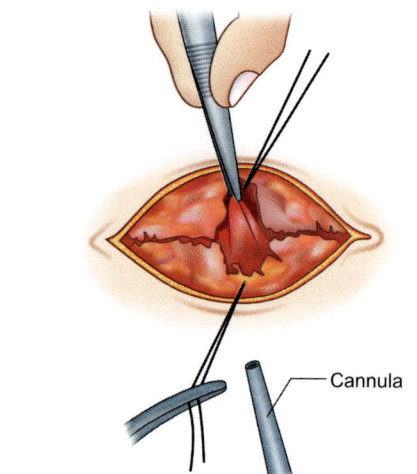

Fig. 5.11C: A catheter is inserted through the nick and the proximal suture taken earlier is tied over the catheter

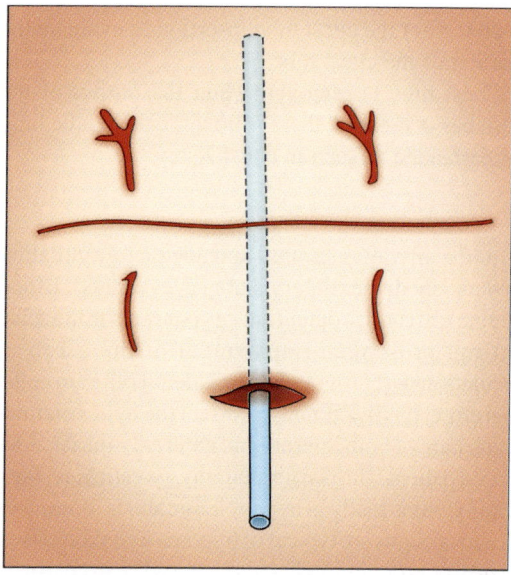

Fig. 5.11D: Skin incision is closed

Apart from hypovolemia other causes for compromised circulation are cardiac tamponade cardiac injuries and myocardial infarction. In cardiac tamponade blood accumulates in the pericardium and it does not allow the heart to get filled up. It should always be suspected in all patients with penetrating injury to the anterior part of left chest. Classical triad (Beck's triad) of cardiac tamponade is muffled heart sounds, distended neck veins and hypotension. It is treated by doing pericardiocentesis (Fig. 5.12).

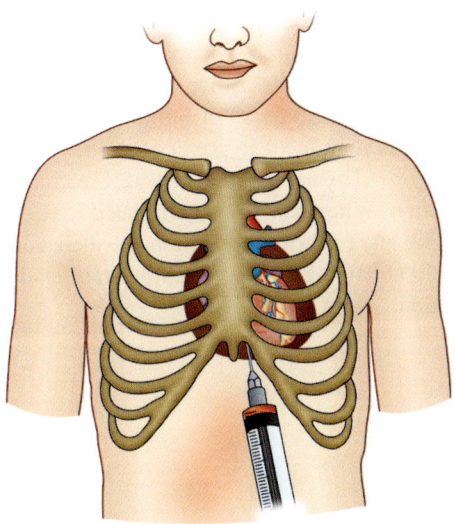

Fig. 5.12: Pericardiocentesis

Pericardiocentesis

- Local anesthesia is infiltrated just below the xiphoid process
- Needle mounted on syringe is inserted through the anesthetized area.
- The needle should be advanced towards the left shoulder at an angle 15–20° from the abdominal wall. While advancing the needle towards maintain negative pressure. Continue to advance the needle until fluid is aspirated in the syringe or the ECG monitor shows ST elevation.
- Withdraw the needle slowly with negative pressure on the syringe if the ECG shows ST elevation.

- Reinsert the needle in a different direction very slowly until fluid is aspirated in the syringe.

Myocardial contusion which is generally seen with thoracic crush injury (steering wheel injury) and usually leads to cardiac rhythm disturbances. ECG monitoring is essential in such circumstances. Myocardial infarction may preceed the traumatic event or can be a result of coronary hypoperfusion as a result of injury. Treatment to be done like any other case of myocardial infarction.

Disability

A quick neurological assessment is performed early. If the patient is talking, he or she must have a clear airway, adequate ventilation, and intact cerebral perfusion. Although this does not give any long-term reassurances, other areas of priority can be assessed.

The neurological status of a patient who is not talking must be evaluated. This is best done by using the AVPU system (Box 5.2). Pupilary reflexes must also be established. Although Glasgow Coma Scale (GCS) is more accurate, it can be approximated to AVPU. A formal assessment using the GCS is done as part of the comprehensive secondary survey (see chapter—Head Injury).

Box 5.2: AVPU
• A—Alert and oriented (GCS 14–15)
• V—Responds to vocal stimuli (GCS 9–13)
• P—Responds to painful stimuli (GCS 4–8)
• U— Unresponsive (GCS 3)

Exposure

By this stage of the initial assessment most of the patient's clothes will have been removed; those that remain should be cut away, leaving the patient fully undressed. This allows a thorough examination (as part of the secondary survey). Take care to keep the patient warm because hypothermia can have devastating consequences.

Secondary Survey

A thorough head to toe assessment is made in secondary survey after the patient has been stabilized with the aim to identify all the injuries sustained. A thorough abdominal and chest examination should be undertaken. During this period additional intravenous access, catheterization, nasogastric tube insertion, basic blood investigations and attachment of monitors are done.

Take a complete history from the patient if possible, or from the ambulance crew or relatives. Key questions stem from the mnemonic AMPLE: **a**llergies, **m**edication, **p**ast medical history, **l**ast meal, and **e**vents and environment related to injury.

Before examining patients with a possible history of blunt trauma, X-ray images of the cervical spine, chest, and pelvis are taken. Examination is then done to look for all possible injuries.

DEFINITIVE CARE

Definitive care begins once the patient has been resuscitated and life-threatening problems are dealt with. During this phase a complete package of care is planned for the patient and includes fracture stabilization, operative intervention or the transfer of the patient to a tertiary referral center.

The initial resuscitation of injured patient needs a team approach. Number of specialists of different discipline working together always have better outcome. The main focus of initial resuscitation is towards prevention of hypoxia at tissue level and that is ensured by maintaining airway, breathing, and circulation. Whenever any patient need to be transported for any further investigation and management, it should always be done after initial stabilization of the patient.

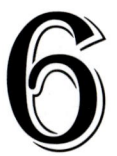

Blunt and Penetrating Abdominal Trauma

INTRODUCTION

Blunt abdominal trauma is a leading cause of morbidity and mortality among all age groups. Identification of serious intra-abdominal pathology is often challenging. Many injuries may not manifest during the initial assessment and treatment period. Many times blunt abdominal trauma is associated with other injuries that may divert the physician's attention from potentially life-threatening intra-abdominal pathology. Patient in following situations carry a fairly high risk for abdominal injuries

- Unexplained hypovolemic shock and hemo-dynamic instability
- Presence of major chest injury and pelvic fractures
- Impaired sensorium with possibility of head injury
- Presence of hematuria
- Objective abdominal findings
- Severe mode of injury.

Abdominal trauma could be either penetrating or blunt. Decision for the treatment in penetrating trauma is considered to be easier than that of blunt abdominal trauma. The frequent coexistence of multiple injuries and at times head injury renders the physical examination unreliable in cases of blunt abdominal trauma. The significant extremity fracture and associated soft tissue injury may distract the patient from noticing the abdominal symptoms.

Approximately 6% of all patients of blunt abdominal trauma will require laparotomy primarily for intra-abdominal hemorrhage. Whereas in majority of the cases of penetrating injury, laparotomy becomes essential.

PATHOPHYSIOLOGY

Injury to intra-abdominal structures can be because of compression or deceleration forces. The liver and spleen are the most frequently injured organs. Small and large intestines are the next most injured organs respectively.

Compression or concussive forces from direct blows or external compression against the spinal column can cause tear and subcapsular hematoma to the solid viscera. These forces may also traumatize hollow organs and transiently increase intraluminal pressure, resulting their perforation. This transient pressure increase is found to be a common mechanism of blunt trauma to the small and large bowel.

Deceleration forces cause stretching and linear shearing between relatively fixed and free objects. Classic deceleration injuries include hepatic tear along the ligamentum teres and injuries to the renal arteries. As bowel loops travel from their mesenteric attachments, mesenteric tears with resultant splanchnic vessel injuries can result.

The penetrating injury of gunshot/missile origin lacerates and crushes the tissues along the missile tract. Gunshot injury of high velocity, in addition to the energy generation also causes a phenomenon known as "cavitation". The extent of cavitation depends upon the density and elasticity of the target organ associated with the injury and may involve many centimeters around the missile tract. Liver may get shattered because of the cavitational forces, whereas little damage is seen in through and through injury to the lung on account of elasticity. Bowel perforations because of gunshot injury need wide excision and anastomosis as treatment.

INITIAL MANAGEMENT

Evaluation and resuscitation should occur simultaneously on the basis of ATLS—Advanced Trauma Life Support (airway, breathing, and circulation). Life-threatening injuries should be identified and treated accordingly. Necessary intravenous fluid resuscitation should be done, blood should be arranged and Foley catheter should be passed. All patients of penetrating gunshot wound of abdomen should be explored by laparotomy. In cases of stab wounds of the abdomen where there is no peritoneal penetration, patients can be safely discharged after primary treatment.

The peritoneal penetration is always checked by local exploration. In case, there is a definite clinical finding suggestive of peritonitis on account of injury to hollow viscus (stomach, small bowel, or colon) the necessary repair of perforation or resection of intestine may be undertaken in hemodynamically stable patients. Many times the diagnosis of peritonitis is not straight forward as some of the patients have local pain at the site of penetration. Such patients need close observation and if generalized peritonitis supervenes then laparotomy should be performed.

Many of the surgeons in case of doubt of peritonitis do prefer to perform the diagnostic peritoneal lavage to confirm the intra-abdominal injury. The red blood cell threshold is typically used as an indication of laparotomy.

In cases of blunt abdominal trauma, diagnostic tests are essential to guide the further line of management along with the findings of clinical examination.

EXAMINATION

Inspection

Examine the abdomen to determine the presence of external signs of injury, patterns of abrasion and/or ecchymotic areas or "seat belt sign", i.e. bruising on the abdomen along the site of the lap portion of the safety belt should be noted. Seat belt sign is associated with high rate of injury to the abdominal organs specially the hollow viscus. Flank bruising and swelling may raise suspicion of retroperitoneal injuries. One should also inspect genitals and perineum for any soft tissue injuries, bleeding, and hematoma.

Palpation

Careful palpation of the abdomen may reveal tenderness, guarding, or rigidity, which can be due to intra-abdominal hemorrhage or associated peritonitis because of bowel perforation. Fullness in the flanks may indicate intra-abdominal hemorrhage. Crepitation or instability of the lower thoracic cage indicates the potential for splenic or hepatic injuries associated with lower rib fractures. Pelvic compression test is done to see for pelvic fracture. Rectal and bimanual vaginal examinations are essential to see for injuries and bleeding.

LABORATORY STUDIES

Initial treatment and resuscitation should not depend on the laboratory findings, but during the period of resuscitation blood sample should be sent for cross matching and rest of the routine investigations like serum glucose, complete blood count (CBC), serum amylase, urinalysis, coagulation studies, arterial blood gas (ABG).

IMAGING STUDIES

The three important diagnostic tests that guide the surgeon in patients of blunt abdominal trauma are FAST (Focused Abdominal Sonogram for Trauma), computed tomography (CT) and diagnostic peritoneal lavage (DPL). Only the DPL and the FAST are suitable and appropriate in hemodynamically unstable patients, whereas the CT scan should only be done in stable patients.

Focused Abdominal Sonogram for Trauma

Bedside ultrasonography in the form of focused abdominal sonogram for trauma (FAST) is used for the evaluation of trauma patients. FAST's diagnostic accuracy is generally equal to that of diagnostic peritoneal lavage (DPL). In the patient with isolated blunt abdominal trauma or multisystem injuries, bedside ultrasonography performed by an experienced sonographer can rapidly detect free intraperitoneal fluid, especially if greater than 200-500 ml. The sensitivity for solid organ encapsulated injury is moderate and hollow viscus injury rarely be identified; however, free fluid may be visualized in these cases also.

FAST evaluation of the abdomen consists of visualization of the pericardium (from a subxiphoid view), the hepatorenal spaces (i.e. Morison pouch), the splenorenal, the paracolic gutters, and the pouch of Douglas in the pelvis in sequential manner (Fig. 6.1). The Morison pouch view has been shown to be the most sensitive, and detection of free fluid in the hepatorenal pouch which indicates hemo-peritoneum, warrants urgent intervention in hemodynamically unstable patients. Though sensitivity and specificity of this study range from 85 to 95%, it cannot be used reliably to grade the solid organ injuries. Therefore, in the hemodyna-mically stable patient, a follow-up CT scan should be obtained if non-operative management is contemplated.

Diagnostic Peritoneal Lavage

DPL is used as a method of rapidly detecting the presence of intraperitoneal blood. DPL is particularly useful in patients who are unstable or has multi-system injuries or abdominal examination is either unreliable (e.g. head injury, alcohol, drug intoxication) or equivocal (e.g. lower rib fractures, pelvic fractures, confounding clinical examination). DPL is also useful for patients in whom serial abdominal examinations cannot be performed (e.g. those in an angiographic suite or operating room during emergent orthopedic or neurosurgical procedures).

The preferred method involves an open or semi-open technique that is performed at an infraumbilical location. In pregnant patients or in patients with particular risk for potential pelvic hematoma, it should be performed above the umbilicus. After insertion of the catheter aspiration is done to see for any blood or intestinal content. If it is negative, 1 L of lactated Ringer solution is infused into the peritoneum and the fluid is allowed to drain by gravity, and laboratory analysis is done for RBC, WBC, and amylase.

Positive DPL Means

- Frank aspiration of blood from the DPL catheter following insertion.
- Presence of more than 100,000 RBC/mm^3 as measured following the collection of the DPL effluent.
- Presence of more than 500 WBC/mm^3, an amylase value more than 175 IU/dl of detection of bile, bacteria, or food fibers.

DPL is absolutely contraindicated if patient requires emergency laparotomy regardless of the findings of DPL. The drawback of DPL is its inability in detecting diaphragmatic tear, retroperitoneal hematoma, renal, pancreatic, duodenal injuries and

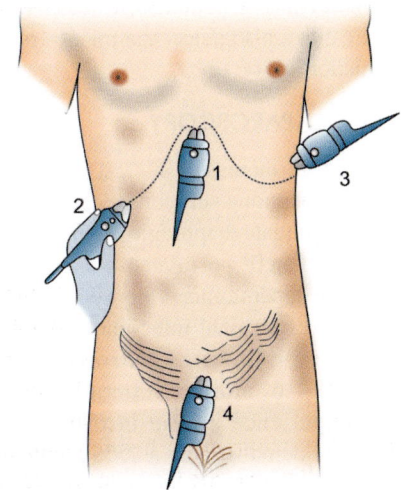

Fig. 6.1: Ultrasound probe positions in FAST

extraperitoneal rupture of bladder. False positive results are seen in cases of pelvic fracture or bleeding from retroperitoneal hematoma.

The overall accuracy of DPL has been reported between 92 and 98%. In an unstable patient grossly positive DPL is an indication for surgery. In microscopically positive DPL condition, the source of the blood loss is usually the abdomen but other sources like pelvic fracture should also be considered. If the DPL fluid during investigation is flowing through the urinary catheter or the chest tube, it indicates bladder or diaphragmatic rupture respectively and laparotomy should be done. Laparotomy for bowel injury is also mandatory in cases of gross enteric content.

CT SCAN

In a stable patient CT scan is the investigation of choice. Although it is time-consuming, CT scan provides the most detailed images of traumatic pathology and assist in determination of operative intervention. It should be performed in hemo-dynamically stable patients. While performing CT scan, close and careful monitoring of vital signs should be done.

The primary advantage of CT scan is its high specificity in diagnosing and grading of the injuries, thereby guiding non-operative management of solid organ injuries. Another advantage of CT scan is its ability to evaluate the retroperitoneal structures (a limitation of both FAST and DPL) and assessment of renal perfusion. CT scan may miss diaphragm injuries, mesenteric trauma, and perforations of the GI tract, especially when CT scan is performed soon after the injury. The best CT imaging requires both oral and intravenous contrast. It has sensitivity between 92 and 97.6% and specificity as high as 98.7%.

Though CT has less sensitivity in detecting hollow viscus injury in penetrating abdominal trauma, presence of following features indicate possibility of bowel injury

- *Signs of Peritoneal Violation*
  - Free Intra-peritoneal air
  - Free intra-peritoneal fluid in the absence of solid organ injury
  - Wound track extending through peritoneum
- *Signs of Bowel Injury*
  - Wound track extending to bowel wall
  - Bowel wall defect
  - Bowel wall thickening
  - Intraluminal contrast leak
- *Other Signs of Intra-peritoneal Injury*
  - Intravenous contrast extravasations
  - Diaphragmatic tear (especially on reformats)

ABDOMINAL RADIOGRAPH

X-ray abdomen may detect free gas in the abdomen suggesting hollow viscus perforation or abdominal contents in the thorax suggesting diaphragmatic injury. Other associated findings in the X-ray like fracture of lower rib cage on the left side may indicate possibility of splenic injury and on the right side for liver injury. Thoraco-abdominal injuries between nipple and costal margin, an X-ray chest is warranted to rule out significant hemothorax or pneumothorax which might represent an immediate threat to life. Presence of pelvic fracture may require urgent fixation in case of hemodynamically unstable patients. In all cases of penetrating abdominal trauma, an abdominal radiograph is mandatory in hemodynamically stable patients. Besides free intra-peritoneal air it can also detect the tract of bullet in cases of gunshot injury.

DIAGNOSTIC LAPAROSCOPY

There has been an increased interest in diagnostic laparoscopy (DL) among surgeons recently. It is the best method to evaluate diaphragmatic injuries. One of the potential benefit postulated is the reduction of nontherapeutic laparotomies where other modality like DPL indicates surgical intervention. Although there are no randomized controlled studies comparing DL to more commonly utilized modalities, experience at one institution using minilaparoscopy demonstrated a 25% incidence of positive findings on DL, which were successfully managed non-operatively.

MANAGEMENT

Out of all the stab wound of the abdomen, about one-third may not have the peritoneal penetration; another third may have peritoneal penetration without any significant abdominal findings. Therefore, wound exploration under local anesthesia is appropriate to determine whether the peritoneum has been breached. All such patients not having peritoneal breach can be discharged after initial wound care and observation. Those having peritoneal breach should can be observed with serial examination like serial hematocrit, frequent examination of vitals and abdominal examination. Any deterioration or evidence of positive abdominal findings (guarding, rigidity) warrants laparotomy.

Although risk of abdominal injury is low in patients with stab injury in flank, a close observation must be done for possible injury of colon, duodenum, kidney, or ureter. On suspicion of colonic injury, CT scan of the abdomen with IV and oral contrast should be done which may detect contrast extravasation from the injured colon.

Diaphragmatic injury should be ruled out by doing laparoscopy in cases of thoraco-abdominal stab where laparotomy is not otherwise indicated. In case the laparotomy is done, a thorough exploration should be carried out to evaluate all solid and hollow viscera.

Every penetrating gunshot wound of the abdomen should always be explored by laparotomy. Prior to the surgery patients must be resuscitated, blood to be arranged and catheter to be passed for monitoring urine output.

Midline incision is to be given. In case of gross blood in the peritoneal cavity, it should be evacuated quickly and abdomen is packed by placing abdominal mops in the following areas:

- Lateral to both descending and ascending colon
- Below the left hemidiaphragm
- Pelvis
- Beneath and over the dome of the liver
- Center of the abdomen.

In all penetrating injury liver, retroperitoneal structures, vascular structures, and mesentery should be examined. A specific search is made for actual source of bleeding by gradual removal of packs and the bleeding sites are controlled either by clamps, sutures or repacking as needed. After the arrest of hemorrhage, a careful examination of all the abdominal contents should be done. In addition to inspecting the liver and spleen, a thorough exploration should be done for anterior/ posterior stomach (by opening the lesser sac) and the entire large and small bowel including the duodenum. Retroperitoneal hematoma in the region of the duodenum requires inspection of posterior duodenal wall by Kocher maneuver. Expanding hematoma surrounding the retroperitoneal parts of the ascending and descending colon may also necessitates exploration by reflecting the right and left hemicolon to view the great vessels (Cattel-Braasch-maneuver). Non-expanding retroperitoneal hematoma over the kidney are to be left undisturbed. The diaphragm, gastrohepatic ligament, the head, body, and tail of the pancreas should also be inspected.

Stomach

Most of the injuries of the stomach are treated by primary closure. Posterior gastric wall should always be checked by opening the lesser sac. Blunt injuries to the stomach are rare. Gastric resection is rarely required.

Duodenum

Clean cut and small lacerations of the duodenum can safely be repaired primarily. Extensive lacerations in the presence of significant tissue contusion (usually in blunt trauma), should be treated by duodenal repair and pyloric exclusion. The procedure consists of closure of pylorus through a gastrotomy and GI continuity is maintained by gastrojejunostomy. Truncal vagotomy is not necessary. Feeding jejunostomy is useful for the provision of enteral nutrition. The Whipple's operation is reserved for massive combined pancreatoduodenal disruption. Duodenal injury has been scaled in five grades (Table 6.1).

Table 6.1: Grades of duodenal injury	
Grade	*Injury*
I	Hematoma and laceration of a single portion of duodenum without perforation.
II	Hematoma or laceration involving more than one portion and disruption of less than 50% of circumference.
III	Lacerations more than 50–75% of D_2, disruption of 50–100% of D_1, D_3, D_4.
IV	Laceration more than 75% of D_2 involving distal CBD or ampulla.
V	Massive disruption of dudeno-pancreatic complex or devascularization of duodenum.

Grade I and II injuries are treated by simple primary repair in the initial six hours. Beyond six hours along with the repair, duodenal decompression is advisable to avoid the risk of any leak, preferably by tube dudenostomy. Grade III injury causing major disruption of duodenal circumference should ideally be treated by primary repair, pyloric exclusion and drainage or alternatively a Roux-en-Y dudenoje-junostomy. Grade IV injuries are difficult to repair. Primary repair of the duodenum, repair of CBD or choledochoenteric anastomosis may be attempted. Pancreaticoduodenectomy although rarely needed, is usually reserved for grade V injuries.

Duodenal fistula is the one of the commonest complication following traumatic rupture of duo-denum. The fistula discharge consists of bile and pancreatic juice, which cause excoriation of skin. Excessive discharge may quickly lead to dehy-dration, electrolyte imbalance and hypoproteinemia. These fistulas are generally managed nonoperatively by

- Total parenteral nutrition till fistula closes may be within 6–8 weeks
- Nasogastric suction with nil per oral
- Protection of skin with aggressive stoma care

About 10–20% of the patients may develop abscess following duodenal fistula which can be managed by percutaneous drainage.

Small Bowel

Small intestinal perforations are either excised and closed transversely or the damaged segment is resected if there are multiple perforations in a short segment. Mesenteric tears may necessitate bowel resection taking care of the vascularity. Resection of large segment of ischemic bowel becomes mandatory at times which may lead to short gut syndrome.

Colon

Lacerations of the colon following the blunt trauma are rare. Usually the areas of serosal damage are seen typically in the caecum and sigmoid colon as they lie in the area of seat belt application.

Right sided colonic laceration can safely be treated by suture repair or resection and primary anastomosis. Occasionally when there is extensive contamination of the peritoneal cavity or patient is hemodynamically unstable, the two cut ends of the bowel is brought to the surface as proximal ileostomy and distal mucosal fistula. On the left sided colonic injury one stage procedure (resection and primary anastomosis) may be undertaken under favorable condition like minimal peritoneal conta-mination, minimal blood loss, hemodynamically stable patients and recent injury within six hours. If the injuries are associated with high-risk factors, the injured colon is either brought out as colostomy or is resected with the proximal end brought out as colostomy and distal end as mucous fistula. In cases where the distal end cannot be brought to the surface, it is closed as in Hartmann's proce-dure.

Rectal Injury

Rectal injuries are uncommon. Mostly these injuries are seen after gunshot or by a fall in a sitting posture on a spiked and blunt pointed object or in association with pelvic fracture. In all suspected cases of rectal injury, anus should be inspected for blood and abdomen should be palpated for guarding and rigidity.

Extra-peritoneal rectal injuries are repaired primarily and a diverting sigmoid loop colostomy is made. Wash out of distal rectal stump and pre-sacral drainage is mandatory. Intraperitoneal rectal injuries are also managed by primary repair, good wash out and diverting colostomy.

Injuries of liver, spleen, pancreas, kidney, ureter and bladder are dealt separately in respective chapters.

DAMAGE CONTROL LAPAROTOMY

Uncontrolled hemorrhage in trauma leads to progressive coagulopathy along with hypothermia and acidosis which eventually leads to death. Based on this, the concept of damage control laparotomy has come up in cases of abdominal injuries with profuse bleeding. Damage control procedure is useful whenever there is difficulty to control the ongoing bleeding like major hepatic injury, retrohepatic venacaval injury and retroperitoneal bleeding because of pelvic fracture. This procedure is also done if the anticipated time for the definitive corrective procedure is long (>90 minutes).

It is pertinent to abort the operation before the coagulopathy sets in. Criteria that predicts the need to pack early in cases of severe intra-abdominal hemorrhage are:

- Coagulopathy PT>19 sec
- Systolic BP <70 mm Hg
- pH< 7.2
- Serum lactate >5 mmol/L
- Temperature <34°C.

Stages of Damage Control Procedure

Intraoperative

Bleeding is stopped by repair or ligation of easily accessible vessels and by packing. Abdomen is closed temporarily with towel clips or plastic bag.

Intensive Care Unit

Patient is then shifted to ICU where coagulopathy, acidosis, hypothermia and hypoxia are all corrected and patient is fully resuscitated. Intra-abdominal pressure should be monitored to avoid the development of abdominal compartment syndrome.

Re-operation

After full stabilization when the organ functions are restored, patient is re-operated after 24–48 hours. Packs are removed and debridement of non-viable tissue is done. At this time definite surgical procedure is carried out for the injuries along with closure of the abdomen.

RETROPERITONEAL HEMATOMA

Major abdominal vascular trauma usually presents clinically as free intra-abdominal hemorrhage or as a contained retroperitoneal hematoma. Mostly the vascular injuries are much more common in gunshot rather than stab injuries. Patient with free intra-peritoneal hemorrhage usually presents in shock, whereas patients with retroperitoneal hematoma may be hemodynamically stable or unstable but usually fluid responsive.

On principle, in cases of penetrating injury causing retroperitoneal hematoma, exploratory laparotomy should be done irrespective of location or size of the hematoma. In blunt trauma abdomen a selective policy can be applied depending on the location of hematoma.

Retroperitoneum is divided into three anatomic zones

- **Zone-I:** Midline retroperitoneum (Fig. 6.2A)
- **Zone II:** Perinephric space (Fig. 6.2B)
- **Zone III:** Pelvic retroperitoneum (Fig. 6.2C).

Hematoma in zone I is centrally located. The supracolic compartment hematoma is located behind the lesser omentum, whereas the infracolic compart-ment involves the root of small bowel mesentery. Supramesocolic hematoma is generally seen because of the injury of supra renal aorta, celiac axis, proximal superior mesenteric artery or proximal renal artery, whereas inframesocolic hematoma is generally due to injury of infrarenal aorta and inferior vena cava (IVC). Any hematoma in zone I mandate the exploration for both penetrating and blunt injury of the abdomen. The proximal control of hemorrhage in supramesocolic compartment is achieved by either

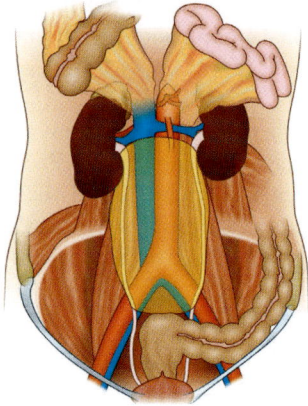

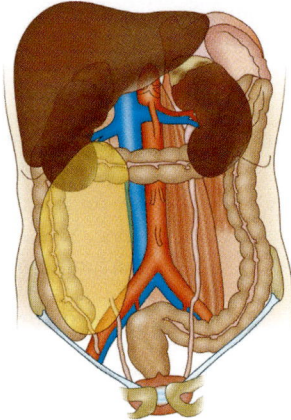

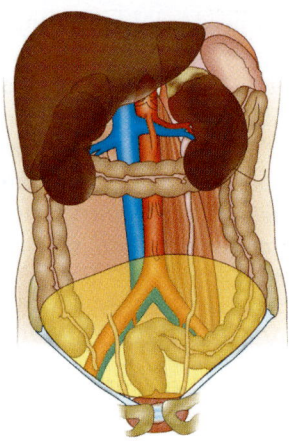

Fig. 6.2A: Midline retroperitoneal hematoma

Fig. 6.2B: Perinephric hematoma

Fig. 6.2C: Pelvic hematoma

compressing or clamping of the aorta at the diaphragmatic hiatus. After this the injured area is exposed and repaired. In inframesocolic compartment control is achieved at the supraceliac aorta.

Hematoma in zone II generally occurs due to injury to the renal vessels or parenchyma. In cases of penetrating trauma it should be explored but a non-expanding stable hematoma resulting from blunt injury of abdomen is better left unexplored. Opening of retroperitoneal hematoma will result in loss of tamponade effect and many times results in profuse bleeding from the damaged kidney.

Zone III: These hematoma results from pelvic fractures and sometimes from injuries to iliac vessels. Blunt traumatic pelvic hematoma should not be explored and are managed conservatively with the control of pelvic fracture or by angiographic embolization. It is important to realize that these hematomas may extend cephalad. Hematoma should not be explored as it may result in the loss of the tamponade effect of the intact peritoneum. All retroperitoneum hematoma (zone III) secondarily to penetrating injury should always be explored to rule out the injury to iliac vessels.

7

Hepatobiliary Injury

INTRODUCTION

Management of liver injury remains a major challenge to surgeons treating injured patients in emergency setup. The liver and the spleen are generally the two most frequently injured solid organs in cases of blunt abdominal trauma. Blunt abdominal trauma can cause extensive destruction of hepatic parenchyma, often in the form of satellite laceration or even major fracture extending across the anatomical planes. At times these may be so severe that it can be fatal. The overall mortality for hepatic trauma continues to be approximately 10–15%.

Liver being the largest solid abdominal organ with relatively fixed position is prone to injury in blunt abdominal trauma despite being well protected underneath the right rib cage. Right lobe is more prone to trauma because it is bigger and relatively fixed than left lobe. More than 90% of blunt hepatic injuries are accompanied by damage to other intra-abdominal organs, especially the spleen, kidney, and intestine. Diaphragm is injured in more than 50% of patients with penetrating injuries to the liver.

The initial management in severely injured patients should be directed towards restoration of adequate ventilation, oxygenation and prompt control of any ongoing blood loss. The ultimate goal of the surgical management of liver injuries should be a live patient with minimal morbidity. Liver injuries range from a trivial to deadly, but majority of these injuries are not so severe to be life-threatening. Most of the problems are caused by hemorrhage, leakage of bile and devitalization of liver tissue.

The single greatest danger following liver injury is severe hemorrhage, leading to hypotension. All such traumatic patients require immediate placement of two large bore intravenous cannula with rapid access to the central venous circulation for resuscitation. The potential hazards of an iatrogenic pneumothorax during the placement of CVP catheter must be kept in mind. Massive intra-abdominal bleeding along with pain in right hypochondrial area with tenderness and guarding at the right upper quadrant are suggestive of liver injury.

Hemodynamically stable patient should be evaluated by ultrasound abdomen after resuscitation. The focused abdominal sonography in trauma (FAST) examination is noninvasive and can be performed in the resuscitation area in short time. In a stable patient without any abdominal signs and a normal ultrasound, no further investigation is required. However, if the ultrasound detects liver injury, then CT scan is done in a stable patient for better characterization and grading of liver injury (Table 7.1).

In the event of nonavailability of ultrasound, diagnostic peritoneal lavage (DPL) can be extremely helpful for evaluating patients with suspected intra-abdominal injuries. The accuracy in detecting blood in the peritoneal cavity in DPL is approximately 90–98%, but it lacks specificity in finding the source of origin of blood. Therefore, it fails to distinguish between significant injuries requiring surgical intervention and insignificant injuries.

Table 7.1: Liver injury scale

	Grade	Injury descriptions
I.	Hematoma	Subcapsular, non-expansible <10% surface area
	Laceration	Capsular tear, non-bleeding <1 cm parenchymal depth
II.	Hematoma	Subcapsular non-expanding 10 to 50% surface, intraparenchymal <10 cm in diameter
	Laceration	<3 cm parenchymal depth, <10 cm in length
III.	Hematoma	Subcapsular >50% surface area
		Ruptured subcapsular or parenchymal hematoma
		Intraparenchymal hematomal >10 cm or expanding
	Laceration	>3 cm parenchymal depth
IV.	Laceration	Parenchymal disruption involving 25–75% of hepatic lobe or 1–3 Couinaud's segments within a single lobe
V.	Laceration	Parenchymal disruption involving >75% of hepatic lobe or >3 Couinaud's segments within a single lobe. Vascular juxtavenous hepatic injuries; i.e. retrohepatic vena cava/central major hepatic veins
VI.	Vascular	Hepatic avulsion

Whenever there is equivocal physical signs and unexplained hypotension, DPL should be done. DPL should not be done if there is a clear indication for laparotomy. In addition, injuries to retroperitoneal structures such as the pancreas and kidney may be missed on DPL. It is for this reasons the CT scan has gained popularity and is considered superior to DPL. There is a high degree of sensitivity and specificity with CT scan in evaluating patients with blunt trauma (Figs 7.1A and B). It is becoming evident that many patients who are stable but have minor hepatic injury, especially those with grade I and grade II injuries would have undergone an unnecessary laparotomy based on positive DPL. Therefore, it seems reasonable that when a hepatic injury is strongly suspected in a stable patient, CT scan should supersede DPL. Both DPL and abdominal CT should be considered complementary rather than competing diagnostic tests in patients

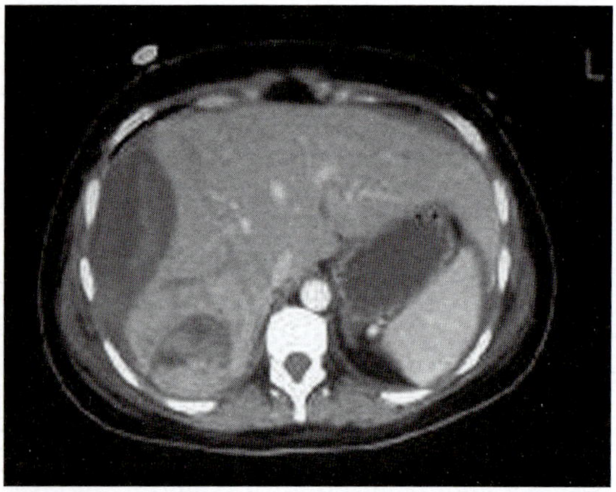

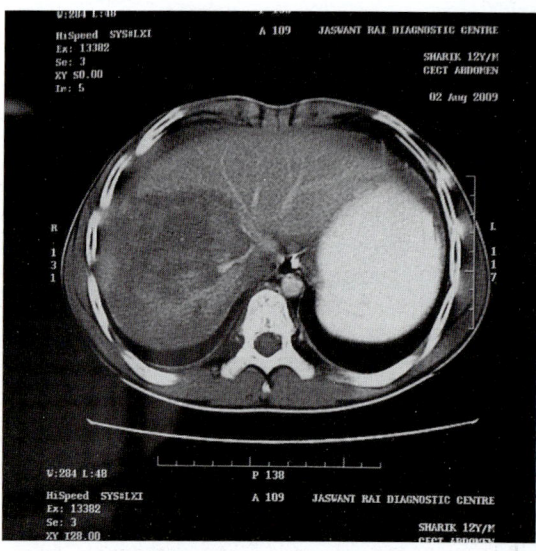

Fig. 7.1A: CT scan showing Grade III liver injury with subcapsular hematoma and liver laceration

Fig. 7.1B: Showing Grade IV lacerated injury involving parenchymal disruption involving 25–75% of hepatic lobe

with abdominal trauma. However, CT scan is the gold standard test for evaluating solid organ injuries.

Careful observation and repeat physical examination are mandatory especially in patients whose liver injuries are to be treated conservatively, as associated injuries like pancreatoduodenal injury can present late.

MANAGEMENT OF BLUNT HEPATIC INJURIES

Non-operative Management

Non-operative management of hemodynamically stable patients with blunt hepatic injuries is now an acceptable form of treatment. The non-operative management should not be viewed as "conservative management" as it is more difficult to manage patients non-operatively than operatively. The key element of the resuscitation should be the availability of adequate blood products—pack red blood cell, platelet, FFP and cryoprecipitate. Role of recombinant factor VIIa has also been used as an adjunctive agent in trauma patients in severe coagulopathic bleeding.

The patients with grade I or grade II hepatic injuries and even those with grade III injury without active bleeding and expanding hematoma, should be considered for non-operative management. Essential part in the management of these patients is close clinical monitoring by frequent recording of vitals. Estimation of hematocrit level should be done at least twice a day. Blood transfusion should be done as per requirement. In the event of deterioration with the fall of blood pressure or hematocrit level, patient should be subjected to exploratory laparotomy with arrangement of adequate blood.

Need of more than 4 units of blood in adults or replacement of more than half of the estimated blood volume in children to maintain stable vital signs, is an indication for surgery in patients with hepatic injury.

In presence of sepsis or development of significant abnormalities in liver function test, patient should be subjected to CT scan. In the presence of abscess or any collection in CT scan, percutaneous ultrasound guided drainage should be done. In case of failure of percutaneous drainage, patient should undergo operative drainage and debridement of non-viable tissue. Bleeding within liver may form large hematoma which is likely to get infected causing abscess or at times it may burst into bile duct causing hematobilia. Biliary leakage may cause biliary peritonitis and subsequent abscess formation.

In a hemodynamically stable patients who had sustained a stab wound which is directly over the liver should be evaluated by CT scan and if scan suggests isolated injury without having any suspicion of other visceral injury, a conservative approach can be taken. Such patient needs a close observation. At any stage, if there is any doubt of generalized peritonitis, a benefit of laparotomy should be given.

Operative Management

Majority of hepatic injuries are found to be minor (grade I and II) during laparotomy and require nothing more than simple suturing, electrocautery or topical hemostatic agents (Figs 7.2A to D). Complex hepatic injuries, which are continuously bleeding remain a challenge to any trauma surgery.

Unstable patients who don't respond to initial resuscitation should undergo urgent laparotomy. The aim of operative management in all liver injuries is the arrest of hemorrhage. Adequate blood products like packed red blood cell, platelet, FFP should be available to deal with coagulopathic bleeding.

Abdomen should be explored by long midline incision for good access to inspect entire abdominal cavity. Liver hemorrhage during surgery should initially be controlled by placing abdominal packs. Another technique is Pringle's maneuver, in which portal triad is occluded at foramen of Winslow usually by applying vascular clamp or pinching with thumb and forefingers to the margins of the hepatoduodenal ligament (Fig. 7.3). This occludes the blood supply to the liver from hepatic artery and portal vein. Bleeding from hepatic vein or inferior vena cava does not stop with Pringle's maneuver. Such clamping at Portal triad must be released after every 15–20 minutes to allow intermittent hepatic

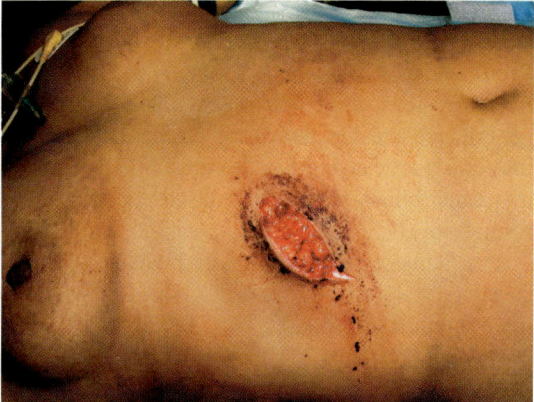

Fig. 7.2A: Site of penetrating injury in right hypochondrium

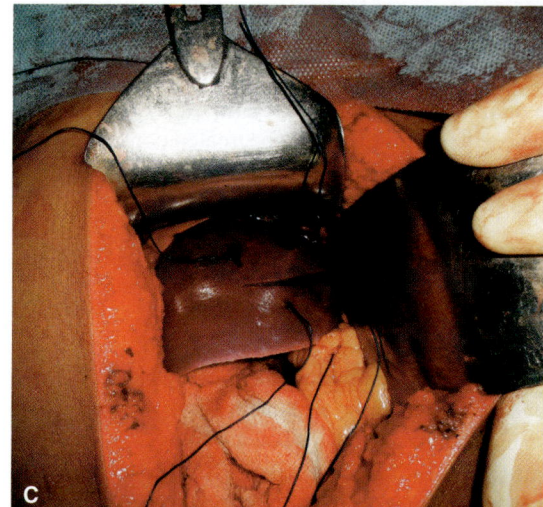

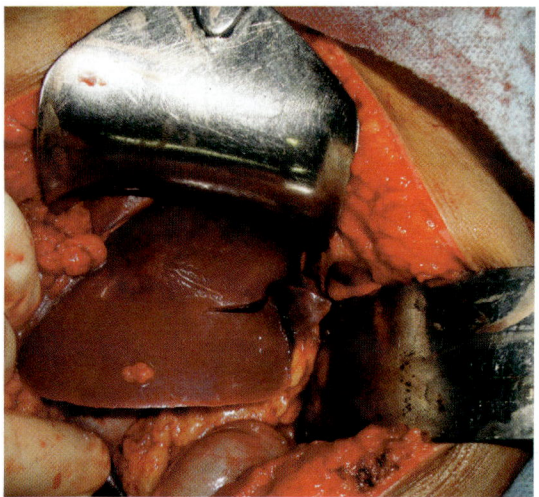

Fig. 7.2B: Laceration in left lobe of liver in the same patient

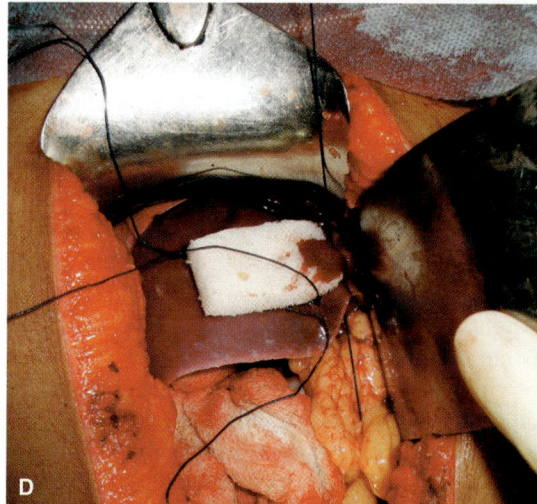

Figs 7.2C and D: Simple closure of liver laceration over a gelfoam)

perfusion. However, it has been observed that occlusion time even up to one hour during elective hepatic surgery are without any untoward effects. Topical hypothermia and large doses of steroids have been tried as a method for prolonging the hypothermic hepatic ischemia. Many advocate the use of topical hypothermia and steroids intravenously prior to performing the Pringle's maneuver.

When Pringle's maneuver provides adequate hemostasis, the vascular clamp is left in place until adequate exposure and local hemostasis at the wound site are accomplished.

In critically unstable patients, perihepatic packing is done as a damage control strategy to save the life of the patient. Perihepatic packing can be employed if bleeding is not controlled by Pringle's maneuver.

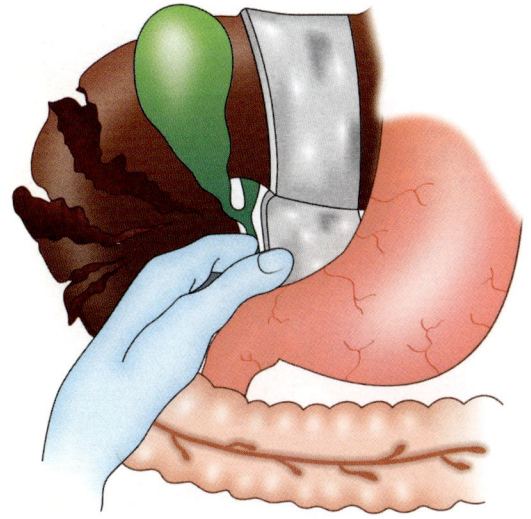

Fig. 7.3: Pringle's maneuver—Occlusion of portal triad at foramen of Winslow by pinching with thumb and forefingers

It is also effective in controlling hemorrhage in patients with caval or hepatic vein injuries. The technique involves approximation of damaged parenchyma followed by placing several dry abdominal packs or single rolled gauze around the liver in a hope to achieve tamponade of the bleeding wound (Figs 7.4A and B). Packing must be employed before the patient has deteriorated, as these patients are coagulopathic and acidotic, and will not tolerate a prolonged operative procedure. The wound should be re-explored after 48 hours, packs removed and hemostasis is achieved. Perihepatic packing and damage control is the most significant surgical advancement in the management of complex liver injuries. It is really effective in controlling life-threatening hemorrhage in severe liver injuries. Packs are removed, as soon as the patient stabilizes and coagulopathy and hypothermia are corrected, which is usually possible within 48 hours, keeping packs for 72 hours do increase the risk of infection.

In case the injury requires mobilization of liver for hemostasis, the following technique should be adopted. Falciform ligament should be divided first (Figs 7.5A and B). The right lobe can be mobilized by dividing the right triangular and coronary ligaments. Thereafter dissection is continued medially dividing the superior and inferior coronary ligaments. The right lobe is then rotated medially in

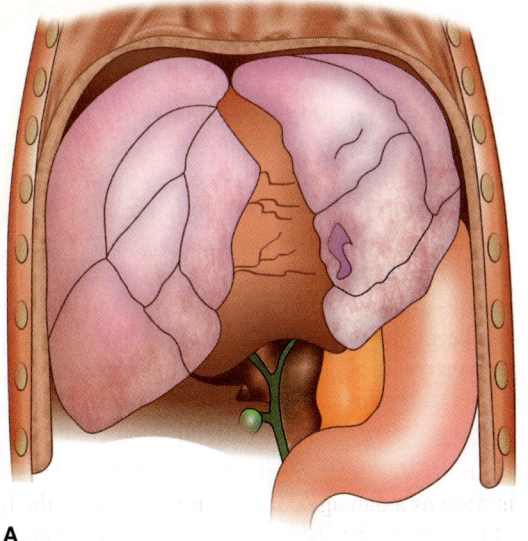

A

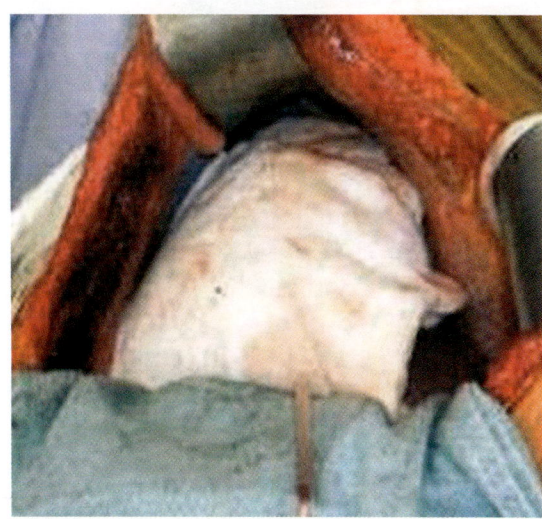

B

Figs 7.4A and B: Perihepatic packing

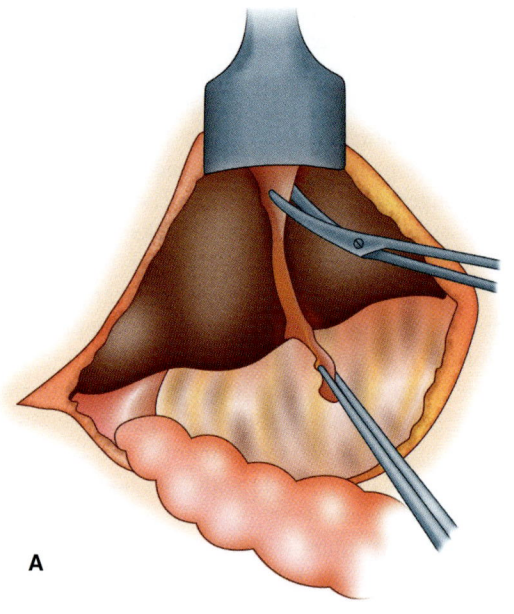

A

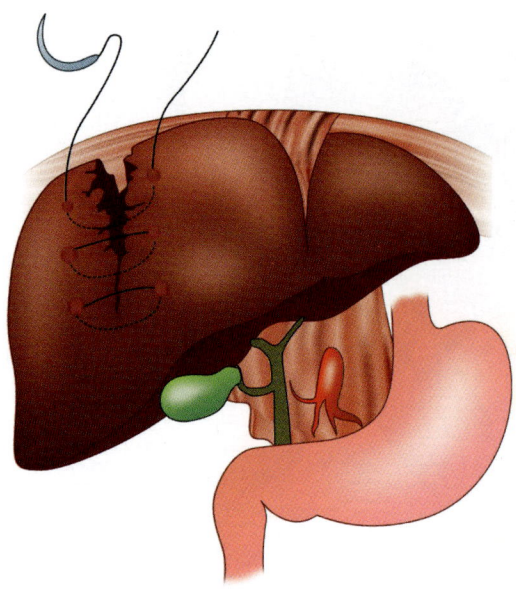

Fig. 7.6: Suturing of superficial laceration

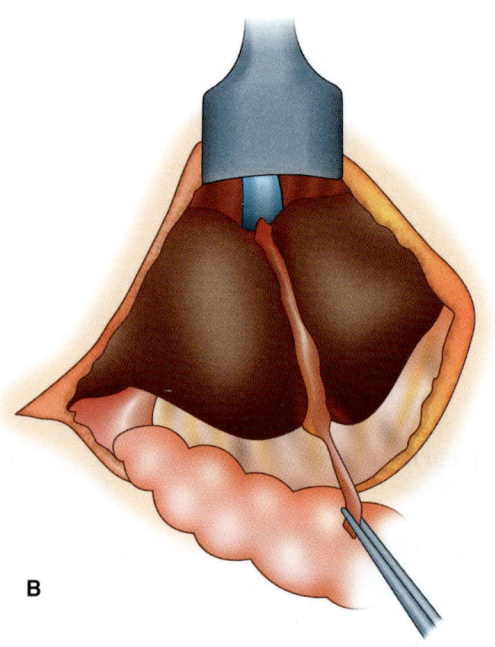

B

Figs 7.5A and B: Division of falciform ligament for hepatic mobilization

the surgical field. The left lobe mobilization is achieved in the same fashion. Care must be taken while dividing the coronary ligaments because of their close proximity to hepatic vein and retrohepatic vena cava.

Liver Suturing

The placement of hepatic sutures to control the bleeding is the most frequently employed hemostatic method by virtue of its simplicity (Fig. 7.6). But the sutures can also cause liver necrosis and may lead to subsequent liver abscess formation. In spite of this many surgeons do recommend deep liver sutures as a life-saving procedure especially in dealing with injuries in inaccessible portion of the liver. However, persistent bleeding form deep liver wounds is usually managed with hepatorrhaphy to control the bleeding, vessel under direct vision. If this is not possible then stuffing the wounds with a viable omentum (Figs 7.7A and B) or perihepatic pack compression should be considered as a damage control procedure.

Blind direct closure of deep laceration of liver should not be done to avoid the formation of abscess

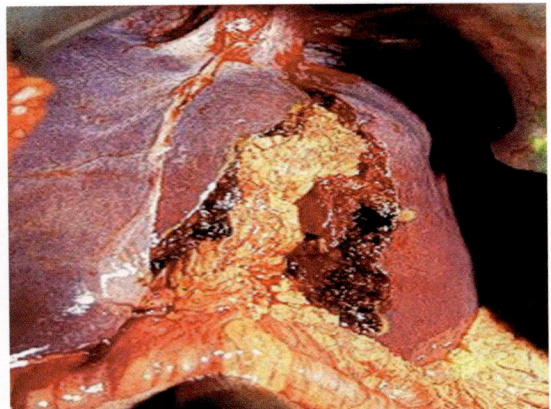

Fig. 7.7A: Placement of omentum in the laceration

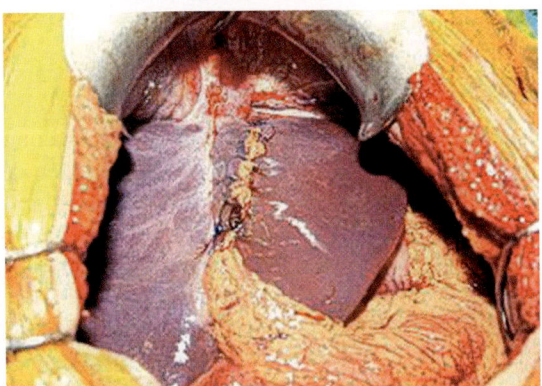

Fig. 7.7B: Suturing of laceration with the omentum stuffed in

and hemobilia. In such situation liver laceration should be extended by finger fracture technique and direct closure of the bleeding vessels should always be done under vision. All efforts must be taken to avoid the injury to right and left hepatic duct while employing the finger fracture technique. After hemostasis has been achieved the vascular clamp applied earlier occluding the portal tract is released. Any additional bleeding points are ligated with 3–0 vicryl sutures. The liver closure should begin from the bottom of wound to avoid the dead space; if the wound cannot be closed without leaving dead space then it should be left open or packed with omentum.

Packing with pedicle omentum nourished either by right or left gastroepiploic vessel has been found to be very useful in obtaining hemostasis in dealing with hepatic wound. The advantages of viable omental pedicle are:

1. The ability to tamponade major bleeding.
2. By filling the large defects within the liver the dead space is obliterated reducing the chance of developing the liver abscess.
3. Omentum is a rich source of macrophages when inserted in the traumatized liver, may be beneficial in combating sepsis.

In order to avoid postoperative, peri-hepatic abscess formation debridement of non-viable tissue must also be performed.

If hemostasis has been adequate and no apparent bile leak exists after repairing in grade I and II injury, drainage is unnecessary, but major complex hepatic injury with considerable parenchymal destruction should always be drained.

Mesh Wrapping

Absorbable polygalactine mesh has been used to wrap the major parenchymal disruption. This procedure does provide the benefit of packing but without a need of re-exploration. The technique is not suitable in juxtacaval or hepatic vein injury.

Hepatic Resection and Selective Hepatic Artery Ligation

Liver possess an ability to replace the lost tissue rapidly by compensatory cellular hypertrophy and hyperplasia. Under elective conditions, hepatic resection can be carried out with a minimum morbidity and mortality, but on the other hand, when such major hepatic resection is carried out for trauma it carries a high mortality.

When bleeding from hepatic wound is not controlled by above techniques, or when bleeding recurs after unclamping the portal triad, selective hepatic artery ligation may provide hemostasis. Acute gangrenous cholecystitis is a well recognized complication of hepatic artery ligation. Therefore cholecystectomy should also be performed, if right hepatic artery is ligated. Hepatic artery ligation has been performed in humans without significant impairment of liver function or development of any subsequent hepatic necrosis.

The hepatic artery ligation is found to be unnecessary in majority of hepatic injury. This is ineffective in controlling the bleeding from major branches of portal or hepatic veins. If hepatic artery ligation is undertaken in a hypotensive patient, it can cause severe hepatic ischemia leading to necrosis and sepsis. Hepatic resection should be reserved for situation in which there is no other reasonable way to control the bleeding.

In general, the indications of hepatic resection include:

a. Total destruction of lobe or segment
b. The injury in which resection is the only method to control hemorrhage.

Adjunctive Hemostatic Agents

Topical agents such as Surgicel (oxidized regenerate cellulose), Avitene (micro fibrillary collagen hemostat) are useful adjuncts for achieving topical hemostasis once major hemorrhage has been controlled. These agents are mostly placed on oozing raw hepatic surface and manually compressed for a period of 1.5 to 2.0 minutes and left undisturbed. For lesser injuries of grade I and II, topical hemostatic agents often suffice as sole means of controlling superficial hemorrhage.

Fibrin Glue

Fibrin glue can be effective in either superficial or deep parenchymal laceration of liver. It can also be used in presence of severe coagulopathy. It can be either sprayed on the injury site or directly injected into torn hepatic parenchyma when deep injuries are present.

Perihepatic Mesh

Use of absorbable mesh to wrap splenic injury has gained support and the technique has also been used in liver trauma as well.

Balloon Tamponade

If the patient has deep penetrating parenchymal injury of the liver and is continuously bleeding, one can insert a Foley catheter with large capacity balloon in the depth of the wound and the balloon is inflated to control the hemorrhage. Hemostatic agents can also be injected through the lumen of the Foley catheter.

When all the techniques fail, the surgeon generally should consider resorting to the placement of perihepatic packs and abdominal closure to prevent death from exsanguinations (damage control). Also when the patient is hemodynamically unstable then damage control approach in form of perihepatic packing should be done without wasting time for controlling the hemorrhage.

Arterial Embolization

Arterial embolization can be used for managing liver injuries when CECT shows extravasation of the contrast in the hepatic parenchyma. Patient should be operated if contrast extravasates to the peritoneum. Angiography is found to be helpful in conjunction with damage control procedure. After the hemorrhage has been control by packing and the subsequent CT shows the pseudoaneurysm of the right hepatic artery, it can be dealt successfully by embolization. Complication of embolization includes hepatic necrosis and gallbladder infarction.

JUXTAHEPATIC VENA CAVA INJURIES

Injury to the hepatic vein or retrohepatic vena cava is usually lethal. A juxtahepatic vena caval bleeding injury should be suspected when there is voluminous dark venous bleeding. There is no consensus on an optimal management strategy in such cases. Total vascular exclusion (clamping of inferior vena cava and suprahepatic vena cava in addition to Pringle's maneuver) may be used. This technique has produced more manuscripts than survival. Packing has been seen to effectively control the bleeding from the retrohepatic area.

COMPLICATIONS OF LIVER INJURY

Complications are similar to those found in any hepatic surgery. Most common is hemorrhage due to coagulopathy and requires correction with FFP and platelet administration. In case the hemorrhage persists, angiography and therapeutic embolization should be undertaken. Among the late complications intra-abdominal abscess and bile leaks are common.

The patients who are at high risk of abscess are those having prolonged shock, extensive parenchymal injuries, associated bowel injuries and the hepatic ischemia due to ligation of major vessels. Leftover non-viable hepatic tissue is also an important cause for postoperative abscess formation. Late deaths due to perihepatic abscess have also been reported. All necrotic materials should be debrided before closure to avoid abscess formation. Biliary leak is generally noticed in grade III and higher hepatic injuries and in those who require hepatic resection or extensive debridement.

BILIARY INJURIES

Extrahepatic biliary injury is exceedingly rare and generally seen in 2% of all the abdominal trauma injuries. Majority of them are on account of penetrating mechanism. Stab wounds typically results in injuries to the gallbladder whereas the gunshot injuries randomly distributed throughout the extrahepatic biliary ductal system.

Patients with bile duct injury generally present days or weeks after the initial trauma. Non- specific symptoms like nausea, vomiting, anorexia or jaundice may be the presenting features.

Sterile bile in the peritoneal cavity seldom leads to early symptoms. Diagnostic tests include USG, CECT, MR/MRCP, and HIDA scan. The bile duct injuries are usually diagnosed during laparotomy.

Management of common bile duct injuries is challenging. Most of them if partial (less than 50% of the circumference) can be repaired primarily, placing a T-tube through a separate choledochotomy. Repair over a T-tube should be avoided. The complete transection of common bile duct will need choledochoenteric (Roux-en-Y) anastomosis. This particular procedure avoids the high incidence of stricture rate in comparison to the primary repair. Many times when the duct is less than 1 cm diameter, a small catheter can be inserted through the jejunal loop to stent the choledochojejunostomy.

The bilateral hepatic duct injuries are repaired by a biliary enteric bypass only when the injury is very proximal. The ligation of unilateral hepatic duct is a viable option provided the remainder of the biliary duct is intact as judged by the intraoperative cholingiogram. Another option is for the proximal unilateral hepatic duct injury is partial hepatectomy or simple drainage alongwith a stent to facilitate the closure of the leak. Most of the gallbladder injury is treated by cholecystectomy.

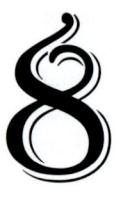

Pancreaticoduodenal Injury

INTRODUCTION

Pancreatic injury is uncommon and mostly occurs in relation with serious blunt abdominal trauma or penetrating trauma. Pancreatic injury constitutes less than 10% of all abdominal injuries. Most of these (70–75%) are caused by penetrating injuries and are associated with injuries to other viscera like spleen, duodenum, liver, kidney, inferior vena cava, aorta, or portal vein. Isolated pancreatic injuries are extremely rare. In blunt trauma, pancreas gets crushed against the vertebral column despite being relatively well protected retroperitoneal organ.

About 50 to 70% patients dying due to pancreatic injury in first 48 hours are due to massive blood loss and other associated injuries. Late mortality is generally a consequence of infection or multiple organ failure.

Prognosis of these cases is influenced by the extent and type of pancreatic injury, duration of shock, amount of blood loss and timing of resuscitation and surgical intervention undertaken. Most minor pancreatic injuries are relatively easier to treat but missed major injuries are responsible for high morbidity and mortality.

The proximity of the larger vessels e.g. portal vein, abdominal aorta, and inferior vena cava (IVC) to the pancreatic head increases the risk of exsanguinating hemorrhage accompanying pancreatic penetrating injury. Exsanguinating hemorrhage due to concomitant vascular injury accounts for the greatest number of deaths in patients with pancreatic injury.

The site of injury of the pancreas is an important factor in the prognosis. An injury of the tail of the pancreas does not usually involve the bowel, whereas the injuries at the pancreatic head are mostly associated with duodenal and biliary tree injury due to their close proximity.

The most common cause of injury is from blow to the epigastrium by a rigid object (steering wheel of car, bicycle handlebars) which generally results in fracture of the pancreas. The mechanism of injury in blunt trauma depends on the magnitude and direction of impact force. The midline force leads to compression of pancreas against the vertebrae. Force on the right causes injury to the head of the pancreas, duodenum and biliary channel, whereas the left sided force leads to the injury of the pancreatic tail, splenic vessels and spleen.

PRESENTATION AND CLASSIFICATION OF INJURIES

Pancreatic injury should be suspected in all significant blunt trauma abdomen especially if seat belt marks or flank ecchymoses are present. Pancreatic injury can be symptom free in early stage and can even be silent because of retroperitoneal location. Minimal findings like tenderness in upper abdomen or rebound tenderness with signs of acute peritonitis can be present.

Spectrum of pancreatic injury is broad and there are number of classifications. The most widely accepted classification is by Lucas.

Modified Lucas Classification for Pancreatic Injury

Class 1: Simple superficial contusion or peripheral laceration with minimal parenchymal damage. Main pancreatic duct is intact.

Class 2: Deep laceration, perforation or transection of neck, body or tail of pancreas with or without pancreatic duct injury.

Class 3: Severe crush, perforation or transection of head with or without ductal injury.

Class 4: Combined pancreatic/duodenal injury, sub classified into
  1. Minor pancreatic injury
  2. Severe pancreatic injury with ductal disruption

The other classification that is used is **American Association for the Surgery of Trauma (AAST)** classification of pancreatic trauma (Table 8.1).

Table 8.1: AAST classification of pancreatic injury

Grade	Injury description
I. Hematoma	Minor contusion without ductal injury
Laceration	Superficial laceration without ductal injury
II. Hematoma	Major contusion without ductal injury or tissue loss
Laceration	Major laceration without ductal injury or tissue loss
III. Laceration	Distal transection or pancreatic parenchymal injury with ductal injury
IV. Laceration	Proximal transection or pancreatic parenchymal injury involving the ampulla
V. Laceration	Massive disruption of the pancreatic head

INVESTIGATIONS

Plain Abdominal Radiograph

A plain abdominal radiograph may reveal retroperitoneal air from duodenal rupture if associated. At times, fracture of transverse process of lumbar vertebrae may indicate significant retroperitoneal injury. Displacement of stomach, transverse colon or generalized ground glass appearance due to intraperitoneal fluid may indicate possibility of pancreatic injury. Upper GI contrast studies can also diagnose duodenal leak secondary to injury.

Ultrasonography

Ultrasound is valuable in detecting free intra-abdominal fluid, usually blood and solid viscous injury But it is not reliable for pancreatic and duodenal injuries, due to associated abdominal injuries, overlying bowel gas, obesity or subcutaneous emphysema.

Computed Tomography

Computed tomography (CT) is good for evaluation of pancreatic injury but patient should not be placed under CT scanner if he is hemodynamically unstable. An increase in the space between duodenum and right kidney, extraluminal gas, duodenal wall thickening, pancreatic edema, enlargement of pancreatic gland on CECT are consistent with pancreatic or duodenal injury. At times, fracture of pancreas may also be visualized (Fig. 8.1). These changes generally took at least 24–48 hrs after injury to develop.

Other non-specific CT findings of pancreatic trauma includes blood or fluid tracking along the mesenteric vessels, fluid in lesser sac, fluid between pancreas and splenic vein.

Overall, sensitivity of CT for detecting pancreatic injury is 80% but for ductal injury sensitivity is only 40%. Ability of CT to demonstrate the pancreatic injury accurately depends on the quality of the CT scanner and experience of the observer.

Diagnostic Peritoneal Lavage

It may detect associated intraperitoneal injury but it is usually not helpful for diagnosis of retroperitoneal injury. A high content of lavage fluid amylase may indicate possibility of pancreatic injury. The incidence of high serum amylase in patients with proven pancreatic trauma ranges from 3 to 75 %.

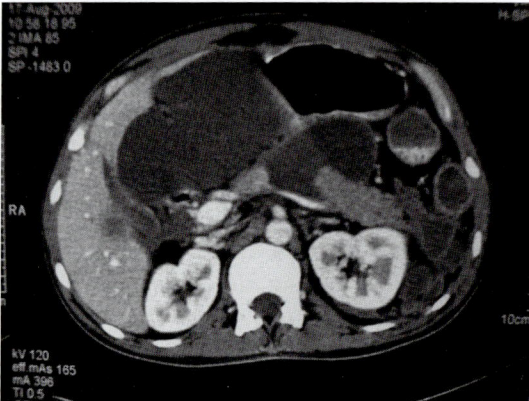

Fig. 8.1: CECT showing transection of neck of pancreas with fluid collection (*Courtesy* Dr D. Mohanty, UCMS, Delhi)

ERCP (Endoscopic Retrograde Cholangiopancreatography)

This can be used to identify ductal injury by demonstrating the extravasation of contrast from the duct but it is seldom practicable in hemodynamically unstable patients, who may require urgent laparotomy for bleeding or associated injuries. This test may be of value in evaluation of patients with delayed presentation or missed injuries.

ERCP is valuable when used in operating room in the patients with an open abdomen to delineate pancreatic duct anatomy, as it may avoid opening the duodenum.

ERCP is an invasive procedure and successful completion of pancreatography is operator dependent and it also has its own complications.

MRCP (Magnetic Resonance cholangiopancreatography)

This is a valuable additional non-invasive imaging modality. Focal disruption of the duct and communication between the duct and intrapancreatic or peripancreatic fluid collection are suggestive of pancreatic ductal injury.

In a stable patient, CT scan is ideal and safest and more comprehensive means of diagnosis of pancreatic injury. This is augmented by careful use of ERCP/ MRCP in selected patients. All hemodynamically unstable patients not responding to conservative management, laparotomy should be undertaken.

APPROACH TO MANAGEMENT

A patient of blunt trauma with stable hemodynamics and CT scan showing no evidence of pancreatic parenchymal tear, hematoma, parenchymal edema, fluid in lesser sac or retroperitoneal hematoma is closely observed for at least 48–72 hours. If clinical findings suggest hemoperitoneum or peritonitis, and patient is hemodynamically unstable, exploratory laparotomy should be done with administration of broad spectrum antibiotics. Before taking up for laparotomy patient should be fully resuscitated.

Following are the principles of emergency surgery in pancreatic trauma:
- A long midline incision provides optimal exposure.
- Thorough and careful evaluation of pancreas is to be done after opening the lesser sac and kocherization of duodenum to provide good exposure of pancreas.
- Evaluation and appropriate management of other associated injuries if present.
- Debridement of devitalized pancreatic tissue.
- Identification and meticulous repair of pancreatic laceration by non-absorbable suture.
- Surgical procedure appropriate for type of pancreatic injury.
- External drainage should always be provided.
- Feeding jejunostomy should be done for postoperative enteral nutrition.
- In case of injury to superior mesenteric artery or vein, portal vein and IVC, effort should be made to repair these vessels first and pancreatic injury is dealt later.
- For evaluation of biliary duct most convenient method is to do an operative cholangiogram through the cystic duct after removing the gallbladder or by inserting the butterfly needle into CBD and pushing the contrast fluid.
- All patients should receive prophylactic antibiotic.
- Intensive postoperative supportive care should be done.

Pancreas is exposed by kocherization and division of gastrohepatic ligament (lesser omentum) to gain access to the lesser sac. Transection of gastrocolic ligament allows inspection of anterior surface of pancreas. For exposure of posterior aspect of the pancreas, transection of the retroperitoneal attachment at the inferior border of pancreas and cephalad rotation of pancreas is done, taking care of great vessels and aorta.

Intraoperative findings which raise suspicion for pancreatoduodenal injury are

- Crepitus along the duodenum
- Bile staining of the paraduodenal area
- Presence of bile leak
- Presence of a right sided retroperitoneal or para- renal hematoma
- Central retroperitoneal hematoma
- Bile staining in the retroperitoneum
- Edema surrounding the pancreas and lesser sac
- Any pancreatic hematoma or laceration.

Class I Injury

Minor contusion and laceration contribute nearly 80% of all the pancreatic injury. These are treated by hemostasis and debridement if necessary and external drainage without repair of capsular laceration.

Abdominal suction drains should be placed in the lesser sac. Drainage tube should be large (30 Fr) to avoid any blockage by secretions and debris. The drain should remain in place till it stops draining and patient starts oral feeding. Continued drainage with high amylase levels persisting beyond 48–72 hours is highly suggestive of a missed ductal injury.

These problems must be treated with workup of the ductal integrity with ERCP or any other modality and may require another operation. Occasionally, a trial of total parenteral nutrition (TPN) or elemental diet through a feeding jejunostomy may result in decreased drainage and closure of the leak.

Class II Injury

Injury to neck, body or tail and no ductal injury can be treated with drainage alone. In case of ductal disruption present on left to the superior mesenteric artery, it can be treated by distal pancreatectomy with splenectomy (Figs 8.2A and B). Pancreatic duct should be identified and ligated separately with non-absorbable suture. Distal end is closed by prolene or silk. External drainage is mandatory. If the splenic vein and splenic artery are normal and patient is hemodynamically stable, preservation of spleen can be tried.

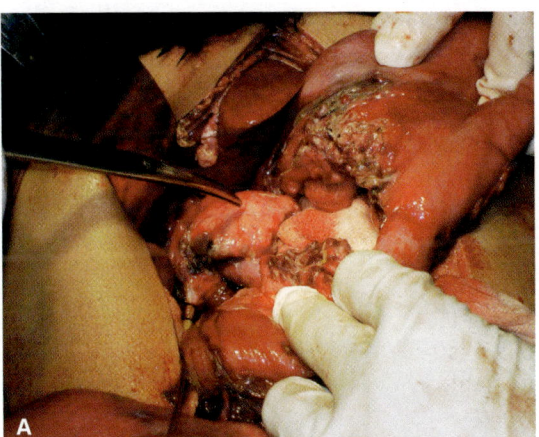

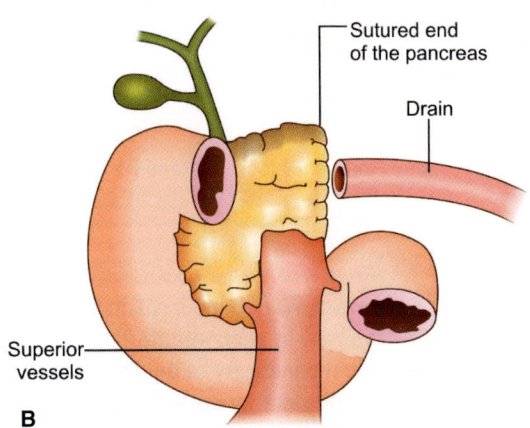

Figs 8.2A and B: (A) A pancreatic transection at the body of pancreas with disruption of pancreatic duct (B) Distal pancreatectomy and drainage

Class III Injury

Injury to the head of pancreas is best managed by simple external drainage. Isolated ductal injury of pancreatic head was used to be earlier treated by Roux-en-Y jejunal loop anastomosis to the injured area in the head of pancreas, but there is high chances of leakage from the anastomosis (Fig. 8.3). In this technique the whole of the injured area can be covered by the open end of Roux loop and sutured to the pancreatic capsule without any attempt to repair the injured area. By this the leaking secretions get diverted to the bowel lumen.

External drainage of injured area is often the safest option. A controlled fistula thus created either settles spontaneously or requires internal drainage later.

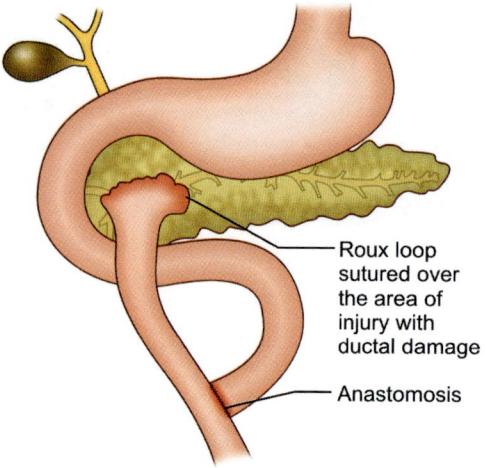

Roux loop sutured over the area of injury with ductal damage

Anastomosis

Fig. 8.3: Onlay Roux-en-Y loop to drain the pancreatic head

Class IV Injury

A combined major pancreaticoduodenal ductal injury is usually uncommon. In such situation, it is very important to define the integrity of the common bile duct (CBD), pancreatic duct, ampulla and the viability of duodenum. At times cholangiogram and pancreatogram is essential to know the intactness of these duct. A variety of procedures are described for grade IV injuries ranging from Roux-en-Y pancrea-

tico-jejunostomy, pancreatico-gastrostomy, pyloric exclusion, duodenal diverticulization and pancreatico-duodenectomy. Recently stenting of the injured pancreatic duct with endoscopic retrograde pancreato-graphy (ERP) has been shown to be effective.

Combined pancreatic and duodenal injury can be treated by pyloric exclusion (Fig. 8.4) or in rare cases duodenal diverticulization (Fig. 8.5) provided duodenum can be repaired primarily. Pancreatico-duodenectomy is a formidable procedure and is generally not recommended.

Duodenal Diversion

It is done when there is an extensive loss of pancreatic head tissue and major duodenal injury. Gastric contents are diverted to promote healing and also to reduce the release of pancreatic and bile secretion. It can be achieved by either pyloric exclusion or by duodenal diverticulization. The duodenal diversion is less time-consuming and technically less demanding than Whipple's procedure.

Pyloric Exclusion

Duodenal injury is repaired, tube gastrostomy is performed in the distal greater curvature and pylorus is closed from inside by polygalactin purse string suture. A gastrojejunostomy is performed at the dependent part of the stomach. This procedure gives temporary diversion of gastric content and within 3 weeks, the pylorus usually reopens and gastro-jejunostomy becomes functionally closed (Fig. 8.4).

Duodenal Diverticulization

It consists of duodenal repair, vagotomy, antrectomy and end-to-side gastrojejunostomy, and duodeno-stomy with T-tube drainage of common bile duct. Aim is total diversion of gastric content and bile from injured area (Fig. 8.5).

Pancreaticoduodenectomy (Whipple's Procedure)

It is only required when there is severe contused injury of duodenum or pancreatic head and injury to distal

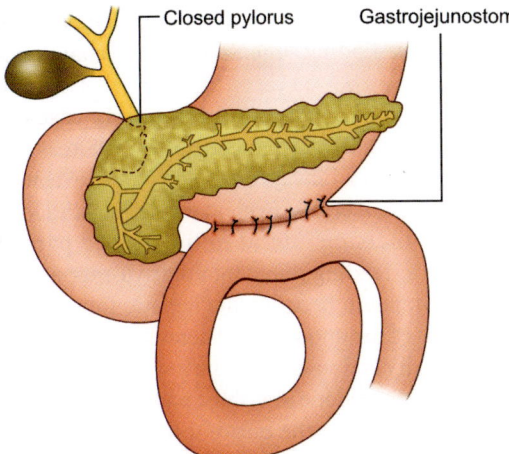

Fig. 8.4: Pyloric exclusion

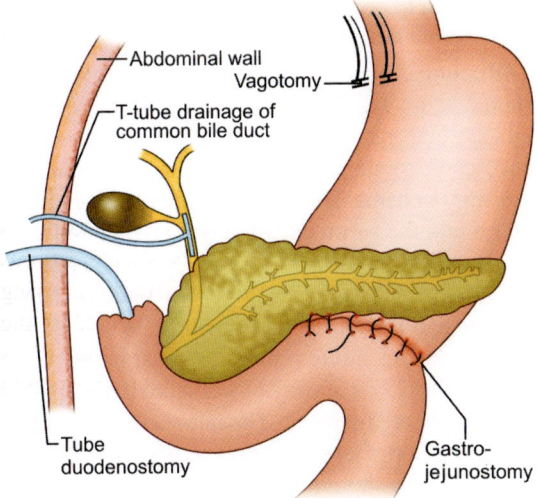

Fig. 8.5: Duodenal diverticulization

CBD, which are unreconstructable or massive uncontrollable hemorrhage is coming from the head of pancreas. Although it has high mortality but has got a definitive place in the management. This surgery may be necessary in 1–2% of isolated pancreatic injuries and in up to 10% of combined pancreatico-duodenal injury. Emergency pancreatoduodenectomy is similar to that of an elective operation.

In all unstable patients with serious associated injuries a simple controlled drainage is done and reconstruction is done at a later stage. At times when patient is actively exsanguinating or when expertise and facility does not exist, the damage control surgery should be done to control the active bleeding and patient is transferred to closest major hospital.

POSTOPERATIVE CARE

Principles of postoperative care are similar to that of any patient with major abdominal injury. Maintenance of intravascular volume, adequate tissue oxygenation, proper nutritional support and early identification of complication is essential. Jejunal feeding should be started after paralytic ileus is over.

COMPLICATION

Pancreatic Fistula

Pancreatic fistula is the most common complication after pancreatic injury and the incidence is around 20–25%. Most of them are minor and resolves spontaneously in one to two weeks of time. Use of octretide 100 mg thrice a day decreases the fistula output and encourages early healing.

High output fistula more than 700 ml/24 hr usually indicates disruption of major pancreatic duct. If such fistula persists for more ten days, then ERCP and transpapillary stent insertion could be helpful. In case of failure, either distal pancreatic resection for leak from pancreatic tail or a Roux-en-Y pancreatico-jejunostomy for proximal leak is undertaken. All efforts should be made to preserve the spleen during distal pancreatectomy.

Pseudopancreatic Cyst

These are often result from inadequate pancreatic drainage or missed ductal injury after abdominal trauma. Surgically the management of traumatic pseudopancreatic cyst depends on the site and nature of the ductal injury, maturity and thickness of cyst wall and lastly the proximity of the pseudocyst to stomach, duodenum or jejunum.

If ERCP/MRCP detects minimal leak from distal duct then USG guided drainage can be done. But if leak is from the major duct it should be drained by endoscopic stenting of pancreatic duct. If it fails or not feasible then surgical decompression by cysto-gastrostomy, cystojejunostomy or cystodudeno-stomy is done. (Also see chapter on Acute Abdomen)

DUODENAL INJURIES

Both blunt and penetrating duodenal trauma is uncommon and account for 3–5% of all abdominal injuries. Overall 78% of duodenal injuries are penetrating on account of gunshot or stab wound. Crush injuries are due to blow to the anterior abdominal wall leading the crush injury of the abdomen against the vertebral column.

The diagnosis of blunt duodenal injury remains challenging. Most of the time the injured patients have only vague or mild complains. Peritonitis becomes evident later, only when the retroperitoneal contents leak into the peritoneal cavity. Duodenal tear must always be suspected whenever blunt injury has occurred to the upper abdomen with persistent vomiting on account of duodenal hematoma leading to complete obstruction. Duodenal injury is invari-ably retroperitoneal, hence DPL and FAST both are unreliable adjuncts for the diagnosis of duodenal injury. Even the laboratory data are also having little diagnostic benefit. Mild elevation of serum amylase can be obtained in duodenal injury. Plain films of the abdomen are equally unhelpful. Free air is seen in less than 10% of cases of duodenal rupture.

The contrast CT scan has got a unique ability to visualize the retroperitoneum and findings consistent with the blunt duodenal injury includes bowel wall thickening or hematoma, extraluminal gas/fluid/contrast medium, retroperitoneal air or edema. The diagnosis of penetrating duodenal injury is often made intraoperatively during laparotomy.

On any suspicion of duodenal rupture or associated concomitant injury to the pancreas, exploratory laparotomy becomes essential.

A long midline incision should be undertaken and intraoperative finding suggestive of duodenal injury as mentioned above (crepitus, bile staining and duodenal hematoma) are to be noted. In cases of staining and hematoma in the region of pancreas and duodenum, it should always be explored by an extended Kocher's maneuver. The maneuver begins with a long semilunar incision lateral to the second part of duodenum extending round into the avasular wedge of the peritoneum between the hepatic flexure and second part of the duodenum. Thereafter the incision turns medially and runs along the lower border of the junction of the second and third part of duodenum. During exploration the entire duodenum is to be inspected and turned to the left across the vena cava and aorta along with the pancreatic head. This technique permits the inspection of the posterior surface of the duodenum to confirm or exclude the rupture in the posterior aspect.

Rupture of the duodenum having been identified, should be managed either by simple suture repair or by some elaborate procedures. The suture repair should be reserved for the smaller injury without surrounding bruising or edema. The wound should be repaired with vicryl and the seromuscular layer is repaired with interrupted silk Lambert sutures. A partial compro-mised duodenal wall should never be repaired as it may lead to high rate of fistula formation. In case of any tension during suture repair, a serosal patch of the neighboring loops of small bowel should to be applied to secure the area of repair. The ante-mesenteric border of the first loop of jejunum serves well in such situation. A sump drain should always be laid down near the suture area.

A large injury with considerable disruption of the duodenal wall should never be repaired primarily. It is advisable to fashion a Roux limb of the first loop of jejunum in a retrocolic fashion and mucosa to mucosa anastomosis to be performed to create an internal drainage. Operation is completed by closed suction drain placed adjacent to the area of repair along with feeding jejunostomy.

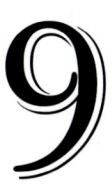

Splenic Injury

Spleen is a highly vascular organ present in the left hypochondrium. Spleen is protected anatomically under the left rib cage but despite this it is frequently injured by blunt external trauma. Earlier, splenectomy was the treatment for splenic injuries but with the realization of the immunological functions of the spleen, the emerging trend is to preserve it whenever possible. Currently most of the splenic injuries are managed successfully on conservative treatment.

WHEN TO SUSPECT SPLENIC INJURY?

Splenic injury should always be considered in patients with blunt trauma abdomen who have got generalized abdominal pain and/or guarding due to hemoperitoneum or who are in shock.

Splenic injury is suspected in presence of
- Left upper quadrant abdominal pain
- Left shoulder pain (referred pain due to irritation of diaphragm by blood—Kehr's sign)
- Left sided lower rib fractures
- Bruising present over left lower chest or left upper abdomen
- Abdominal distention, guarding and tenderness because of peritonism due to blood in peritoneal cavity
- Shifting dullness in the flanks due to hemo-peritoneum. In about 25% of patients Balance's sign may be positive. (Balance's sign—both flanks are dull on percussion. On the right side the dullness can be made to shift while on the left side it is constant. It indicates that there is hemoperitoneum in the abdomen but the blood in the perisplenic area has coagulated.)

- Rectal examination may reveal tenderness and soft bogginess anteriorly because of blood in the rectovesical pouch.

Features which Suggest Splenic Injury on Plain Abdominal X-ray

- Obliteration of splenic outline
- Obliteration of psoas shadow
- Indentation of the left side of the gastric air bubble
- Elevation of the left side of the diaphragm
- Free fluid between gas filled intestinal loops.

EVALUATION AND MANAGEMENT OF PATIENT WITH SPLENIC INJURY

Scenario 1: Patient is Hemodynamically Unstable
Patient is resuscitated on the lines of ATLS (advanced trauma life support). Intravenous lines are placed and ringer lactate infusion is started. Blood is sent for cross-match. If patient does not respond to the initial resuscitation and cause of the shock is bleeding in the abdomen, then patient is planned for emergency exploratory laparotomy. If facility is available then FAST (focused abdominal sonography in trauma) is done in the casualty. No other imaging investigation is to be done in a hemodynamically unstable patient. If the patient responds to the initial resuscitation then he is to be managed as a hemodynamically stable patient as in scenario 2.

Scenario 2: Hemodynamically Stable Patient
Patients who are hemodynamically stable should undergo CECT (contrast enhanced computed tomogram) of abdomen after initial resuscitation (Fig. 9.1). Splenic injury is graded based on the findings

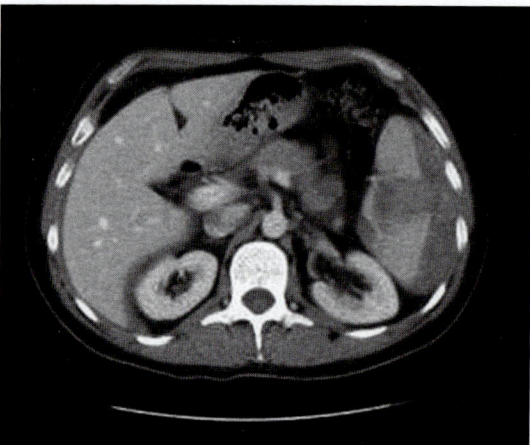

Fig. 9.1: CECT showing splenic laceration and hematoma

of CECT of abdomen (Table 9.1). Injuries to any other intra-abdominal organs are also looked for. Hemodynamically stable patients with Grade I to Grade III injuries can be managed conservatively. If CECT abdomen shows Grade IV or V injuries (shattered spleen or hilar vascular injury) then patient

Table 9.1: Splenic Injury Scale		
Grade	*Injury*	*Description*
I	Hematoma	Subcapsular, <10% surface area
	Laceration	Capsular tear, <1 cm parenchymal depth
II	Hematoma	Subcapsular, 10–50% surface area Intraparenchymal, <5 cm diameter
	Laceration	1–3 cm parenchymal depth not involving a parenchymal vessel
III	Hematoma	Subcapsular, >50% surface area or expanding Raptured subcapsular or parenchymal hematoma Intraparenchymal hematoma >5 cm
	Laceration	>3 cm parenchymal depth or involving trabecular vessels
IV	Laceration	Laceration of segmental or hilar vessels producing major devascularization (>25% of spleen)
V	Laceration	Completely shattered spleen
	Vascular	Hilar vascular injury with devascularized spleen

should be planned for exploratory laparotomy at the earliest.

Patients who are being managed conservatively should be examined serially so that any deterioration can be detected early.

Serial Examination

Following parameters are to be checked at least every four hourly:
- Pulse rate
- Blood pressure
- Abdominal examination
- Abdominal girth measurement
- Urine output
- Hematocrit estimation (every 12 hourly). Hematocrit estimation is better than hemoglobin because hemoglobin level can be falsely elevated because of dehydration.

Tachycardia, fall in blood pressure, increase in abdominal girth, decreased urine output, fall in hematocrit and ongoing requirement of blood transfusion are evidences of ongoing bleeding from the injured spleen. In such scenario conservative management should be abandoned and patient should be taken up for exploratory laparotomy.

It is important to remember that conservative management should be attempted only if it is possible to monitor the patient properly and facilities for operation in emergency are available.

Operative Management of Splenic Injury

Exploratory laparotomy is carried out by an upper midline incision. After opening the peritoneal cavity blood is suctioned and surface of spleen and liver is palpated for any lacerations. Areas of obvious palpable injury are packed and rest of the abdomen is examined to see for any other source of bleeding and injuries to any other organs.

Salvage of spleen is not considered if patient is hemodynamically unstable or other life-threatening injuries are present. Splenectomy is mandatory in such situations. Splenectomy is also the only option in cases where spleen is completely shattered or there is avulsion of the splenic pedicle.

Splenectomy in Trauma

After suctioning out the blood, spleen is quickly mobilized by passing hand around the outer surface of spleen and rotating it medially. Posterior layer of lienorenal ligament and phrenicosplenic ligament is divided and spleen is brought at main abdominal incision (Fig. 9.2). Abdominal pads are placed in the splenic fossa. Splenic vessels are then quickly ligated, preferably vein and artery separately taking care not to include the pancreatic tail in the sutures. Gastrosplenic ligament is then divided after careful ligation of short gastric arteries contained in it. Spleen is finally removed by dividing lienocolic ligament.

Splenic Salvage

After fully mobilizing the spleen and delivering out of the abdominal incision, spleen is evaluated regarding the possibility of splenic preservation (Fig. 9.3). Temporary occlusion of splenic vessels is sometimes helpful in achieving hemostasis. Various modalities used for splenic salvage are as follows:

Topical Hemostasis

If a superficial avulsion has stopped bleeding spontaneously, no further treatment is required. If

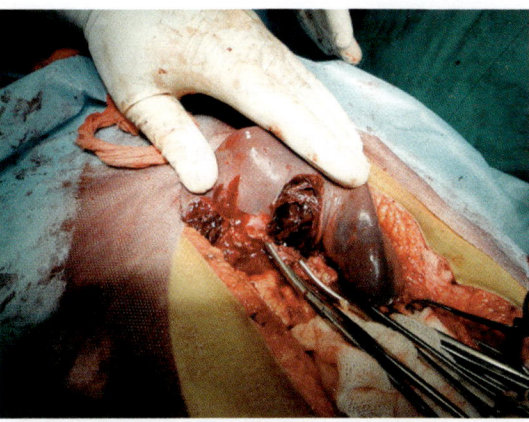

Fig. 9.3: Spleen is delivered out of the abdominal incision after mobilization. In this case splenic hilum was lacerated and hence splenectomy was done

the bleeding persists topical hemostatic agents are applied at the bleeding surface of spleen and gentle pressure is applied for 5–10 minutes. Topical hemostatic agents include Surgicel, Gelfoam, topical thrombin and fibrin glue. Argon beam laser is also effective in controlling the bleeding from the surface of the spleen.

Suturing

In case of actively bleeding parenchymal laceration of the spleen, attempt is made to localize and directly

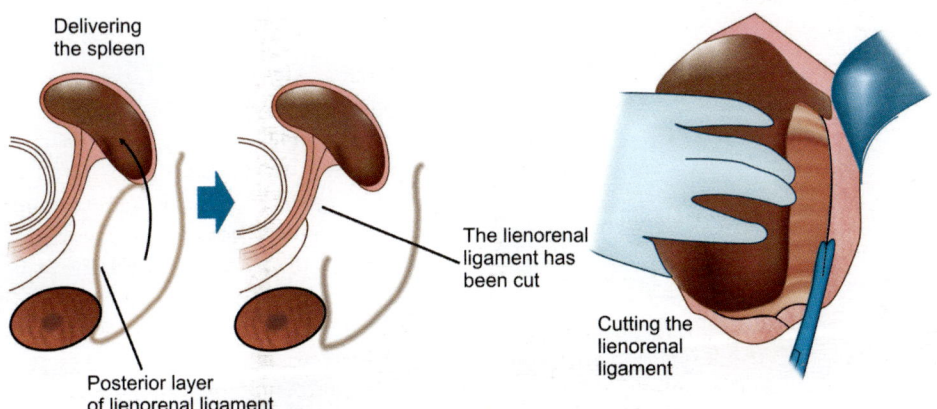

Fig. 9.2: Cutting the lienorenal ligament to mobilize the spleen

suture the bleeding vessel. Diffuse bleeding is controlled by application of horizontal mattress sutures (Fig. 9.4). In children relatively thick capsule of spleen permits the direct suturing but in adults pledgets of Surgicel or Gelfoam are used to reduce the tendency of horizontal mattress sutures to cut through the splenic tissue.

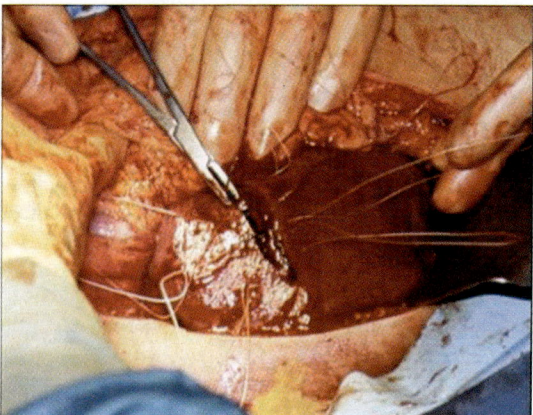

Fig. 9.4: Horizontal mattress sutures being applied on the splenic laceration

Omentum can also be placed in the lacerated part and the splenic tissue is sutured over it to achieve hemostasis (Fig. 9.5).

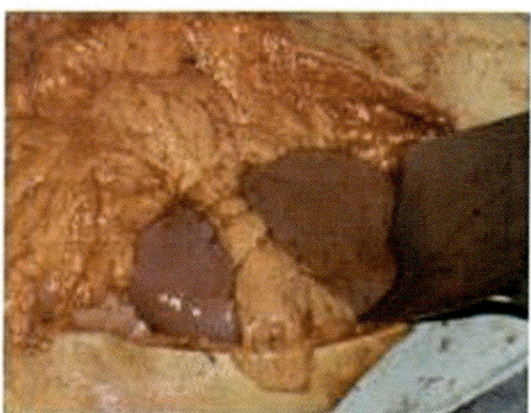

Fig. 9.5: Omentum placed in the lacerated part of the spleen

Splenic Wrap

Splenic wrap using vicryl mesh is an effective technique to control bleeding in splenic injuries with deep or multiple lacerations (Fig. 9.6). A slit is made in vicryl mesh to accommodate the splenic artery and vein. The mobilized spleen is enveloped in the mesh by approximating the free edges of the mesh with absorbable suture.

Partial Splenectomy

Partial splenectomy is required in complex splenic laceration with deep parenchymal injuries and injuries which cannot be managed by suturing techniques or splenic wrap. Spleen is composed of 4–6 segments, each of which has its own blood supply. Segmental arteries of the part of the spleen to be resected are first ligated, which demarcates the avascular intersegmental plane in the parenchyma. Thereafter that avascular segment of spleen is removed.

Splenic Artery Embolization in Splenic Injury

If facility of angiographic embolization is available then splenic artery embolization can be used as an alternative to operative intervention in hemodynamically stable patients with grade IV or V splenic injury, active contrast extravasation or vascular injury determined by CECT abdomen.

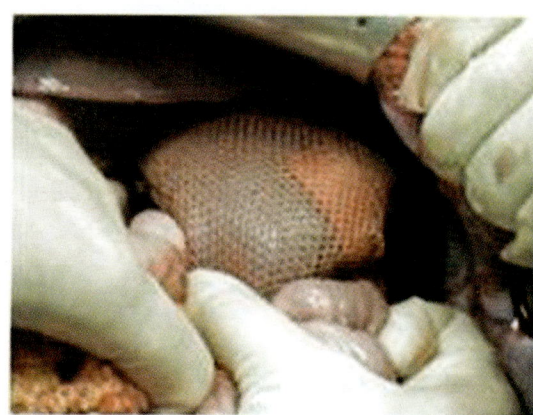

Fig. 9.6: Splenic wrap done with vicryl mesh

Two primary techniques of splenic artery embolization have been described: proximal splenic artery embolization (PSAE) and superselective distal embolization. In PSAE, embolic coils are placed in the splenic artery beyond the origin of dorsal pancreatic artery. Proximal splenic artery embolization promotes hemostasis by causing a reduction in intrasplenic blood flow, which may facilitate clot formation and the healing of the spleen. Splenic perfusion is likely to be maintained through a collateral arterial network, which develops rapidly after embolization.

In distal embolization, a microcatheter is advanced as close as possible to the site of vascular injury. Embolization is then performed using one or more small coils and/or pledgets of Gelfoam. This technique achieves hemostasis to the injured parts while preserving perfusion to the remainder of the spleen.

Distal splenic artery embolization is associated with higher failure rates and also area of splenic infarct is larger compared to the proximal splenic embolization. For these reasons, proximal embolization has been used more extensively than distal embolization for the management of blunt splenic injuries. Studies have reported more than 90% success rate of conservative management by splenic artery embolization. Long-term effect of arterial embolization on splenic functions is yet to be evaluated.

POSTOPERATIVE COMPLICATIONS OF SPLENECTOMY

- *Hemorrhage:* It can occur because of slippage of ligature from the splenic vessels.

- *Gastric dilatation:* This can be prevented by placing nasogastric tube for 24 hours postoperatively.
- Hematemesis can rarely occur because of mucosal damage to the stomach while ligating the short gastric vessels.
- Left basal atelectasis due to damage or irritation of left hemidiaphragm.
- Pancreatic fistula due to damage of the pancreatic tail while ligating the splenic vessels.
- Thrombocytosis in postsplenectomy patient may increase the risk of thrombosis.
- Gastric fistula may occur due to gastric damage while ligating short gastric vessels.
- OPSI (overwhelming postsplenectomy infection)—This occurs due to reduced antibody production in postsplenectomy patient. Patients become susceptible to capsulated bacterial infection like *S. pneumoniae*, *H. influenzae,* and *N. meningitidis*. Risk of OPSI is high in children, in those who undergo splenectomy for hematological conditions or malignancy and in immunocompromised patients. Adult patients who had undergone splenectomy for traumatic injuries have the lowest risk for OPSI. OPSI carries a mortality of about 50%. Patient should be vaccinated against pneumococcus, *H. influenzae* and meningococcus within two weeks of splenectomy as a preventive measure. In children penicillin prophylaxis is usually given for few years after splenectomy. Available data does not support the use of prophylactic antibiotic in adults. However, patients should be instructed to take antibiotics (amoxicillin) in case of fever, sore throat, or respiratory infections.

Urogenital Trauma

RENAL TRAUMA

Renal injuries are more common due to blunt trauma (road traffic accident, fall from height and assaults) and some times as a result of penetrating injury (stab injury or gunshot injury). Severe renal injuries are commonly associated with injuries to the other organs also.

WHEN TO SUSPECT A RENAL INJURY

Hematuria is the best indicator of traumatic urinary system injury. Both gross and microscopic hematuria indicate urinary tract injury. Microscopic hematuria can be detected by urine microscopy or dipstick analysis. Besides this, fractures of lower ribs, upper lumbar and lower thoracic vertebrae fracture and bruising over flanks (Fig. 10.1) are likely to be associated with renal injuries. Renal injuries should always be suspected in cases of penetrating injuries at lumbar area.

There may be pain at the lumbar area with fullness and tenderness at renal angle on abdominal examination. Abdominal distention may appear after a day or two of the accident on account of retroperitoneal hematoma irritating the splanchnic nerves which is known as meteorism.

IMAGING FOR EVALUATION OF RENAL INJURIES

Contrast Enhanced CT scan

Contrast-enhanced CT scan (CECT) is the gold standard investigation to evaluate renal injuries.

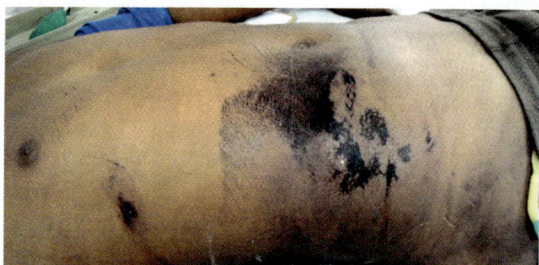

Fig. 10.1: Bruising over the flank—Renal injury should be suspected

CECT scan delineates grade of injury (Table 10.1, Fig. 10.2), shows infarcted segments of kidney and also images the whole abdomen and retroperitoneum (Fig. 10.3).

Indications of doing CECT scan are:
1. Gross hematuria
2. Microscopic hematuria (>5 RBC/ high power field) and shock in a patient with blunt trauma
3. Any degree of hematuria in penetrating injury.

Table 10.1: Grades of renal injury	
Grade	*Injury*
i.	Renal contusion; non-expanding subcapsular hematoma
ii.	Laceration < 1 cm in depth sparing the renal medulla and collecting system; non-expanding retroperitoneal hematoma
iii.	Laceration > 1 cm sparing the collecting system
iv.	Laceration > 1 cm involving the collecting system; renal vessel injury with hemorrhage
v.	Shattered kidney or avulsed renal vessels

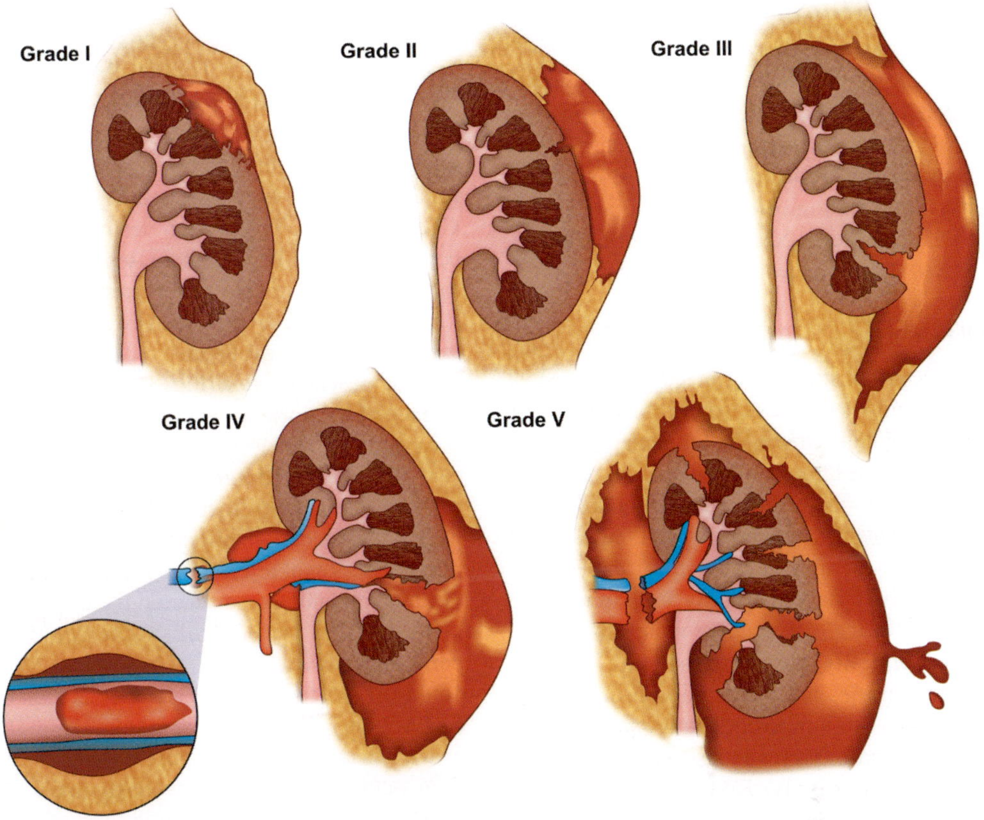

Grade I   Grade II   Grade III

Grade IV   Grade V

Fig. 10.2: Grades of renal injury

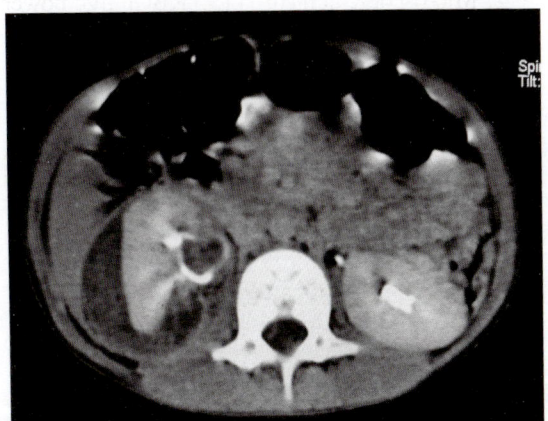

Fig. 10.3: Contrast-enhanced CT scan showing right perinephric hematoma

4. Perirenal hematoma found on ultrasound of abdomen.

Patient must be fully resuscitated and stabilized before CT scan is undertaken. During CECT scan both arterial and venous phase scanning is necessary to detect renal vascular injuries which are diagnosed just after injection of contrast medium. Injuries to renal collecting system may be missed by this first evaluation, so a repeat scan 10–20 minutes after the injection is recommended.

If CT scan is not available then single shot intra-venous urography can be done to find out extra-vasation of the dye indicating renal injury. Both these investigations also give information about the uninvolved opposite kidney, whether functional, non-functional or absent.

Ultrasonography

Focused assessment sonography for trauma (FAST) has been shown to successfully identify free intraperitoneal fluid and possible organ injury in blunt abdominal trauma. But it cannot differentiate between blood, extravasated urine or other types of free fluid. It is observed that majority of the isolated renal injuries will not have associated free fluid. Therefore, FAST is less sensitive then CECT for renal injury

MANAGEMENT

Basic resuscitation should be carried out first. Most of the renal injuries can be managed conservatively. An operation could remove the tamponading effect of a hematoma, resulting in torrential hemorrhage and many a time one ends up doing nephrectomy. Only in a few selected patients surgical intervention is required. A hemodynamically stable patient and renal injury well staged by CECT abdomen are prerequisites for the conservative management.

Hemodynamically stable patients with Grade I, II, III renal injuries are managed conservatively. Urinary extravasation from collecting system injury in Grade IV renal injury can also be successfully managed conservatively. Renal injury patients require strict bed rest until gross hematuria has resolved. Segmental renal artery injury and injuries associated with more than 20% area of non-viable renal tissue, avulsion of the pelviureteric junction are relative indications for renal exploration. Hemodynamically unstable patient and Grade V renal injury should be operated.

If perirenal retroperitoneal hematoma is found during laparotomy then indications of renal exploration are

1. Persistent renal bleeding
2. Expanding perirenal hematoma
3. Pulsatile renal hematoma.

Surgery—Renal Exploration

The aims of surgery are to control hemorrhage and to preserve renal tissue. Adequate blood should be arranged prior to exploration. Exploration is done by a midline laparotomy which allows inspection of all the intra-abdominal organs and the opposite kidney. Proximal control of the renal artery and vein should be achieved before the mobilization of the colon and opening of Gerota's fascia. This helps to quickly control the hemorrhage by occluding the renal vessels if bleeding occurs on opening the Gerota's fascia. It has been seen that early initial control of renal vessels increases the rate of renal salvage and lowers the nephrectomy rate.

Renal vessels are exposed by giving a vertical incision on the peritoneum over the aorta medial to inferior mesenteric vein (Figs 10.4A and B). Anterior surface of the aorta is exposed and left renal vein is seen crossing the aorta anteriorly. Right renal vein can also be secured through this incision, however, if there is difficulty then reflection of the second part of the duodenum provides exposure to the right renal vein. Renal arteries are present on either side of the aorta and can be secured there.

Following the control of the renal vessels, peritoneum lateral to the colon is incised and the colon is reflected medially. Kidney is then exposed by incising the Gerota's fascia. Hematoma is evacuated and kidney is exposed. If there is bleeding then occlusion of the previously isolated renal vessels is done. Warm ischemia time of the kidney is 20 minutes and acute tubular necrosis develops after this. Non-viable renal tissue is then debrided, hemostasis is achieved by suturing the bleeding vessel and open collecting system is sutured by absorbable suture (Figs 10.5A and B). If possible margins of the laceration are approximated using renal capsule (Fig. 10.5C), otherwise an omental flap is placed over the defect (Fig. 10.6). This procedure is known as renal reconstruction or renorrhaphy. If renal reconstruction is not possible then partial nephrectomy is done for polar injuries.

Nephrectomy is indicated in the shattered kidney or renal pedicle injury in an unstable patient (Fig. 10.7). The pedicle vessels are ligated separately, to avoid later arteriovenous fistula formation. Before doing the nephrectomy, presence of the opposite kidney should always be confirmed by palpation if CECT/ IVP has not been done.

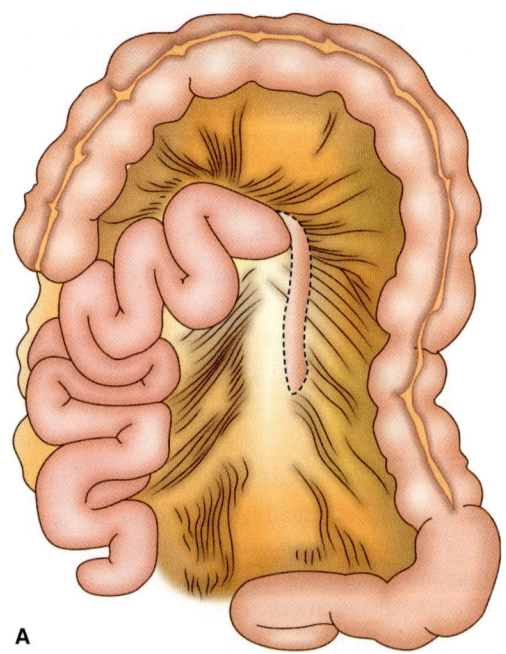

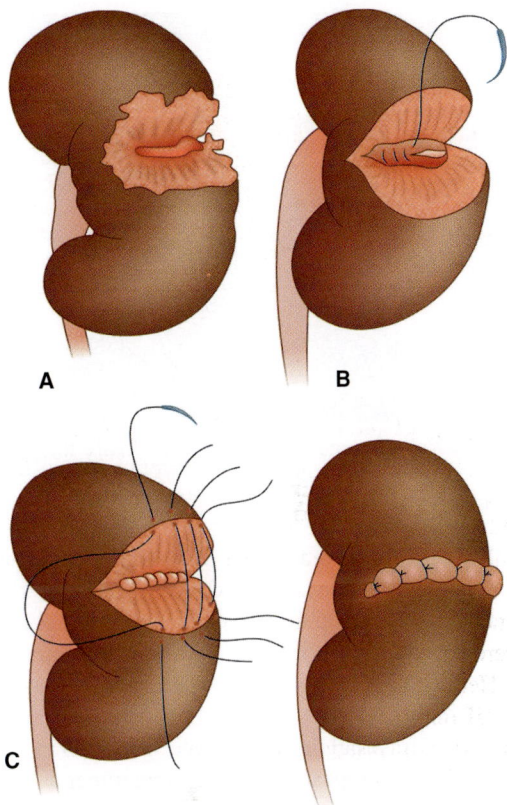

A B

C

Figs 10.5A to C: (A) Debridement of the devitalized tissue, (B) Closure of the collecting system, (C) Approximation of renal capsule

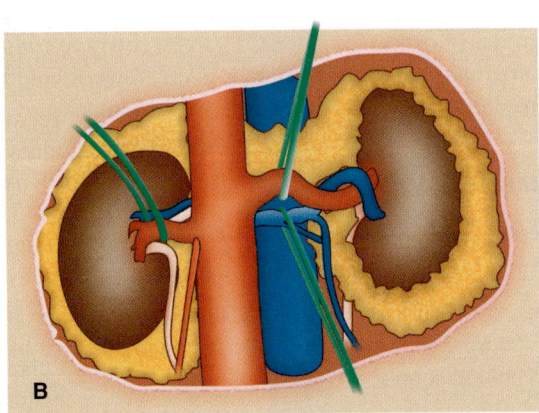

B

Figs 10.4A and B: (A) Incision over the peritoneum medial to inferior mesenteric vessels for the exposure of renal vessels, (B) Control of renal vessels

If solitary kidney is sufficiently damaged to necessitate exploration all efforts are made to repair the kidney, failing which wound should be packed to control the bleeding and also with the hope that the ruptured kidney may heal.

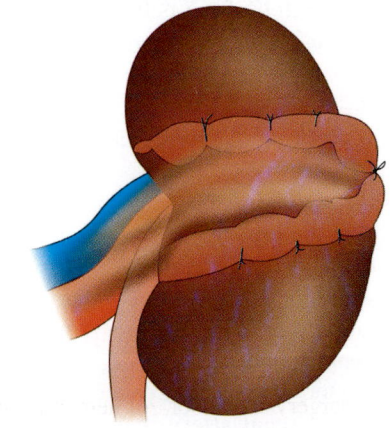

Fig. 10.6: Omentum placed over the lacerated area

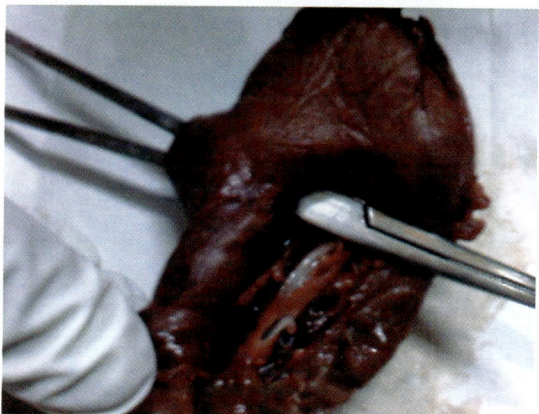

Fig. 10.7: Nephrectomy done for stab injury that had lacerated the kidney and the renal vein. Artery forcep is showing the laceration

Retroperitoneal drainage is necessary after partial or total nephrectomy. If the collecting system has been repaired, a nephrostomy tube and/or double-J stent should be placed. Injuries to other abdominal organs should be looked for and are managed accordingly.

If severe renal injuries have been managed conservatively repeat imaging is recommended in order to identify urinary extravasation, ongoing significant hemorrhage and rare complication like pseudoaneurysm.

COMPLICATIONS OF RENAL INJURIES

- *Clot retention in bladder:* It can be cleared by irrigation by three-way Foley catheter and bladder wash out.
- *Urinoma:* Collection of the extravasated urine in the lumbar area
- *Perinephric abscess:* It occurs because of the infection of the urinoma. It can be managed by ultrasound guided aspiration
- *Hypertension:* It may occur as delayed complication due to renal fibrosis which may require nephrectomy at a later stage if it is found to be refractory to medical treatment.
- Aneurysm of renal artery may occur as late complication.

URETERIC INJURY

Traumatic ureteral injuries are uncommon as ureter is well-protected in the retroperitoneum by the bony pelvis, psoas muscle and vertebrae. Therefore, ureter is damaged more commonly in penetrating injuries (stab or gunshot) rather than blunt trauma.

Ureteral injuries are commonly found to be associated with injuries to other surrounding organs as well. Iatrogenic injury to the ureter is also known to occur in gynecological, urological and colorectal injuries.

PRESENTATION

Ureteric injury is usually not evident at the early stage. Hematuria is an unreliable sign of ureteric trauma and its absence does not exclude the injury. Delayed presentation can be in the form of prolonged ileus, urinary leakage (urinoma), prolonged high urinary output in drain postoperatively, fever, sepsis or deranged renal function. In all such cases further investigations like CECT, IVU (intravenous urography) or RGP (retrograde pyelography) should be done to evaluate the integrity of the ureter.

MANAGEMENT

Key Points Regarding Operative Repair of Ureteric Injuries

- Adventitia of the ureter should be preserved during mobilization of the ureter to preserve its blood supply.
- Non-viable ureteric tissue are debrided until the edges bleed.
- Edges of the ureter are spatulated and repaired with 4–O/5–O absorbable suture under magnification.
- Repair should be done over an internal stent (Double-J stent)
- Anastomosis should be watertight and tension-free.

Successful methods of ureteric repair are based on injury location and extent of ureteric loss. Options according to the site of injury are:

- Pelviureteric junction injury—ureteropyelostomy
- Proximal and mid-ureteric injury—when there is no loss or very short segment loss, ureteric injuries can be repaired primarily as uretero-ureterostomy (Fig. 10.8)
- Distal ureter—Uretero-neocystostomy with or without psoas bladder hitch.

Partial Transection

Partial transection of the ureteral wall after blunt injury or stab wound may be managed with primary closure. However, gunshot injuries require wide debridement, as the associated microvascular injuries extend up to 2 cm beyond the areas of gross injury.

Major Transection

Appropriate management of profound ureteral loss which cannot be managed by the simple procedures, is to ligate the ureter and drain the kidney with a percutaneous nephrostomy tube. This will allow the patient to recover from the injury and more complex repair can be performed in planned setting at a later date. The options are

Vesicopsoas Hitch and Ureteric Reimplantation

This is the treatment of choice for lower ureteral injuries. This procedure involves mobilizing the bladder and pulling it superiorly and laterally by fixing it to the psoas tendon with an absorbable suture (Fig. 10.9). This technique can be used to bridge a 6 to 8 cm defect and it helps in reimplanting the ureter to the bladder.

Boari Bladder Flap

Boari bladder flap is made for lower ureteric injuries where the segment loss is too long to be managed with the psoas hitch. Boari flap provides an

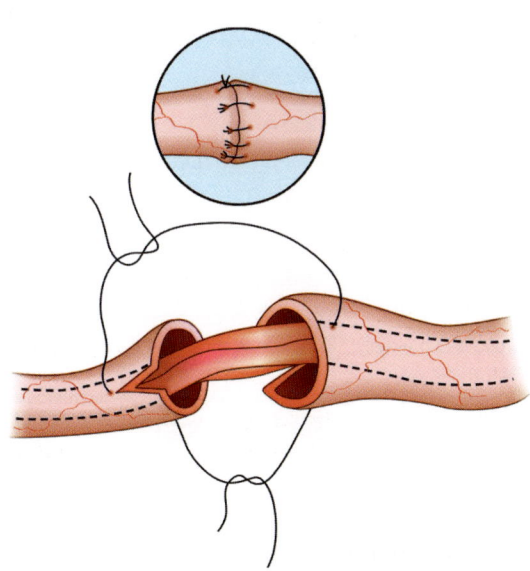

Fig. 10.8: Ends of the ureter spatulated and repaired over a double-J stent

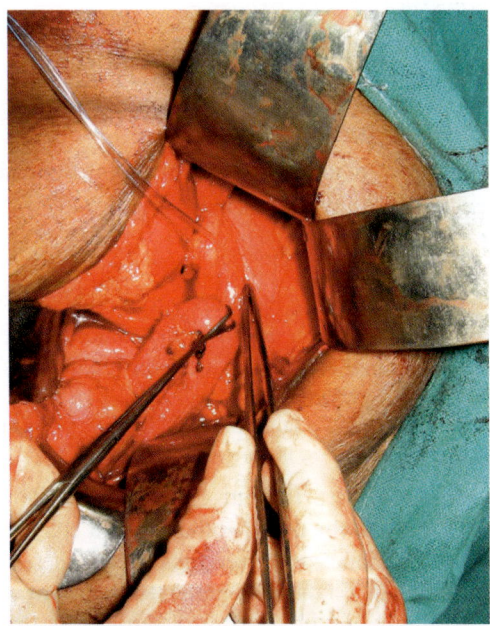

Fig. 10.9: Bladder sutured to the psoas tendon (psoas hitch)

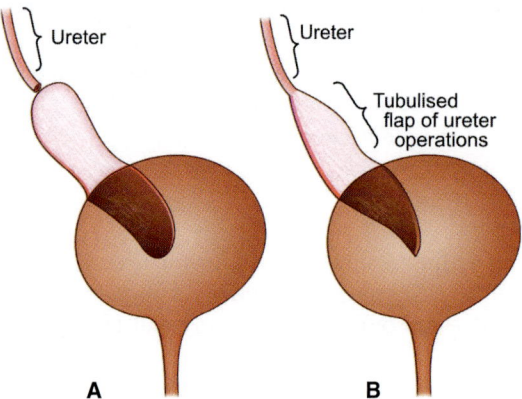

Figs 10.10A and B: Boari bladder flap: (A) Dotted area shows the flap of bladder, (B) Proximal end of the ureter reimplanted in the bladder and flap is closed

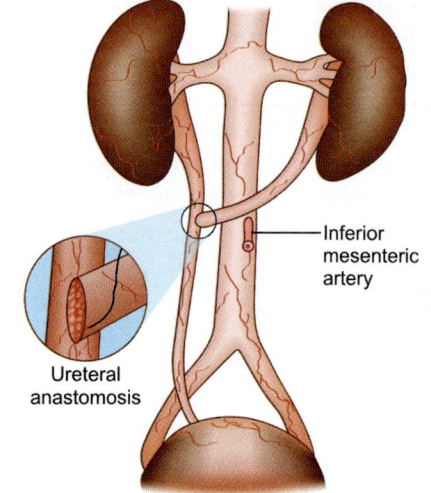

Fig. 10.11: Transureteroureterostomy

additional 12–15 cm of length. In this procedure, a pedicle of bladder is swung cephalad and tubularized to bridge the gap to the injured ureter (Fig. 10.10).

Transureteroureterostomy

In this procedure the ureter is anastomosed end to side to the opposite ureter (Fig.10.11)

Ileal Interposition

In this a segment of the ileum is anastomosed between the kidney and bladder (Fig. 10.12)

Autotransplantation

It involves relocating the kidney to the pelvis. The renal artery and vein are then anastomosed to the iliac vessels and the healthy ureter or renal pelvis is anastomosed to the bladder.

Ureteroileostomy or Ureterosigmoidostomy

In this procedure the cut end of the ureter is anastomosed to the ileum or the sigmoid colon.

If ureteric injury is missed initially and there is a delayed diagnosis then the preferred treatment will be percutaneous nephrostomy with or without antegrade stenting. Definite repair is undertaken when the acute inflammation is settled.

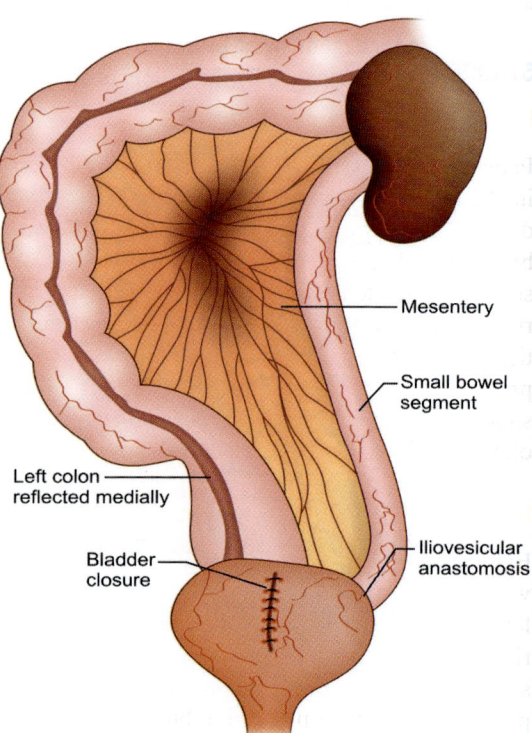

Fig. 10.12: Ileal interposition

LATE COMPLICATIONS OF URETERIC INJURY

Stricture: Ischemic ureter heals with formation of scar and development of stricture. Open segmental resection and repair is necessary in these cases.
Fistula: Ureterovaginal and ureterovesical fistula can develop rarely.

BLADDER INJURIES

Rupture of bladder may be intraperitoneal (20%) or extraperitoneal (80%). Intraperitoneal rupture may be secondary to a blow, kick or fall on a fully distended bladder. The increased pressure results in rupture of the dome which is the weakest part of the bladder (Fig. 10.13A).

Extraperitoneal rupture is usually found in association with fracture pelvis (Fig. 10.13B).

SYMPTOMS AND SIGNS

Intraperitoneal Rupture of Bladder

Patient will have a history of sudden agonizing pain in the hypogastrium and he would not have any desire to micturate. On abdominal examination bladder will not be palpable and there will be suprapubic tenderness. There will be guarding and rigidity because of the peritonitis caused by urine in the peritoneal cavity. Shifting dullness may be present. If the urine is sterile then symptoms and signs of peritonitis is delayed. Rectal examination often reveals bulging of the rectovesical pouch.

Extraperitoneal Rupture of Bladder

Extraperitoneal rupture are commonly associated with fracture pelvis. The bladder is usually torn at lateral wall near the base by distortion of the pelvic rim. Occasionally bladder can also get torn by the sharp fractured edges of the pelvic bone. Although patient may want to pass urine but is able to pass only small amount of blood. Blood and urine gets accumulated in the prevesical space and tracks

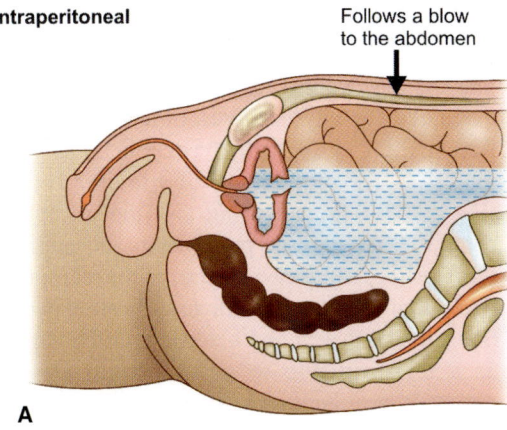

Intraperitoneal   Follows a blow to the abdomen

A

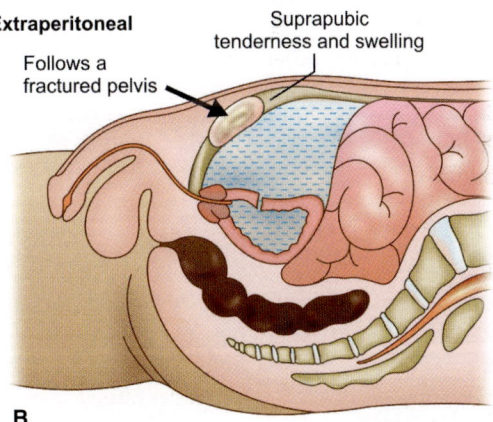

Extraperitoneal   Suprapubic tenderness and swelling

Follows a fractured pelvis

B

Figs 10.13A and B: Intraperitoneal rupture of bladder (B) Extraperitoneal rupture of bladder

between the peritoneum and transversalis fascia. They infiltrate laterally towards the anterosuperior iliac spines. If left untreated, this mixture of blood and urine gets infected and ultimately reaches the thigh through sacrosciatic notches and obturator foramina. Sometimes it is difficult to differentiate extraperitoneal rupture from posterior urethral rupture.

INVESTIGATIONS

- Retrograde cystography is the investigation of choice. With careful asepsis a 14 Fr catheter is passed. A solution made from 60 ml of urograffin with 120 ml of sterile isotonic saline is pushed into the bladder and radiographs are taken and evaluated for any extravasation (Fig. 10.14). Recently, CT cystography has come up as good modality for evaluation of bladder injury (Fig. 10.15). In case of intraperitoneal rupture contrast leaks into the peritoneum and outlines the intestines. Whereas in extraperitoneal rupture flame-shaped areas of extravasation are noted in the perivesical area and bladder is often appear as a teardrop due to compression by the retroperitoneal hematoma (teardrop deformity).

- Plain X-ray in the erect position may show the ground-glass appearance of fluid in the lower abdomen.

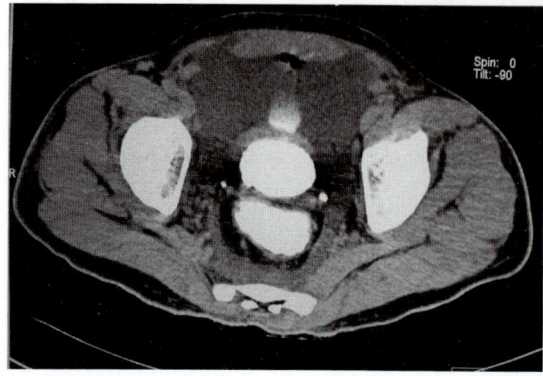

Fig. 10.15: CT scan showing rupture of bladder as evident by extravasation of contrast

- Intravenous urography (IVU) may confirm a leak from the bladder.
- A peritoneal tap may be of value if facilities for radiological examination are not available. Aspiration of urine will indicate the bladder injury.

TREATMENT

Intraperitoneal Rupture

The standard treatment is to perform a lower midline laparotomy. Urine from peritoneum is removed by suction. The edges of the rent of the bladder, which are usually situated in the dome of the bladder, are trimmed and sutured with two layers of interrupted vicryl stitches, and the operation is completed by placement of a suprapubic malecot catheter and insertion of Foley catheter in the urethra. The perineum should be irrigated with copious amounts of warm saline and abdomen is closed by keeping an abdominal drain.

Extraperitoneal Rupture

Usually uncomplicated extraperitoneal bladder rupture is managed conservatively with urethral catheter drainage and administration of antibiotics. Cystography is done after two weeks and if there is no extravasation then Foley is removed.

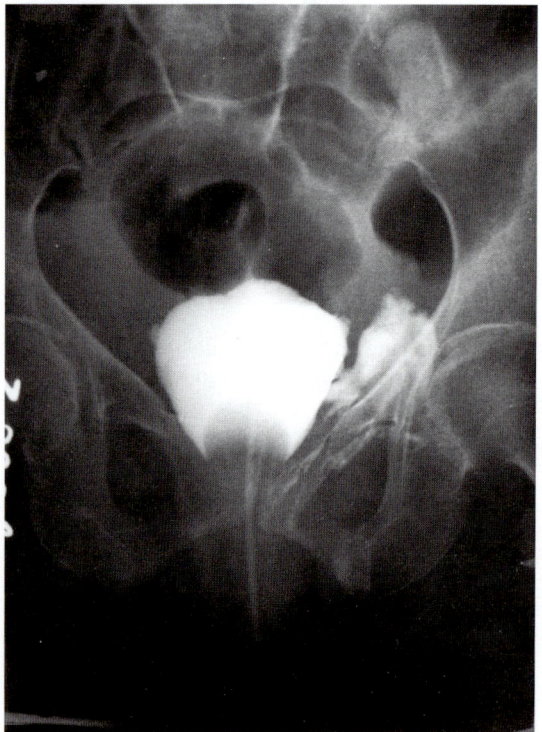

Fig. 10.14: Retrograde cystography showing extraperitoneal rupture of bladder with extravasation of contrast

Open repair of extraperitoneal bladder injuries is done if it is associated with bladder neck injury, rectal or vaginal injury, open pelvic fracture, bone fragments projecting into the bladder, if there is inadequate bladder drainage or clots in the urine.

Complications of simple rupture of bladder are rare. But if the trauma involving the bladder neck, vagina or rectum and not repaired promptly can result in incontinence, fistula and stricture formation.

URETHRAL TRAUMA

ANATOMY OF URETHRA

The male urethra is divided into posterior and anterior urethra (Fig. 10.16). The posterior urethra includes prostatic urethra and membranous urethra. Prostatic urethra extends from the bladder neck through the prostate gland and joins the membranous urethra, which lies between the prostatic apex and the perineal membrane. Distal to membranous urethra is the anterior urethra which is conventionally divided into the penile (or pendulous) and bulbous parts at the penoscrotal junction. The pendulous portion terminates in the glans penis to form the fossa navicularis.

ETIOLOGY

Causes of Anterior Urethral Injury

- Blunt trauma, fall astride/kicks in the perineum.
- Penetrating trauma like gunshot and stab injury
- Vigorous sexual act, penile fracture, urethral foreign body
- Iatrogenic injuries like endoscopic instrumentation.

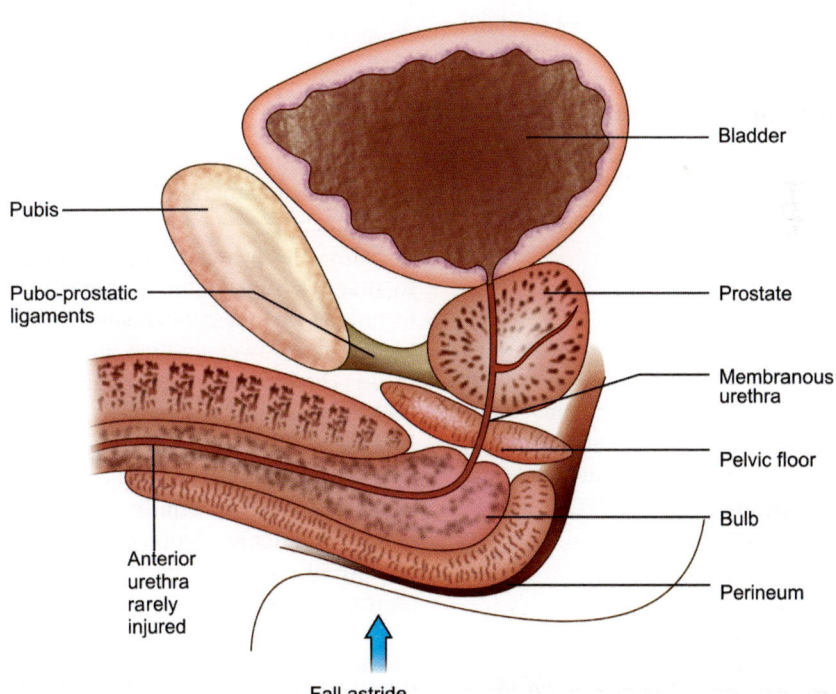

Fig. 10.16: Anatomy of male urethra

Causes of Posterior Urethral Injury

It is usually associated with major trauma like
- Urethral injury associated with pelvic fracture (road traffic accident, fall from height, industrial accidents)
- Penetrating injury, i.e. stab injury
- Gunshot injury
- Iatrogenic injury e.g. complication of endoscopic surgery particularly TURP and in cases of radical prostatectomy.

CLASSIFICATION

Blunt urethral trauma is traditionally classified as anterior or posterior injury. Posterior urethral injury usually is caused by a crushing force to the pelvis (e.g. from a high-speed automobile accident) and is associated with pelvic fractures. The prostatic urethra is fixed in position because of the attachments of the puboprostatic ligaments. Displacement of the bony pelvis from a fracture can thus lead to either tearing or stretching of the membranous urethra.

Anterior urethral injury usually results from a straddle injury (e.g. falling on a bicycle cross bar) and is most often isolated.

Injuries are also classified as complete or incomplete which relates to the circumference of urethral wall.

CLINICAL FEATURES

Blood at the urethral meatus, inability to pass urine and palpable urinary bladder are the cardinal features of urethral injury. Additional signs of membranous urethral injury include perineal, scrotal, and penile ecchymosis, and a high-riding prostate on rectal examination.

Sign of membranous urethral injury are:
- Pelvic fracture
- Perineal bruising
- Blood at the meatus
- Inability to pass urine
- High riding prostate.

The extravasation of urine can be present in complete rupture of bulbar urethra. Urine can extravasate into the scrotum, beneath the superficial fascia of penis and up the abdominal wall beneath the deep layer of superficial fascia.

TREATMENT

When faced with urethral trauma, initial management decisions must be made in the context of other injuries and patient stability. Life-threatening injuries must be corrected first.

Posterior Urethral Injuries

A urethral Foley catheter must not be inserted as it may aggravate the injury converting a partial disruption into a complete one.

If signs of urethral injury are present then retrograde urethrogram should be done. A Foley catheter (16 Fr) is placed from the external urethral meatus for about one cm and the balloon is filled with 1 ml of saline to snug the catheter in the urethra. It is best to conduct the study under fluoroscopy. 25 ml of contrast (urograffin) is gently injected and extravasation of the contrast indicating urethral injury is looked for (Fig. 10.17). If fluoroscopy is not available then oblique X-ray films are taken after injection of contrast. If there is no extravasation of contrast on urethrogram then nothing else is required to be done.

Safest management for posterior urethral tear is to insert a suprapubic catheter either by open technique or under ultrasound guidance. In open technique a lower midline abdominal incision is made. The bladder is opened in the midline and it should be carefully inspected. Bladder lacerations if present are closed from within with absorbable suture (2.0 vicryl) and a malecot tube inserted for urinary drainage. Definitive repair is carried out 6–8 weeks after resolution of hematoma, which can be carried out either by perineal approach or be transapubic approach.

Early realignment of urethra (rail roading) is also a treatment option which is carried out at the time of injury by using interlocking urethral sounds (Figs 10.18 and 10.19A to E). Foley catheter is placed for 4 to 6 weeks along with suprapubic cystostomy

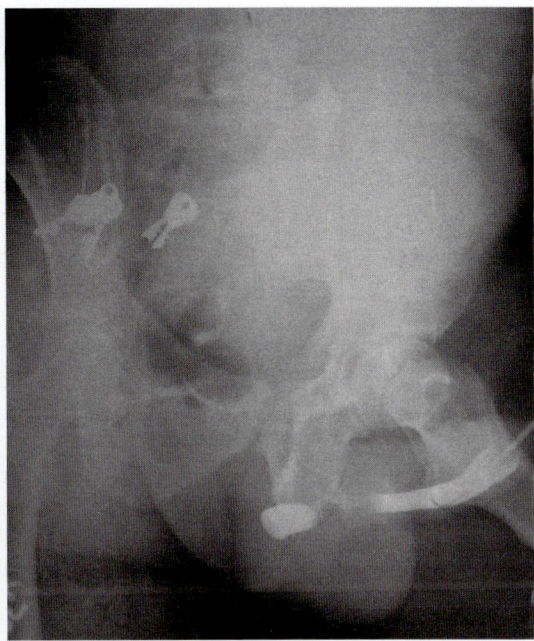

Fig. 10.17: Retrograde urethrography showing complete urethral rupture

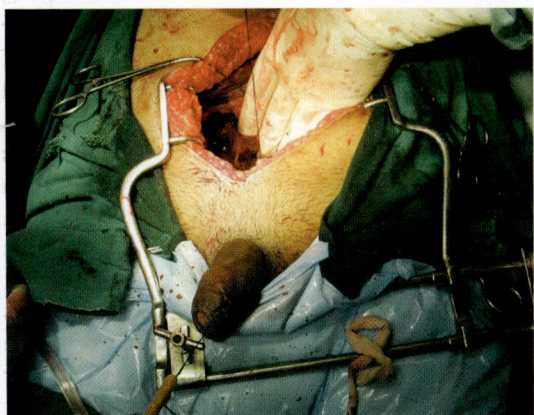

Fig. 10.18: Railroading for urethral injury to lays thread attched to the Foley catheter is being pulled to place the catheter in the urinary bladder

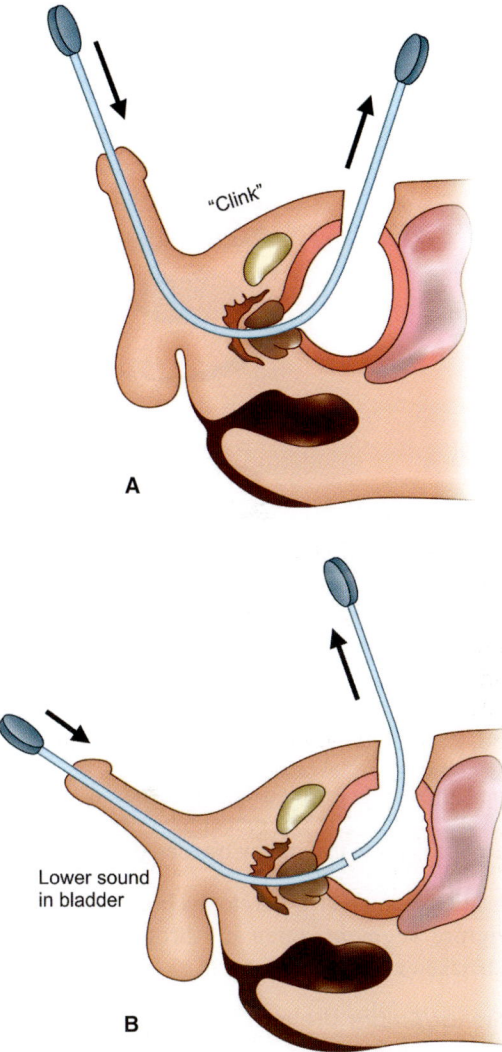

Figs 10.19A and B: Railroading with sounds: (A) One sound is placed from the external urinary meatus and second from the cystostomy. The two sounds meeting in the patient's retropubic space, (B) The lower sound has entered the bladder

as many patients despite urethral realignment develop posterior urethral stenosis. If the patients voids satisfactorily after the removal of the Foley catheter, then suprapubic cystostomy is removed.

Urethral stricture will develop in most of the patients undergoing primary urethral alignment, however, stricture segment in these cases will be of shorter length which can be managed by urethral

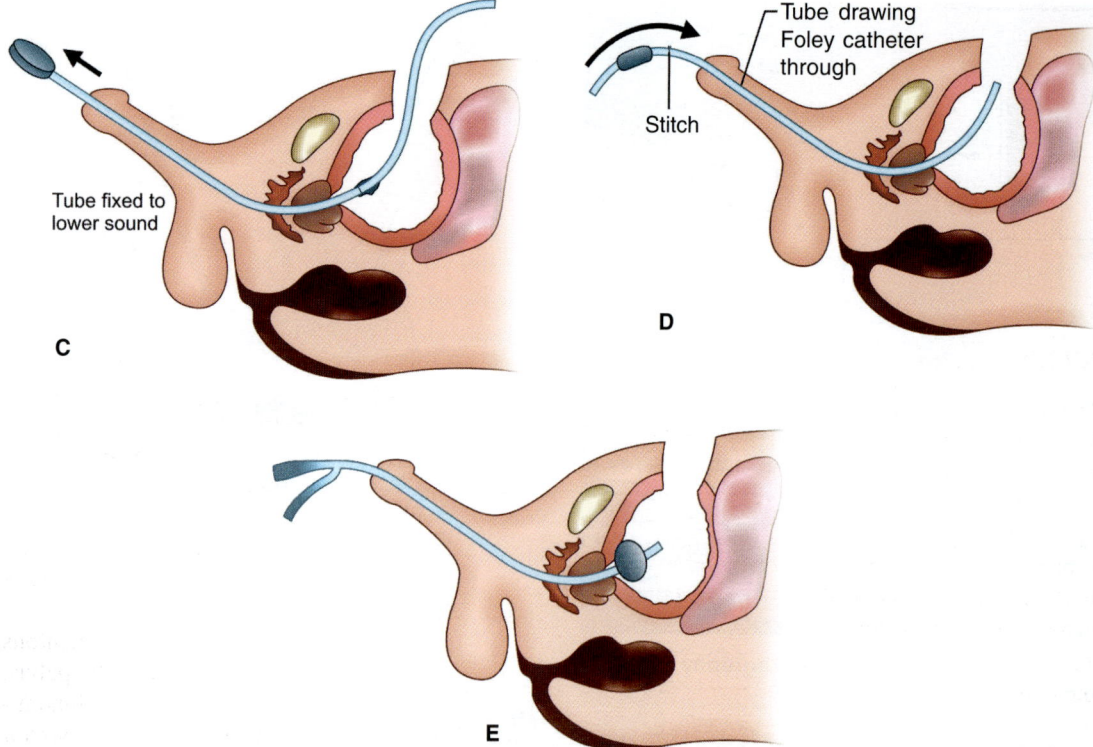

Figs 10.19C to E: Railroading with sounds: (C) A rubber tube is fitted on the lower sound and is drawn through the patient's urethra, (D) The rubber tube has been stitched to the Foley catheter and the rubber tube is pulled to place the Foley in the urinary bladder, (E) Bulb of the Foley is inflated in the urinary bladder

dilatation or internal urethrotomy. In cases of longer stricture segment, open urethroplasty can be undertaken at a later date.

Anterior/Bulbar Urethral Injury

Patients with bulbar urethral injury have perineal bruising, blood at the urinary meatus and retention of urine. A urethral catheter must not be passed as it may aggravate the injury. If the patient passes urine, he should be given antibiotics and followed up. Patients with urinary retention should be treated by inserting a suprapubic catheter. Antibiotics are given and urethrography is performed after about five days. If the patients develops stricture later on then it is managed by either urethral dilatation or endoscopic urethrotomy for incomplete stricture or urethroplasty for complete stricture.

Penetrating Anterior Urethral Injury

This type of injury should be explored. Devitalized tissue should be debrided carefully to minimize tissue loss. Defects up to 2.0 cm in the bulbar urethra and up to 1.5 cm in the penile urethra can be repaired primarily by direct anastomosis over a catheter with fine absorbable sutures. Longer defects are reconstructed at a later date.

11 Management of Pelvic Fracture

INTRODUCTION

Pelvic fractures are life-threatening injuries. Approximately 15 to 30% of patients with high-energy pelvic injuries are hemodynamically unstable, which may be directly related to blood loss from the pelvic injury. Hemorrhage remains the leading cause of death in patients with pelvic fractures, with an overall mortality rate between 6 and 35% in large series of high-energy pelvic fractures. Bleeding associated with pelvic fractures requires efficient evaluation and rapid intervention. To optimize outcome, evaluation and treatment of patients with pelvic fractures necessitates a multidisciplinary approach. It is important for the patient with pelvic fracture that the orthopedic surgeon be involved in every phase of treatment, including primary resuscitation. Early assessment by an orthopedic surgeon familiar with pelvic fracture patterns allows the treatment team to establish diagnostic and treatment priorities. A thorough understanding of potential sources of bleeding and an awareness of treatment options are essential for all physicians involved.

Pelvic fracture confers a mortality risk which may exceed 25%, depending on the severity of the fracture and the frequently associated injuries. High-energy impact from motor vehicle accidents or falls from heights are the most common causes of these multiple comminuted fractures within the normally very stable and solid pelvic ring.

ANATOMY (Figs 11.1 and 11.2)

The pelvis is a ring-like structure made up of three bones: the sacrum and two innominate bone each comprising of ilium, ischium, and pubis. The innominate bones join the sacrum posteriorly at the two sacroiliac joints; anteriorly, these bones are joined at the pubic symphysis. The symphysis acts as a strut during weight bearing to maintain the structure of the pelvic ring. The symphysis is reinforced inferiorly by muscle insertions and the arcuate ligament. The thickest portion of this fibrous joint is usually superior and anterior.

The strongest and most important ligamentous structures are in the posterior aspect of the pelvis. These ligaments connect the sacrum to the innominate bones. The stability provided by the posterior ligaments must withstand the forces of weight-bearing transmitted across the sacroiliac joints from the lower extremities to the spine. The posterior sacroiliac ligaments are divided into two components: short and long. The short posterior ligaments are oblique and run from the posterior ridge of the sacrum to the posterior–superior and posterior–inferior spines of the ilium. The long posterior ligaments are longitudinal fibers that run from the lateral aspect of the sacrum to the posterior–superior iliac spines (PSIS) and merge with the sacrotuberous ligament. The long ligaments lie posterior and superficial to the short ligaments. The anterior sacroiliac ligaments run from the ilium to the sacrum. This structure provides some stability, but less than that provided by the posterior ligaments.

The sacrotuberous ligament is a strong band that runs from the posterolateral sacrum and dorsal aspect of the posterior iliac spine to the ischial tuberosity. This ligament, along with the posterior sacroiliac ligaments, provides vertical stability to

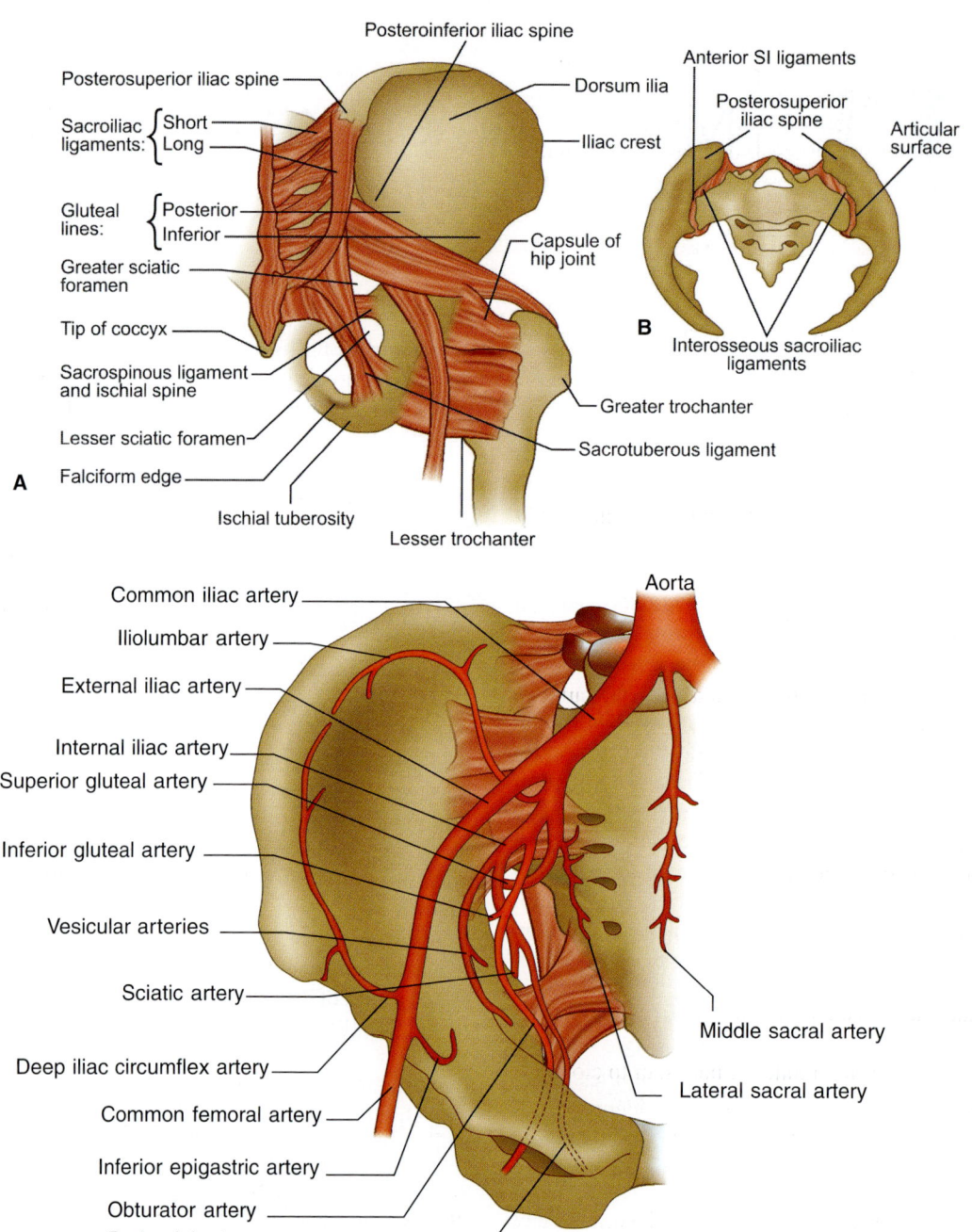

Figs 11.1 and 11.2: Anatomy of pelvis

the pelvis. The sacrospinous ligament runs from the lateral edge of the sacrum and coccyx to the sacrotuberous ligament and inserts onto the ischial spine. The iliolumbar ligaments run from the fourth and fifth lumbar transverse processes to the posterior iliac crest; the lumbosacral ligaments run from the fifth lumbar transverse process to the sacral ala.

Major blood vessels lie on the innerwall of the pelvis. The common iliac artery divides, giving off the external iliac artery, which exits the pelvis anteriorly over the pelvic brim. The internal iliac artery lies over the pelvic brim. It courses anterior and in close proximity to the sacroiliac joint. The posterior branches of the internal iliac artery include the iliolumbar, superior gluteal, and lateral sacral arteries. The superior gluteal artery sweeps around to exit the greater sciatic notch, where it lies directly on bone. Anterior branches of the internal iliac artery include the obturator, umbilical, vesical, pudendal, inferior gluteal, rectal, and hemorrhoidal arteries. The pudendal and obturator arteries are anatomically related to the pubic rami and can be injured with fractures or injuries to these structures. These arteries and their associated veins can all be injured during pelvic disruption. An understanding of pelvic anatomy will help the surgeon recognize which fracture patterns are more likely to cause direct damage to major vessels and result in significant retroperitoneal bleeding.

MECHANISM OF INJURY

For the pelvis, the instability is defined by two displacements: rotational and vertical. The forces, caused by rotational displacements, tend either to open and externally rotate the pelvis, or to close and internally rotate it. Vertical instability indicates disruption of the posterior tension band and implies craniocaudal, rotational and antero-posterior displacement. Three basic mechanisms lead to pelvic ring disruptions. They are based on the direction of the force imparted to the pelvis at the time of injury. (Table 11.1 and Fig. 11.3)

Table 11.1: Types of pelvic fracture	
Anteroposterior compression	
Type I	Disruption of the pubis symphysis of <2.5 cm of diastasis; no significant posterior pelvic injury
Type II	Disruption of the pubis symphysis of >2.5 cm, with tearing of the anterior sacroiliac and sacrospinous and sacrotuberous ligaments
Type III	Complete disruption of the pubic symphysis and posterior ligament complexes, with hemipelvic displacement
Lateral compression	
Type I	Posterior compression of the sacroiliac joint without ligament disruption; oblique pubic ramus fracture
Type II	Rupture of the posterior sacroiliac ligament; pivotal internal rotation of hemipelvis on the anterior SI joint with a crush injury of the sacrum and an oblique pubic ramus fracture
Type III	Finding in type II injury with evidence of an anteroposterior compression injury to the contralateral hemipelvis

Antero-posterior Compression

The antero-posterior (AP) compression injury (Fig. 11.4) pattern is due to a force directly applied to the pubis or to the posterior pelvis and results in iliac external rotation deformity. The symphyseal separation suggests damage to the ligamentous structures and possible instability. The presence of a vertical obturator ring fracture, a diastasis of both the symphysis pubis and the sacroiliac joint are important points of this pattern and serve as stability hallmarks.

Lateral Compression

The lateral compression injury pattern or iliac internal rotation injury is the result of a lateral blow to the side of the pelvis (Fig.11.5). This fracture affects either one or both sides of the pelvis ring. Anteriorly, the fracture fragments frequently override the adjacent fragments. Posteriorly, the

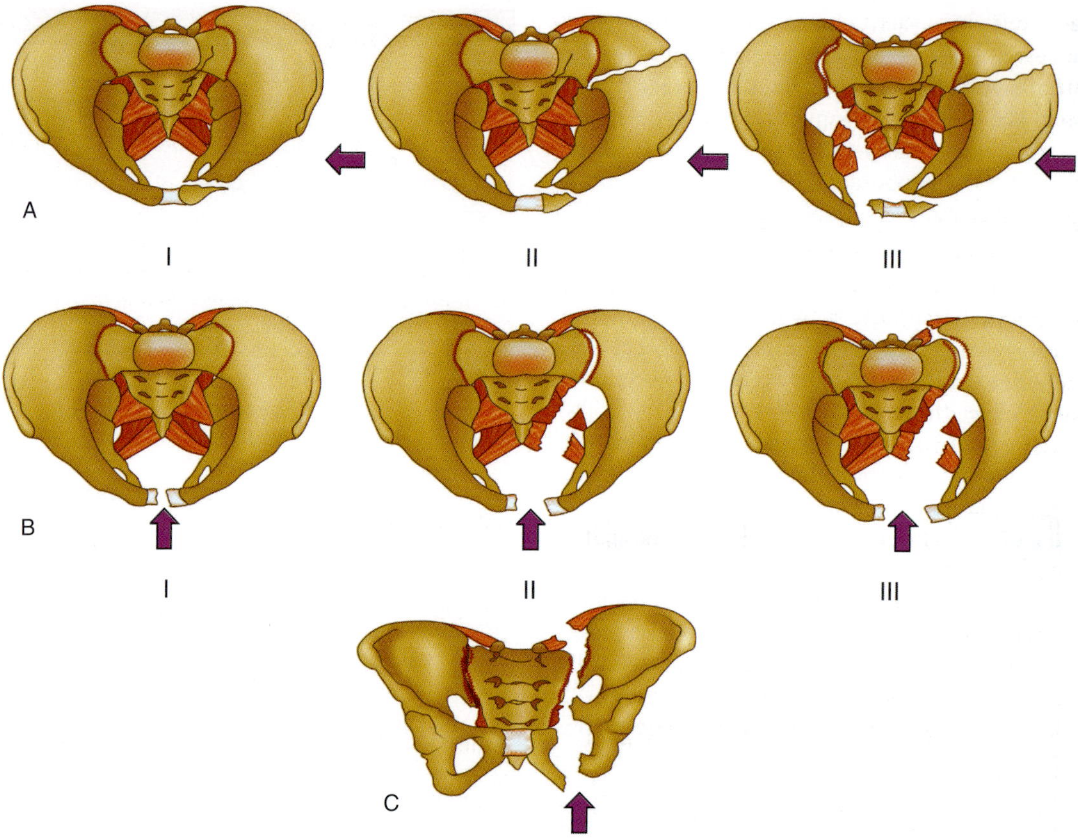

A

I   II   III

B

I   II   III

C

Fig. 11.3: Types of fracture according to the impact

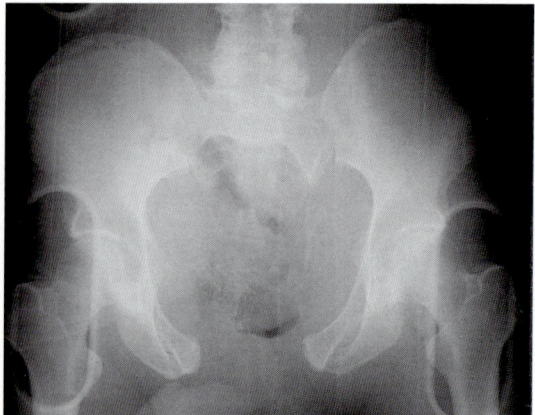

Fig. 11.4: Antero-posterior compression

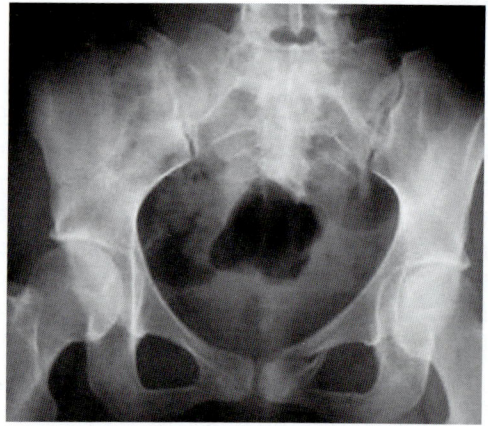

Fig. 11.5: Lateral compression

fracture fragments are impacted (mainly in elderly patients), or there is a diastasis of the sacroiliac joint (mainly in the younger patients, sometimes associated with ligamentous disruption).

Vertical Shear

The vertical shear pattern is often an unstable state, when it appears after a vertical axial fall, with presence of anterior and posterior fractures of the pubic rami, fractures of the sacrum, sacroiliac diastasis, or iliac wing fracture (Fig. 11.6). A typical finding is always present as a superior and usually asymmetric displacement of the involved hemi-pelvis secondary to the vertical axial fall.

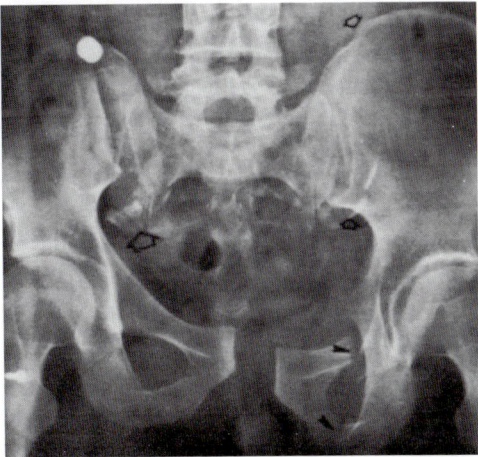

Fig. 11.6: Vertical shear

COMPREHENSIVE PELVIC CLASSIFICATION (MODIFIED AFTER TILE)

The classification combines the mechanism of injury and the degree of pelvic stability. It harmonizes the prognosis and treatment options. Pelvic fractures are classified into three main categories: A, B and C.

Type-A fracture

Type-A fracture is an incomplete fracture with neither disruption of the pelvic ring nor lesion of the posterior band.

Type A1 corresponds to an avulsion fracture of the pelvic ring. The avulsion of the anterior–superior spine is caused by the sudden contraction of the sartorius, whereas that of the anterior–inferior spine is caused by the contraction of the rectus femoris. The avulsion of the pubic tubercle is caused by the contraction of the pectineus.

Type A2.1 corresponds to a stable iliac wing fracture caused by direct blow on the ilium and does not involve pelvic ring which remains stable.

Type A2.2 relates to a stable, minimally, or undisplaced fracture of the pelvic ring and usually affects elderly women with osteoporosis after a fall. The mechanism corresponds to a lateral compression, cracking the pubic rami.

Type A2.3 relates to anterior ring fractures or four pillar fractures and involves the four pubic rami frontally, without posterior injury. These fractures are caused by a direct blow or by a high-energy trauma of shearing or lateral compression.

Type A3 are sacral or coccygeal fractures.

Type A3.1 implies fractures of the coccyx or sacrococcygeal dislocation which is common after a sitting fall and may be the source of prolonged pain, but no neurological disability is observed. The transverse fractures of the sacrum distal to the gluteal line do not involve the pelvic ring.

Type A3.2 relates to undisplaced fractures and rarely causes neurological deficit.

Type A3.3 corresponds to displaced and translated fractures with injury to the sacral nerve roots.

Type-B fracture

Type-B fracture relates to disruption (or fracture) of the symphysis pubis, associated with anterior sacroiliac joint disruption (unilateral or bilateral). The posterior sacroiliac ligaments, responsible for the vertical stability, remain untouched. The typical lesion is caused by an AP compression applied to the anterior–superior iliac spines of the fixed pelvis. A posterior blow against the posterior–superior iliac spines may produce a similar fracture. Displacement of the symphysis pubis is an important feature of this type. If the splitting of the symphysis pubis is smaller than 2.5 cm, it cannot be associated with a disruption of either the pelvic floor or the sacro-spinous ligament. But if it is wider than 2.5 cm, then it is often associated with a disruption of either the pelvic floor or the sacro-spinous ligament. In the latter case, a much higher occurrence of visceral injury is observed.

Type B1 relates to a unilateral "open-book" injury usually caused by a violent external rotation of one femur. The typical situation is that of the motorcyclist who puts out a leg for balance and gets caught by a stationary object such as a road panel or a tree. The external rotation force usually disrupts the symphysis pubis first, and as the external rotation goes on, a disruption of the pelvic floor, of the fascia, of the sacrospinous, and of anterior sacroiliac ligaments follows. The variants include B1.1 (sacroiliac joint anterior disruption) and B1.2 (sacral fractures).

Type B2 relates to lateral compression injuries characterized by unilateral partial disruption of the posterior arch maintaining the vertical or posterior stability (internal rotation). A lateral compressive force directed at the pelvic ring may cause two types of injury, the first in which the anterior and posterior lesions occurs on the same side of the pelvis, and the second in which the displacement is shown on the opposite side. In the latter case, the relative stability is maintained by the osseous impaction (no muscle or ligament tears). Variants include B2.1 (anterior crush fracture of the sacrum), B2.2 (partial sacroiliac joint fracture/subluxation), and B2.3 (incomplete iliac fracture).

Type B3 stands for the classical bilateral "open-book" injury. Despite the relative stability of the pelvic ring, maintained by the posterior sacroiliac ligaments, the pelvic floor disruption causes visceral injuries. Variants include B3.1 (bilateral B1), B3.2 (B1 on one side and B2 on the other side), and B3.3 (bilateral B2).

Type-C Fracture

Type-C fracture relates to unstable injuries with complete disruption of the posterior–sacroiliac complex, involving vertical shearing forces. These unilateral or bilateral fractures are almost always caused by severe trauma such as falls from heights, crushing injuries, or motor vehicle accidents. They cause massive disruption of both the pelvic ring and the surrounding soft tissues.

Type C1 corresponds to unilateral injuries of the hemi-pelvis.

Type C1.1 relates to shear fractures of the ilium, which begin at the inferior part of the sacroiliac joint and run to the iliac crest at the rear.

Type C1.2 stands for sacroiliac dislocations. These fractures can only be associated with extreme violence, as the sacroiliac ligaments are the strongest in the human body.

Type C1.3 deals with fractures of the sacrum caused by high-energy shearing forces.

Type C2 stands for bilateral injuries of the pelvis ring in which one side remains partially stable and thus corresponds to a type-B injury, e.g., in sacral fractures, whereas the opposite relates to an unstable type-C injury such as an iliac fracture.

Type C3 deals with bilateral injuries in which both hemi-pelves are unstable.

Type-A lesions represent up to 52%, type B up to 27%, and type C up to 21% of all cases.

SOURCES OF BLEEDING IN PELVIC FRACTURE

Both the arteries and veins traversing the pelvis conduct among the highest volume in the body. These include the iliac vessels and their branches to the inferior abdominal viscera and pelvic organs, as well as the blood supply to the lower extremities. It is reasonable to assume that arterial bleeding contributes substantially to the hemorrhage associated with pelvic fractures. Arterial injuries are frequently identified during pelvic angiography after trauma, and there is some evidence that embolization of these vessels reduces mortality. For example, in the series by Agolini et al, of 806 patients admitted with pelvic fractures, 35 underwent pelvic angiography; 15 (1.9%) required embolization and embolization successfully stopped bleeding in all of these patients.

Similarly, numerous authors have implicated venous bleeding in exsanguinating blood loss associated with pelvic fractures. For example, Connolly and Hedberg analyzed a series of 200 pelvic fractures treated at Sydney Hospital. Five of the thirty deaths in this series were thought to have resulted from intrapelvic hemorrhage. They noted that the source of bleeding was usually the "plexus of veins and arteries lining the side walls of the pelvis," and they pointed out that both vessel tearing and puncture by bone fragments contribute to bleeding.

Unfortunately, it is difficult to know the proportional contributions of venous and arterial bleeding to the overall pelvic hemorrhage. Venography would be unlikely to distinguish major venous from minor venous injury. Arteriography gives no information about the veins and, since arterial embolization does not always stop bleeding, it is likely that some other source is present. The literature includes one attempt to localize the source of bleeding at autopsies of people who had died from exsanguination following pelvic injury. Huittinen and Slatis in their study in 1973 dissected the cadavers of 27 such accident victims. The cadavers were examined with plain X-ray films, contrast arteriography and dissection. Contrast leakage in the injured area occurred in 23 of 27 cadavers, all near the posterior pelvic ring. Bleeding was unilateral in 17, bilateral in 6, and leakage from more than 2 sites was seen in 15. Comparing the X-ray evidence and sites of arteriographic contrast leakage with direct observation at dissection yielded three important results. Firstly, the extent of bony and vascular damage was almost always greater than the plain films had suggested. Secondly, "leakage" from fractured cancellous bone of the sacrum in posterior fractures was a major source of bleeding, even in "minor" fractures. Thirdly, identification of torn major arteries was possible in only 3/17. Based on these data, the authors suggested "accurate reposition of the dislocated pelvic fracture is preferable to ligation of the hypogastric arteries for control of severe hemorrhage from pelvic fractures."

Although bone is certainly a potential source of blood loss, it seems unlikely to be as important as suggested by this study. Minor sacral fractures resulting from lateral compression injuries occur frequently and rarely result in significant blood loss. Unstable sacroiliac disruptions often bleed, despite the absence of fractures, and acetabular fractures that expose large areas of cancellous bone rarely cause significant blood loss. This can be true even when the fractures are not caused by impaction, in which case it would be intuitive to expect them to bleedless.

In summary, three types of bleeding are noted in pelvic fracture: arterial bleeding that result from disruption of any of the arteries in the pelvis, venous bleeding that result from tearing or shearing, of veins, especially in the posterior venous plexus and bleeding directly from fractured cancellous bone. It is clear that the management of each of these bleeding sources would ideally be different. Moreover, it is likely that pelvic hemorrhage results from injuries to both arteries and veins. Since it is not possible to determine the major source for a particular injury, it is important to address both systems. Certainly, the most important step in this process is to optimize the patient's ability to coagulate the bleeding vessels. Beyond that, arterial injuries are best managed by embolization and venous injuries are best managed by providing some form of tamponade.

PATIENT EVALUATION AND INITIAL MANAGEMENT

All patients sustaining high-energy blunt trauma should be assumed to have a pelvic fracture until proven otherwise. Often, if awake and alert, patients will complain of pelvic pain. However, complaints may not be specific and may include reports of hip or lower abdominal pain. Vehicular crashes are the most common cause of pelvic injury. These are followed in order of frequency by automobile-pedestrian collisions, falls from a height, motorcycle crashes, and crush injuries.

Complete clinical evaluation of the patient with a high-energy pelvic fracture is essential because this is rarely an isolated injury. The same forces that lead to disruption of the pelvic ring are frequently associated with abdominal, head, and thoracic injury. In addition to these injuries, 60 to 80% of patients with a high-energy pelvic fracture have other associated musculoskeletal injuries, 12% have urogenital injuries, and 8% have lumbosacral plexus injuries. Physical findings seen commonly in patients with pelvic fractures include abrasions, contusions, or hematomas over the bony prominences of the pelvis. An examination of the perineum is important to identify scrotal or vulval hematoma. A rectal exam should be performed, as well as a vaginal exam in women. These are particularly important in patients with perineal lacerations, as rectal or vaginal lacerations often accompany open pelvic fractures.

A plan for simultaneous assessment and treatment of a patient with a high-energy pelvic fracture is required. An interdisciplinary team, including a general surgeon, an orthopedic surgeon, a representative from the blood bank, and an interventional radiologist, is equipped to promptly assess and manage the spectrum of injuries associated with pelvic fractures. The initial management of the patient with multiple injuries and suspected pelvic fracture largely follows Advanced Trauma Life Support (ATLS) guidelines of the American College of Surgeons Committee on Trauma. During primary survey, an airway is secured and resuscitation begun with intravenous crystalloid solutions while deliberate hypotension is maintained until all sources of hemorrhage have been identified and controlled. The most important factor in the survival of patients with pelvic fracture is urgent hemostasis thus limiting the detrimental effects of both shock and high volume resuscitation.

Hypotension is associated with an increased risk of mortality, adult respiratory distress syndrome, and multiple organ failure. Hypotension associated with blunt trauma may result from a variety of insults, including hypovolemic, septic, cardiac, or neurologic compromise. A rapid and systematic search for the source of the hypotension must be undertaken.

Hemorrhagic shock is the most common cause of hypotension in blunt trauma patients. There are five cavities into which patients can lose large quantities of blood: the thorax, abdomen, muscle compartments, retroperitoneum, and "the street". A patient can be hypotensive from blood loss associated with one bleeding site or a combination of many bleeding sites.

Physical examination, chest radiographs, and tube thoracostomy will detect the presence and severity of intrathoracic blood loss.

Physical examination of the abdomen may be unremarkable in the unresponsive patient. Abdominal injury is the associated injury that most substantially affects patient outcome, and its diagnosis is difficult in the hypotensive patient with pelvic fractures. The presence of intra-abdominal hemorrhage can be evaluated by ultrasound, diagnostic peritoneal lavage (DPL) and/or CT scanning. When performed by properly accredited staff as part of the Focused Assessment with Sonography for Trauma (FAST), abdominal ultrasound is a rapid and accurate means of diagnosing hemoperitoneum and should serve as the primary screening modality in the emergency department. Additionally, it may be repeated for serial assessment of the patient after transfer to an angiography suite or intensive care unit (ICU). Supra-umbilical DPL may be used in cases of equivocal ultrasound findings, which may be caused by anatomic distortions of the retroperitoneum from injury, or to differentiate hemoperitoneum from uroperitoneum, as between 4 to 8% of patients with pelvic fracture may have an associated bladder injury.

Bleeding from the pelvic fracture site is seldom the only cause of blood loss in the patient with multiple injuries, and massive bleeding from a pelvic fracture alone is uncommon. Nevertheless, pelvic fracture must be considered among the most prominent sites of significant bleeding in a hemodynamically unstable patient, particularly when initial attempts to control bleeding from other sources fail to stabilize the patient. In cases of suspected pelvic fracture bleeding, provisional pelvic stabilization should occur immediately during initial evaluation and resuscitation. Provisional stabilization may consist of a pelvic binder or a simple sheet wrapped securely around the pelvis and secured with a sturdy clamp.

The severity of blood loss can be determined on initial evaluation by assessing pulse, blood pressure, and capillary refill. The ATLS classification system of the American College of Surgeons is useful for understanding the manifestations associated with hemorrhagic shock in adults. Blood volume is estimated at 7% of ideal body weight, or approximately 4,900 ml in a patient weighing 70 kg (155 lb).

Class I hemorrhage, defined as blood loss of <15% of total blood volume, leads to no measurable changes in heart or respiratory rates, blood pressure, or pulse pressure and requires little or no treatment.

Class II hemorrhage is defined as blood loss of 15 to 30% of blood volume (750 to 1,500 mL), with clinical signs including tachycardia and tachypnea. Systolic blood pressure may be only slightly decreased, especially when the patient is in the supine position, but the pulse pressure is narrowed. Urine output is only slightly reduced (i.e. to 20 to 30 mL/hr). The patient with a class II hemorrhage can usually be resuscitated with a crystalloid solution alone, but some patients may require blood transfusion.

Class III hemorrhage is defined as loss of 30 to 40% (1,500–2,000 mL) of blood volume. Inadequate perfusion in patients with class III hemorrhage results in marked tachycardia and tachypnea, cold extremities with significantly delayed capillary refill, hypotension, and significant negative changes in mental status. Class III hemorrhage represents the smallest volume of blood loss that consistently produces a decrease in systemic blood pressure. The resuscitation of these patients frequently requires blood transfusion in addition to administration of crystalloid solutions.

Class IV hemorrhage is defined as blood loss >40% of blood volume (>2,000 ml), representing life-threatening hemorrhage. Signs include marked tachycardia, significantly depressed systolic blood pressure, and narrowed pulse pressure or unobtainable diastolic blood pressure. The skin is cold and pale, and the mental status is severely depressed. Urine output is negligible. These patients require immediate transfusion for resuscitation and frequently need immediate surgical intervention.

Clinically, a palpable hematoma above the inguinal ligament, on the proximal thigh, and/or over the perineum (Destot sign) may indicate pelvic fracture with associated bleeding; ecchymosis about the flank (Grey Turner's sign) is associated with retroperitoneal hemorrhage. The practice of grasping the iliac crests in search of palpable instability lacks sensitivity and specificity and rarely provide information that cannot be obtained on a single antero-posterior pelvic radiograph. Additionally, it may dislodge adherent clot further exacerbating hemorrhage, is painful to the conscious patient and should therefore be avoided.

Gross posterior disruption of the pelvis is usually evident on AP view when the pelvis is fractured. Inlet and outlet views of the pelvis, which can provide more information about the presence and location of posterior ring injuries, should be obtained only after the patient has achieved hemodynamic stability. A rapid CT is extremely valuable for defining posterior ring instability. The information from this study often helps direct early management because it may aid in defining the magnitude of the posterior ring injury. However, prolonged CT scanning in the acutely hypotensive patient should be avoided. Additional thin cut CT scans may be indicated to further evaluate pelvic or acetabular fractures, but only after the patient is stabilized. Contrast-enhanced CT imaging of the pelvis, which is often done in the hemodynamically stable trauma patient, is a noninvasive technique that has proved to be reasonably accurate in determining the presence or absence of ongoing pelvic hemorrhage. In a study comparing this methodology with findings on pelvic angiography, CT detected bleeding in 16 of 19 patients who had extravasation or vascular injury demonstrated by angiography, with a sensitivity of 84%. Results of pelvic angiography were negative in 11 patients, and no patient had evidence of bleeding on pre-angiographic CT scans. Two sites of contrast-agent extravasation identified by CT imaging in two patients did not show bleeding at angiography, for a specificity of 85% for the detection of bleeding. The overall accuracy of CT for determining the presence or absence of bleeding in this study was 90%.

FLUID RESUSCITATION AND PATIENT MONITORING

Hemoglobin and/or hematocrit levels measured within minutes of patient arrival in the trauma bay may be a reliable marker of ongoing hemorrhage and need for massive transfusion, and an admission hematocrit of 30% or less has been shown to be a predictor of major pelvic hemorrhage. Once resuscitation is begun, however, both hemoglobin and hematocrit are potentially spurious and should not be trusted to determine amount of blood lost. Furthermore, neither is an end-point of resuscitation. High base deficits and lactate levels have correlated with mortality in pelvic trauma and those with base deficits of more than 5 mmol/l on arrival are more likely to die. Sequential measurements of base deficit and blood lactate in early period of resuscitation may be a more rapid and reliable measurement of blood loss and further transfusion requirements than other more commonly used hemodynamic and/or laboratory parameters. Additionally, improvement in base deficit and blood lactate signals amelioration of oxygen debt and reversal of the shock state. This attests to a positive response to resuscitative measures. Once the pelvis is shown to be the major source of hemorrhage, component therapy simulating whole blood (i.e. hemostatic or damage control resuscitation) is promptly administered with transfusion of packed red blood cells (PRBC), fresh frozen plasma (FFP) and platelets ideally in a 1:1:1 (pack) ratio. As a result of tissue damage/destruction and resultant hypoperfusion, trauma-induced coagulopathy may be present in 25% of patients on Emergency Department (ED) admission and appears to increase linearly with ISS and risk of death. Using this ratio of blood products has been shown to improve survival of patients requiring massive transfusions and may reduce the overall volume of blood transfused. The on-call orthopedic surgeon,

blood bank, operating room (OR) and interventional radiologist (IR) are immediately notified and a massive transfusion protocol activated. Crystalloid use is then significantly limited and should serve mainly as a carrier to keep lines open between blood products. Early transfusion of platelets as six packs to keep platelet counts above 100,000/mL during massive transfusion appears to provide a survival advantage. Cryoprecipitate and recombinant factor VIIa (rFVIIa) may be used as adjuncts to hemostatic resuscitation especially in those patients who are coagulopathic as a result of delayed presentation or ongoing hemorrhage with simultaneous correction of pH and acid-base deficits. Furthermore, every effort should be made to maintain the patient at normothermia either by passive means (warm trauma bay, warm blankets, space blanket, Bair Hugger) or active means (Rapid infusers).

End-points of resuscitation are determined based on the combination of laboratory data and physiologic signs. A hemoglobin level reading is known to be inaccurate during the acute phase of resuscitation. The commonly considered end-points of resuscitation include normal blood pressure, decreased heart rate, adequate urine output (> 30 ml/hr), and normal central venous pressure. However, even after normalization of these parameters, inadequate tissue oxygenation may persist. Additional laboratory measures that can be used to evaluate tissue oxygenation include base deficit, bicarbonate, and lactate. All of these assess anerobic glycolysis. A normal base deficit is 0-3 mmol/l; this is routinely measured with an arterial blood gas analysis. A persistent base deficit suggests insufficient resuscitation.

METHODS TO CONTROL BLEEDING (INVASIVE AND NON-INVASIVE)

Non-Invasive

MAST

Military antishock trousers can achieve direct compression and immobilization of the pelvic ring and lower extremity via pneumatic pressure. Use of MAST was advocated in 1970s and 1980s to induce pelvic tamponade and increase venous return. However, several studies have not shown a survival benefit for use of pre-hospital MAST although none have focused on pelvic fractures. The device is also associated with inherent complications, such as lower extremity ischemia/reperfusion, development of compartment syndrome, and skin necrosis.

Pelvic Binder or Sheet Wrapping

Over the past decade, simple devices, such as bed sheets have been used as an alternative to MAST, tied around the greater trochanter to apply pressure with internal rotation of the legs. Sheeting facilitates closing the pelvis in open-book pelvic injuries but avoids lower extremity ischemia. Commercial pelvic binders have been devised which permit tension adjustment to 140–200 N. These circumferential pelvic sheets or binders are advantageous because of their ease of application, relative safety, cost-effectiveness, and non-invasive character. They also minimize the movement of the fracture site during transport and provide pain relief for patients. The application of a pelvic binder should be considered as early as possible. Patients in the pre-hospital setting in particular, may benefit because maintaining the fractured pelvis' stability prevents disruption of hemostatic clots and consumption of clotting factors which can lead to coagulopathy. Potential complications are the development of pressure ulceration, skin necrosis, or slough. Another disadvantage is these devices compromise access for laparotomy or pelvic packing as well as prevent monitoring of the skin around the pelvis. Sheet wrapping and pelvic binders are less rigid than external fixators, and fracture reduction and restoration of bone contact is tenuous except in cases of simple open-book injuries. These external pelvic interventions can only provide a temporary solution in serious situations, buying doctors time to carry out hemostatic treatment. Pelvic binders or sheets should be considered as temporary measures bridging acute injury towards more rigid stabilization. If the binder appears to be effective and longer application is needed, other definitive means, such as external fixation or internal fixation should be planned.

Invasive

External Fixation (Figs 11.7 and 11.8)

In conjunction with the development of clinically useful fracture classifications based on the stability of the pelvic ring, immediate external fixation of unstable pelvic fractures has been a mainstay in the treatment of hemodynamically unstable patients for

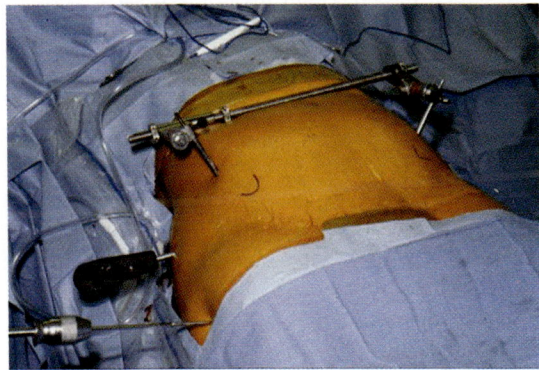

Fig. 11.7: A simple external fixator in situ

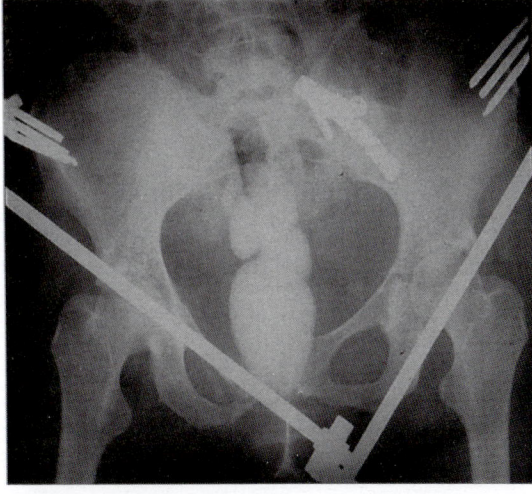

Fig. 11.8: Radiograph with external fixator in situ

the past three decades. External fixation controls bleeding by providing tamponade and reduces the displaced fracture and allows the hemostatic pathway to control bleeding from raw bony surfaces. An external fixator can be applied in 15–20 min by an orthopedic surgeon experienced in this procedure. External fixation can be performed either by placing the pin in the iliac crest under direct palpation without fluoroscopy or placing the pin in the supra-acetabular bones with fluoroscopy. Biomechanical studies show that supra-acetabular pin placement has greater rigidity and pull-out strength. However, for the patient in shock and undergoing resuscitation, iliac crest placement is quicker and requires less equipment. Because early frame application, often before laparotomy, is advocated, the frame construct must provide easy access to the abdomen and allow for subsequent abdominal distension. In the emergent application of a pelvic external fixator, the following basic technical principles must be observed: adequate soft tissue protection via guide sleeves for drilling and pin insertion; skin incisions at 90° angles to the iliac crest and large enough to accommodate guide sleeves; 5 mm or larger blunt ½ pin, 180 mm in length or longer; 2 or 3 pins clusters per hemipelvis; converging pin placement into the anterior 1/3 of the iliac wing; a frame construct which provides clearance from and access to the abdomen; and dual frame construct to allow independent free manipulation without loss of pelvic reduction.

Pins can be placed percutaneously or via an open technique. Percutaneously, the anterosuperior iliac spines are palpated along with the greater trochanters. Transverse stab incisions are made in the skin approximately 2 cm posterior to the anterosuperior iliac spine. Trochar tip drill guides are placed in the stab wounds and seated on the iliac crest. The drill guide can be moved medially and laterally to obtain a feel for the center of the iliac crest. Remembering that there is an overhang to the outer table of the hemipelvis, the drill guide is to be placed along the inner 2/3 of the crest. While aiming

the drill guide toward the greater trochanter, the drill bit is used to open the cortex of the iliac crest. Next, a blunt tipped ½ pin is hand tightened into position with a drill brace aiming the pin toward the greater trochanter, allowing the pin to find its way between the tables of the hemipelvis. With an open technique, a longer transverse skin incision is made which allows placement of a palpating finger or Kirschner wire along the inner table to aid pin direction parallel to the inner table and still aiming toward the greater trochanter. These techniques diminish the chances of cortical penetration. One or two additional ½ pin can be placed with similar technique along the iliac crest. Again, the pins should be placed in a converging configuration. Attention to detail and careful ½ pin placement are of paramount importance. Well placed pins assure maximal bone/ pin interface, which provides the stable foundation on which an anterior frame can be constructed. Two upright bars are applied to each pin cluster and are connected to 2 cross bars, thereby creating a rectangular frame construct. Each independent frame can be loosened subsequently and manipulated, thereby allowing access to the abdomen.

Once the pins are in position and the frame is constructed, before tightening, the displaced pelvic ring injury can be reduced. It is important that injury type is recognized so that appropriate reduction maneuvers can be performed. Tile B injuries require relatively simple maneuvers. Open-book type requires closure of the book; lateral compression injuries require opening the book. Remembering that Tile C injuries are unstable posteriorly, simple closing the book maneuvers can further displace the disrupted posterior pelvic anatomy. Therefore, bilateral compressive forces need to be applied to the pelvic ring posteriorly. With intact hips, compressive forces can be applied at the greater trochanters before frame tightening. If associated with vertical displacement, longitudinal traction should be applied simultaneously. Anterior external fixation is not stable enough to neutralize hemipelvic migration. Therefore, longitudinal traction can be applied by proximal tibial or distal femoral skeletal traction until definitive internal fixation can be carried out. This traction helps neutralize the displacing forces upon the unstable pelvis. The adequacy of reduction is monitored by fluoroscopy or plain film radiography.

Experimental studies have shown that external fixation provides only a small volume change within the true pelvis even if applied to open-book pelvic fractures. Thus, an external fixator is thought to contribute to hemostasis primarily by decreasing bony motion at the fracture site, re-opposing the cancellous bone surface, and allowing stable clot formation as well as maintaining a reduced pelvic volume and not by tamponade as previously thought.

The disadvantage of external fixators is they do not provide posterior stability and can potentially increase displacement of the fractured pelvis in a vertically unstable fracture configuration. Additionally, pin sites if they become infected, can compromise subsequent definitive open reduction and fixation. It is recommended that simple external fixation should be placed quickly during resuscitation procedures, with conversion to definitive internal or more stable external fixation when the patient is hemodynamically stable.

C-Clamp (Fig. 11.9)

Pelvic C-clamps are a form of external fixation. They can be placed quickly without fluoroscopic control when used as anterior–external fixators. The anterior placement sites are supra and lateral acetabulum and have been well established. One advantage of a pelvic C-clamp is that it can be used posteriorly for direct reduction of vertically and rotationally unstable fractures. By inserting a wide pin bilaterally in the region of the sacroiliac joints, C-clamps offer a distinct biomechanical advantage over anterior–external fixators because they can exert transverse compression directly across the sacroiliac joint with a significant force. C-clamps can be assembled and applied in a very short duration. Thus, they can provide prompt stabilization of the posterior pelvic ring and can be

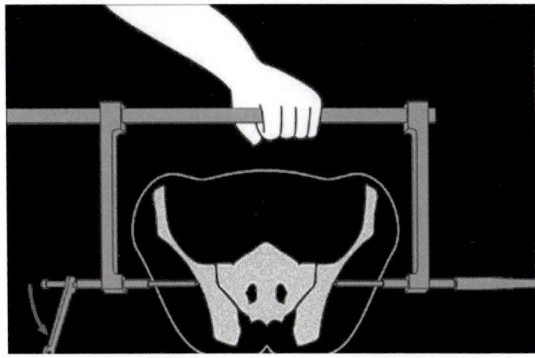

Fig. 11.9: Illustration of a C-clamp

effective in case of complete disruption of the posterior ring. Because the clamp can be rotated cephalad and caudad, access to the abdomen and perineum is not limited. The C-clamp can be applied in the emergency department in hemodynamically unstable patient status based on an antero-posterior pelvis X-ray. However, it is not applicable in iliac fractures and transiliac fracture dislocations. Also, pelvic penetration or misplacement through the greater sciatic notch that caused iatrogenic nerve and vascular injuries has been reported.

Therefore, C-clamps should be applied by an experienced surgeon after careful evaluation of radiographs, and, if possible, with the aid of fluoroscopy in the case of posterior placement.

A C-clamp or external fixator should be considered before or concomitantly with emergent laparotomy because the anterior abdominal wall contributes to limiting the degree of pubic diastasis through a tension band effect on the iliac wings, and the pelvic volume will increase if the pelvis is not stabilized prior to laparotomy. The application of these devices is also necessary when pelvic packing is performed for the mechanically unstable pelvis because the fracture must be stabilized during this procedure in order to provide a stable wall against which to pack. Without ring stability the pelvic space can increase tremendously, preventing tamponade and, thus, having limited impact on bleeding and related coagulopathy.

Angiography and Embolization

Pelvic angiography with therapeutic embolization of the internal iliac arteries for pelvic fractures was reported in 1972. As experience increased, this less-invasive procedure became widely accepted as a safe and efficacious substitute for direct surgical intervention. Pelvic angiography consists of a non-selective injection of contrast medium just above the aortic bifurcation followed by selective injection of the branches of the internal iliac arteries. However, branches of other arterial systems, such as the lumbar artery, median sacral artery, deep iliac circumflex artery, and corona mortis, are possible sources of bleeding, which may be amenable for selective catheterization. Angiographic evidence of extra-luminal contrast extravasation indicates ongoing arterial bleeding and hemostasis is obtained by catheter embolization with gelatin sponge and/or coils.

Generally, patients who remain hemodynamically unstable after appropriate fluid resuscitation with PRBC and FFP and mechanical stabilization of the pelvis, are possible candidates for pelvic angio-graphy. The other indications for pelvic angiography include the incidental discovery of extravasation of contrast medium on the arterial phase of computed tomography (CT) scans. Arterial extravasation seen on the CT scan is considered an indication of active arterial bleeding. CT scans are also useful in gauging the amount and location of pelvic hemorrhage, both of which may predict arterial injuries.

Pelvic arterial embolization requires arterial access, frequently via an arterial introducer (4 or 5 Fr), positioned via the femoral route on the side contra-lateral to the suspected fracture and hemorrhagic vascular lesion. Tomodensitometry should be performed if the hemodynamic status is stable or stabilized, to localize arterial bleeding, and to guide the rapid and selective catheterization of arteries that are likely to be damaged. Embolization is sequential. The first angiogram is performed in the common iliac artery of the presumed traumatic/hemorrhagic side. During angiography one looks for signs of macrovascular lesions, based on extravasation of

contrast product (false aneurysms), missing arteries and arteries with wall irregularities, or arterial or venous stagnation of contrast product. The arteries most frequently involved in hemorrhages associated with pelvic fractures are (in descending order of frequency) superior gluteal, lateral sacral, iliolumbar, obturator, vesical and inferior gluteal. A wide range of embolization materials has been developed. Embolic agents function by inducing direct mechani-cal obstruction and providing a skeleton for continuous thrombus formation and closing of a vessel, and are classified as either temporary or permanent according to their properties. The most commonly used temporary embolic material is gelatine sponge, either as a torpedo or cut into small pledges and mixed with contrast medium. Gelatine sponge is biodegradable, with a durability lasting for days to weeks; after this period there is a possibility of recanalization of the vessels.

Early angiography and subsequent embolization have been recommended by multiple authors to improve patient outcomes. Agolini et al. showed embolization within 3 hours of arrival resulted in a significantly greater survival rate. Balogh et al. described that their protocol including pelvic angiography within 90 min after admission improved mortality. Thus, it is desirable that availability of 24 hours angiography on an emergent basis is ensured for treatment of persistently unstable patients with pelvic fractures.

Angiography for pelvic fractures allow both selective embolization of bleeding arteries and non-selective embolization of bilateral internal iliac arteries. Ideally, selective embolization is preferable. In patients who are hemodynamically stable or who responded to an initial fluid resuscitation, and who have extravasation from a single branch, selective embolization offers a non-invasive method of treatment that may remove the need for further intervention or blood transfusion. On the other hand, hemodynamically unstable patients should not undergo selective embolization.

Critically injured patients who undergo angiography often do not show active bleeding in spite of the presence of arterial injuries due to vasospasm of injured arteries, temporal clotting, and/ or low perfusion secondary to hypotension. These factors can lead to intermittent bleeding distally due to changing coagulation status, blood pressure, and motion of fracture sites. Multiple bleeding sites from bilateral internal iliac artery branches can often be observed in hemodynamically unstable patients. In such cases, non-selective bilateral internal iliac artery embolization with gelatin sponge from the internal iliac artery trunk has been advocated by numerous authors. This non-selective embolization is time-saving compared to selective embolization. Moreover, this technique is theoretically supported by the fact that there are generous collateral pathways and anastomoses between each artery and cross circulation from the contralateral side. The collateral arteries may supply the ruptured arteries from the opposite side. In order to truly stop significant bleeding, these potential collateral vessels should be considered as multiple communicating channels and need to be embolized at their common trunk.

Disadvantages of Arterial Embolization

Even with aggressive resuscitation, mechanical stabilization, and successful embolization, mortality remains high. Evers et al. reported that 88.9% of patients treated with embolization eventually died. Several authors have reported that the mortality of patients treated with embolization was around 50% despite successful control of arterial bleeding. Anatomic studies as well as clinical series show that the majority of patients who die with pelvic fractures, die of blood loss, without major arterial injury. These facts imply that arterial embolization does not always stop bleeding due to pelvic fractures, and it is likely that other significant sources are present within the pelvic ring. It is still difficult to know the proportional contributions of arterial, fracture site, and venous bleeding to the overall pelvic hemorrhage in a particular case.

There are several downsides reported in performing angiography. In some patients, access to the femoral artery is difficult due to obesity, hematoma, hypotension, or degloving injuries. Arteriosclerosis and other arterial occlusive diseases can cause arterial stenosis and occlusion that precludes catheterization of bleeding arteries. Complications, such as hematoma at the arterial puncture site, femoral artery thrombosis, subintimal dissection, and pseudo-aneurysm have been reported. The issue of radiation is inevitable, and the dose in a single pelvic embolization procedure is reported to be as much as 3 Gy at the skin level. The incidence of side effects with contrast materials ranges from 3 to 13%. Allergic reaction to the contrast material, serum creatinine level increase, or renal failure may not be noticed in severely injured patients due to concomitant hypotension, but will compromise patient survival. There is also concern that high-pressure injection of contrast medium through a catheter can cause fragmentation of primary hemostatic thrombus leading to further extravasation form a ruptured artery. Recurrent pelvic arterial bleeding may also occur several hours after successful embolization or after a negative initial angiography. CT scans are the only definitive way to detect arterial bleeding before angiography. However, the utility of these findings is questionable since unstable patients are not considered for CT scanning and stable patients with a pelvic arterial blush on CT probably do not benefit from angiography.

The lack of readily available experts in angiography can limit emergent hemostasis. Furthermore, angiography and embolization can be time-consuming and simultaneous treatment of other associated injuries during the procedure is delayed. Successful embolization rates for arterial injuries have been reported to be 85–100%. However, in the reported studies, success has been defined as cessation of angiographically identified bleeding and not stabilization of hypotension. Furthermore, several authors have reported spontaneous cessation of arterial bleeding without embolization. Just because an arterial injury is found, it does not mean it requires embolization. There is still controversy regarding the utility of angiography in small vessel arterial bleeding and risk/benefit ratio of spending prolonged periods of time attempting selective embolization in hypotensive patients.

If a large amount of gelatin sponge is used for successful embolization, tissue necrosis may occur. Necrosis and ischemia of tissues due to embolization of internal iliac arteries have been reported in various types of tissues, such as sacral skin, bladder wall, uterus, femoral head, gluteal muscle, and colon with complications including paresis of the lower extremity, acute ischemia of the lower extremity, impotence, and rectal stenosis. Tissue necrosis is more extensive following massive embolization of overlapping arterial areas. Therefore, some tissue necrosis may be unavoidable and the risk/benefit ratio must be considered for a given patient scenario.

Pelvic Packing

Historically open surgical exploration and ligation of arterial bleeding from internal iliac arteries was advocated in the treatment of pelvic fractures. However, because of the difficulty of accessing the arteries and ineffectiveness due to widely distributed anastomoses, this procedure often produced massive, uncontrollable bleeding resulting in fatalities. Therefore, instead of ligating internal iliac arteries, pelvic packing was employed. Packing was performed after an exploratory laparotomy when the contained intrapelvic hematoma ruptured intra-peritoneally. However, performing laparotomy may increase pelvic volume and directly aggravate pelvic hemorrhage due to decompression of the retroperi-toneum. Incision of the intact peritoneum and disruption of the pelvic hematoma can also disrupt the tamponade effect of the retroperitoneal space. Furthermore, there was also concern about an increased risk of infection in the pelvic hematoma following transabdominal pelvic packing.

To minimize the disadvantages of pelvic packing via the transabdominal approach, a more controlled, retroperitoneal method has been described. This technique can facilitate control of retroperitoneal bleeding through a small incision which does not violate the intraperitoneal space and leaves the peritoneum intact. First a simple external fixator or C-clamp is placed to stabilize the pelvic ring for packing. Then, using an 8 cm midline incision of the lower abdomen, direct access to the bleeding retroperitoneal space is possible, and the pre-sacral area and paravesicle region is packed with surgical lap packs (usually 3 per side in adults). The key to this maneuver is packing of the true pelvis, below the pelvic brim and not the false pelvis, above the pelvic brim. Since the major venous bleeding occurs in the plexus of vessels in the true pelvis, packing above the pelvic brim has minimal tamponade effect. Afterwards, the skin incision is closed with running fascial sutures and skin staples. The total time for the packing procedure can be less than 20 min, and operative blood loss is minimal. If laparotomy is required, it should follow the closure of the retroperitoneal fascia to preserve the anatomic integrity of the compartments and to allow for tamponade in the retroperitoneum. The packing is changed or removed 24–48 h after the injury. This newer version of pelvic packing is different from earlier attempts at direct surgical control. The procedure is quick, easy to perform, and less invasive, requiring a short time with minimal blood loss. Therefore, it is appropriate for patients with a variety of severity of hemodynamic instability, and can reduce unnecessary angiography. Cothren et al. showed no deaths as a result of acute blood loss in persistent hemodynamically unstable patients treated with direct packing. They reported that only 4 of 24 (16.7%) non-responders required subsequent embolization, and concluded that packing is a method that can quickly control hemorrhage and serve as a specific triage tool for emergent angiography.

One of the disadvantages of packing is that it is a relatively invasive procedure compared to angio-graphy, and infection at the incision site may occur after pelvic packing. Pelvic packing may also increase the possibility of abdominal compartment syndrome. Packing may not be effective for treatment of bleeding from a large-bore artery, especially those ruptured outside the true pelvis. Therefore, it is imperative that the use of pelvic packing does not supplant angiography. Packing should be considered a quick, effective tool for diminishing venous bleeding and can usually be accomplished while waiting for the angiographic team to set up. Additionally, the necessity of a reoperation to remove the surgical lap packs at 24–48 h is a theoretical disadvantage though most of these patients have high injury severity and require multiple operating room treatments. In most cases, however, internal fixation of the anterior pelvis can be performed at the time of packing removal through the packing incision and a C-clamp or external fixation can then be removed as well.

In the treatment of open pelvic fractures, it has been shown that the only effective hemostatic technique for torrential external bleeding is packing of the open wound. The only difference between an open pelvic fracture and a closed displaced pelvic fracture where the tamponade effect is lost, is whether the bleeding is visible or not. **Therefore, it is reasonable that pelvic packing should be the first line of treatment for persistent hemodynamically unstable patients with pelvic fractures.** During pelvic packing, associated injuries that contribute to mortality, such as closed head injuries, intra-abdominal hemorrhage, and hemothorax can be simultaneously assessed and treated with damage control techniques. In patients with significant hemodynamic instability, arterial bleeding may accompany venous and fracture-site bleeding. Thus, angiography may be required following pelvic packing if there is persistent hypotension or ongoing hemorrhage suspected. It is clear that pelvic packing can be an intervention that provides stabilization of the hemodynamically unstable patient in the operating room and can allow the patient to be transported to the angiography suite for selective embolization. The packing procedure can also provide time for the emergent angiography preparations. Initial angiography prior to pelvic packing may be indicated in cases where hemodynamic stability with volume replacement can be achieved but in which ongoing pelvic hemorrhage is suspected.

Role of Pelvic Venous Bleed

Pelvic vein injuries have received little attention. One reason for this may be that the retroperitoneum is considered a closed space that can usually provide a tamponade for bleeding from a pelvic fracture. Most bleeding from venous injuries arises from small- and medium-sized torn veins and can stop naturally if the patient's cardiovascular function, blood volume, and coagulation status are kept within acceptable limits.

The true pelvic volume is estimated at approximately 1.5 L, and 4–6 units of red blood cells transfused may be enough to tamponade venous bleeding within a stable or stabilized pelvic ring. However, the space available to accommodate blood loss from pelvic fractures is much greater than the true pelvis volume measured in anatomy experiments. Furthermore, tamponade ability is lost in the case of severe pelvic fractures due to traumatic disruption of parapelvic fascia, and hemostasis may not be attained by the tamponade effect, despite placement of binders or external fixators. This is especially true for injuries with significant posterior displacement, such as sacroiliac dislocations, sacral fractures, and sacroiliac fracture dislocations crescent fractures. In other words, hemorrhage from pelvic fracture is essentially bleeding into a free space, potentially capable of accommodating the patient's entire blood volume without gaining sufficient pressure-dependent tamponade. This can lead rapidly to the requirement of massive transfusion with the risk of exsanguination, despite an absence of arterial injury. In these patients, time spent in angiography may be life-threatening.

Many current treatment algorithms appear to disregard the presence of venous injuries, perhaps because an adequate method to detect injuries in the low-pressure venous system has not been established. However, venous structures are more fragile to external trauma force than are arteries, and therefore, venous injuries and bleeding are likely to occur more frequently than arterial injury. Even when arterial bleeding is clearly present, the likelihood of concomitant venous bleeding is probably close to 100%. Most treatment approaches grossly overestimate the significance and incidence of arterial bleeding while underestimating the significance of venous bleeding. This miscalculation likely contributes to the ongoing high mortality for pelvic fracture patients who fail to respond during initial resuscitation.

MANAGEMENT OF OPEN PELVIC FRACTURES

Open pelvic fractures consist of open iliac wing fractures that do not destabilize the pelvic ring and open wounds associated with pelvic ring injuries. Whereas the iliac wing fractures tend not to cause damage to deep vasculature and organs, the open pelvic ring injuries can be devastating. While they can vary in severity, there are few situations more challenging than a patient with severe soft tissue, bony, and vascular injury located within or adjacent to the pelvis. Because of the severity of these injuries, many of these patients do not survive to reach medical attention.

Richardson et al. advocated four important treatment priorities for these devastating injuries: (a) control of hemorrhage, (b) debridement and management of the concomitant soft tissue injury, (c) recognition and treatment of associated injuries, and (d) treatment of the pelvic fracture itself. Despite advances in the treatment of pelvic fractures and the associated injuries, a mortality rate of 45% for patients with open pelvic fracture was published in a recent series (Fig. 11.10). Deaths from open pelvic

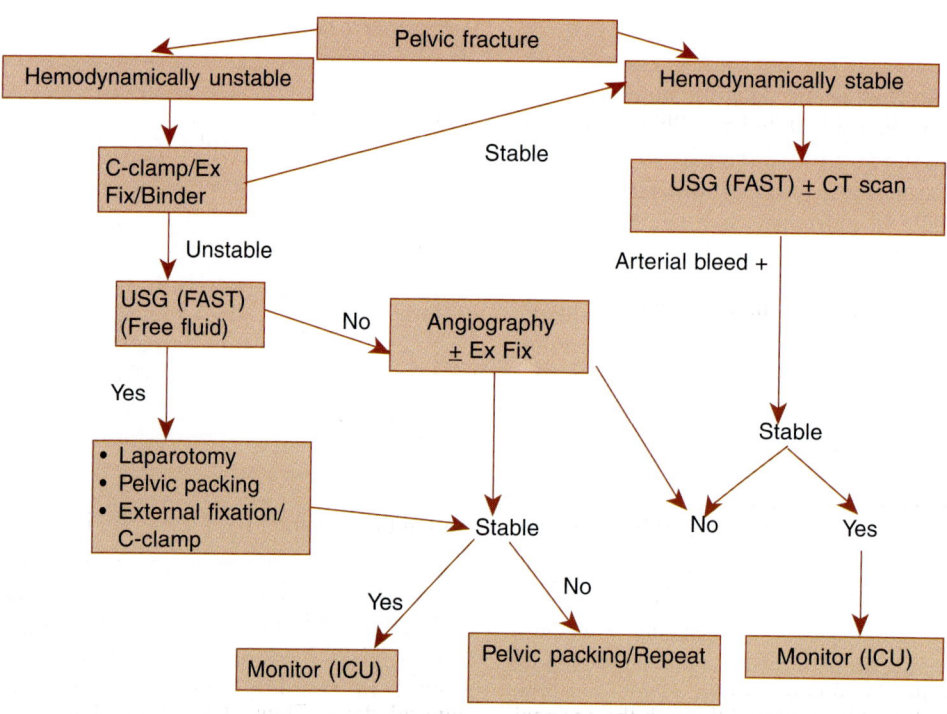

Fig. 11.10: Suggested algorithm for bleeding control and management of pelvic fractures

fractures occur either early (<24 hours) secondary to exsanguination, or late (days to weeks following injury) secondary to sepsis and multiple organ dysfunction.

The major difference in the treatment priorities of patients with open pelvic fractures concerns the evaluation and treatment of the patient with hemorrhage. By definition, open pelvic fractures involve a communication between the fracture and the skin. This may include other perineal structures such as the vagina or the rectum. Arterial bleeding out of the wound can be massive. Presentation to the emergency department can be quite dramatic, especially if the patient has severe open soft tissue injury. Because of the direct communication to the environment, there is no longer any tamponade afforded by the peritoneum or any increase in intra-abdominal pressure. Thus, free blood loss will continue until the patient exsanguinates.

Direct compression is probably the best manner of achieving temporary vascular control. Depending on the size of the skin laceration, a variety of materials can be used to help tamponade blood loss. Simple gauze packing may suffice if the skin opening is relatively small. This can be supplemented with temporary skin closure to increase the tamponade effect. Patients with large perineal lacerations and soft tissue injuries may require larger packing such as laparotomy pads or towels. Skin closure may not be technically feasible for these patients, and direct hand pressure may be the only way to control blood loss.

Once bleeding is controlled temporarily, the patient should be resuscitated and plans made to provide more definitive hemostasis. One option is to take the patient directly to the operating room. Local wound exploration and hemorrhage control in the ED should never be employed. This maneuver requires good lighting, retractor systems, and deep instruments as well as skilled technicians. Blind manipulation in the ED may only compound an already desperate situation. In the operating room, the patient should be explored through the perineal wound and injured blood vessels individually identified and ligated. For all the aforementioned reasons, an approach via laparotomy will seldom result in adequate hemostasis. It is also important to remember that hemostasis may be incomplete even if it appears adequate after perineal exploration. Injured vessels may be difficult to expose via this approach. Once the patient is resuscitated, bleeding may again ensue.

The one time when a direct approach via laparotomy may be helpful, is in the patient with near-total amputation at the level of the pelvis or hip. These patients generally present in extremis with obvious exsanguination. They often have major arterial injury at the level of the common iliac, proximal hypogastric, or external iliac artery. Vascular control via the perineal injury may be impossible. Laparotomy can be life-saving in these patients. Concomitant bony, nervous, and soft tissue injuries may make these patients candidates for hemipelvectomy. Most reports concerning pelvic fractures contain small numbers of these types of patients. There are some case reports of patients who have undergone hemipelvectomy for this particular injury and survived.

Angiographic embolization can be quite beneficial for patients with open pelvic fractures. The angiography service should be alerted at the time of patient presentation even if the patient is going to be transferred to the operating room in an effort to surgically control blood loss. Following attempts at hemostasis, the wound should be packed tightly with skin closure if possible. Patients can then be transferred to the angiography suite to evaluate for undiagnosed vascular injuries as a supplement to surgical hemostasis. One should avoid large dissections or prolonged attempts to control blood loss in the operating room. Obvious injuries should be treated and the wound be packed and then taken to the angiography suite as quickly as possible.

Once hemostasis is secured, the soft tissue injury should be addressed. While this is a very high priority, pelvic sepsis is unlikely to be an issue for several days. Thus, if the patient has not been completely evaluated for potentially life-threatening associated injuries; this should take priority and be completed in order to allow proper sequencing of further diagnostics and therapeutics. All patients should have been evaluated with DPL or FAST to rule out intra-abdominal blood loss. The urinary system should be imaged completely. CT scanning should be considered at this point to examine the kidneys, bladder, and other retroperitoneal structures. A complete evaluation of the perineum is then necessary. This includes a sigmoidoscopy in all patients and a pelvic exam in women. Associated injuries to the rectum and the genitourinary system are quite common, and must be fully evaluated. Rectal or vaginal lacerations should be repaired at this time. The abdomen should be explored and a diverting colostomy performed. This will help prevent subsequent pelvic sepsis. The wounds are packed open and the packing changed frequently.

DEFINITIVE TREATMENT OF PELVIC RING DISRUPTIONS

Definitive therapy of mechanically unstable pelvic fractures does not necessarily mean early rigid internal fixation. Definitive therapy may be, in fact, the continuation of external fixation. Conversely, external fixation may not be appropriate if early internal fixation is planned. Certain conditions such as open pelvic fractures make long-term external fixation the therapy of choice, particularly when there is substantial soiling from open bowel injuries. In addition, severe comminution of strategic portions of the pelvis, such as the pubic rami, may indicate that the patient would be better served by external rather than internal fixation. The choice of fixation in patients that need fixation is, therefore based on the specifics of the pelvic disruption, the patient's soft tissue envelope, and other injuries.

Management of the APC injuries is relatively straightforward. An APC1 fracture is a very rare pattern that is mechanically stable and the patient typically can bear weight as tolerated with no intervention. APC2 fractures are an open-book injury that is hinged on the strong posterior SI ligaments. These injuries need surgery to restore a "tension band" in the front of the pelvis, and therefore can often be treated by addressing the anterior injury only. The options for this are plate and screw fixation or external fixation. Plate fixation is usually used when the disruption is at or near the symphysis, and external fixation is used more when the anterior displacement is through rami fractures or there are other reasons why external fixation is desirable. In the obese patient, or when fixation anteriorly is weak, the anterior fixation can be augmented with posterior fixation (percutaneous sacro-iliac screws). APC3 injuries typically need posterior fixation (SI screws or plate and screws) in addition to anterior fixation.

Management of LC injuries is less straightforward because even though the LC1 type is the most common, it is also the most heterogeneous. LC1 injuries are divided into "good" and "bad" LCls. Good LCls have a minor "sacral crunch" or incomplete sacral fractures. These are typically managed non-operatively with no limitations to ambulation. Bad LCls have complete sacral fractures and can have significant anterior injuries. These injuries are mechanically unstable and need at least posterior SI screws, protected weight bearing, and sometimes even anterior fixation or iliac wing fixation. LC3 fractures are managed by the strategy for the individual APC and LC injuries on each side. Vertical shear injuries are treated like APC3 injuries.

Bladder rupture merits separate consideration as it may change management strategy and this injury is relatively common. If the patient has a pelvic injury that would typically be treated with a plate anteriorly, bladder rupture must be repaired to prevent bathing the plate in urine, even for extra-peritoneal bladder ruptures that could heal without treatment. A bladder rupture is therefore a relative contraindication to plate fixation and may push the balance toward external fixation.

TIMING OF OPERATIVE TREATMENT OF PELVIC RING DISRUPTIONS

The timing of surgery is often determined by associated injuries and their complications, such as pulmonary compromise and central nervous system injury. In some patients, very early internal fixation may be the best option. For instance, a patient with an open-book pelvic injury and a simple symphyseal disruption with intact posterior SI ligaments (APC II) who needs a laparotomy may be best served by laparotomy followed by symphyseal plating. Recent work indicates that ORIF at the time of laparotomy for acute treatment of unstable pelvic fractures may be as safe as external fixator application and does not appear to be associated with any increased morbidity.

In patients who do not need an emergent laparotomy, there is more flexibility regarding operative timing. The best management of pelvic ring injuries that require fixation may be staged surgery. If the patient is hemodynamically stable, the pelvic fracture that otherwise requires surgery does not necessarily require definitive fixation on the first day. For reasons of hemodynamic stability, coagulopathy, and hypothermia, surgery may be best delayed. However, most severe pelvic injuries require some type of surgical intervention early in the treatment regimen, whereas definitive and more rigid fixation may be more appropriately applied later when resuscitation is complete and management of other injuries have been addressed. This should be balanced against the advantages of earlier definitive fixation that allows for early patient mobilization which may benefit the patient in facilitating pulmonary toilet, terminating mechanical ventilation, and providing more aggressive early rehabilitation.

In general, open reduction of the anterior pelvis is typically attempted after some time (24 to 48 hours) has been allowed for clot to stabilize. Immediate plating is associated with increased blood loss and should not be entered into lightly in the patient who was previously hemodynamically unstable. However external fixation can be performed immediately with little blood loss. The advantage of immediate external fixation is that it allows for the removal of the binder in patients who needed a binder for hemodynamic compromise, particularly if the patient has ramus fractures that

are not easily treated with plates and screws. Percutaneous fixation of the SI joint or iliac wing fractures can also be performed immediately as there is only minimal blood loss with these injuries. Problem with early posterior fixation is that percutaneous techniques require good fluoroscopic images and these may be difficult to obtain in the acute setting due to contrast from CT scans.

METHODS OF FIXATION

In mechanically unstable pelvic ring disruptions, fixation options can be thought of addressing either the anterior ring or the posterior ring. The anterior ring is fixed with either an external fixator or with plate and screw fixation. Posterior ring injuries are either treated with percutaneous screw fixation or with open plating techniques, depending on the injury pattern and the soft tissue injuries.

There are two standard approaches for attaining access to the pubic symphysis for anterior plate and screw fixation. One is through the continuation of a midline laparotomy incision created for abdominal surgery. The second approach is through a Pfannenstiel incision two fingerbreadths cephalad to the superior pubic rami. Whichever skin approach is used, the plane of injury is then approached through the rectus abdominis muscle (one-half of which is almost always disconnected at its insertion to the symphysis). The non-disrupted portion of the rectus abdominis muscle is then elevated gently forward, and retractors are placed behind the remaining rectus to provide access to the superior portions of both pubic bones.

Fluoroscopic guidance is useful to verify reduction. Anterior fixation of the pelvis has been achieved with various plates and screw constructs.

Definitive operative techniques for posterior pelvic ring injury are varied. One approach is simply a surgical incision over the iliac crest with most of the reduction maneuvers occurring on the medial surface of the ilium after retraction of the iliacus. Exposure can be gained to address fractures of the iliac wing (LC2) as well as disruptions running all the way back to the SI joint (APC2, APC3). Open fixation of the SI joint can be done through this approach and offers the advantage of direct visualization of the SI joint. Two perpendicular two-hole plates are traditionally used for fixation of the SI joint through this approach. Another option to address posterior ring disruptions is a posterior approach to the ilium in a lateral or prone position with exposure made from the external surface of the ilium. This approach is needed to reduce certain "complete" sacral fractures. Large posterior approaches, and plating across the posterior pelvis (or "sacral bars") have been associated with high rates of wound complication and should be avoided if possible. Whenever possible, it is advantageous to perform percutaneous fixation of the posterior ring. The advantage is the minimal blood loss and small surgical incisions. Open reduction techniques have the advantage of direct visualization, accuracy of reduction, and potentially more rigid fixation. However, in situations involving compromised skin and in patients whose other medical conditions do not permit certain surgical positioning, these techniques have considerable potential for complications. In addition, the wide exposure necessary for the benefit of direct visualization has the disadvantage of devascularization secondary to periosteal elevation, with all the attendant problems with wound infections.

The advantages of image-guided indirect reduction and percutaneous fixation of the posterior pelvic ring are best realized when the reduction can be accurately achieved. This relies on fluoroscopic visualization so the patient must not have contrast obscuring the radiographic views or be too obese to obtain good images. Disruptions of the SI joint, fractures of the sacrum, and certain iliac wing fractures are candidates for percutaneous fixation.

ASSOCIATED INJURIES

Traumatic brain injury is common in patients with pelvic fractures. CT scanning is the "gold standard" for the diagnosis and management of patients with closed-head injuries. Unfortunately, the hemodynamic status of patients may preclude safe transport to the CT scanner. Hypotension can substantially worsen long-term outcome from brain injury, even if transient. Thus, the first priority must be resuscitation and treatment of hemorrhage. One option for patients who are not able to have CT scanning is to have blind placement of intracranial pressure monitors. While this does give the clinician some measure of comfort about the patient's neurologic status, the information may not change the therapy. Patients who have CT scans that demonstrate lesions requiring craniotomy can have that procedure performed concurrently with laparotomy or application of external pelvic fixation. Patients with retroperitoneal hemorrhage, hypotension, and brain injury requiring craniotomy represent a special subset. A decision must be made as to whether the patients can be stabilized with transfusions long enough to allow a full craniotomy or whether they are better served by angiography followed by craniotomy. Unfortunately, there is no cookbook way to approach this decision, but rather should be made at the level of best clinical judgment. After hemorrhage and life-threatening brain injuries are addressed, the next priority is the repair of visceral injuries that are not accompanied by hemorrhage. Examples include intraperitoneal bladder rupture or a diaphragmatic injury. Occasionally, repair of these injuries must be staged in a manner similar to that of the patient treated with damage control techniques. For instance, patients with pelvic fractures and hypotension with positive FAST for free fluid should be taken to the operating room. Small bowel injuries can be stapled and bladder injuries temporized with sutures. If patients have ongoing pelvic hemorrhage, they should be rapidly taken to angiography and undergo embolization or have operative pelvic packing possibly followed by adjunctive angiography. Postembolization, patients can be returned to the operating room for a more complete exploration that allows for definitive management of important but non-life-threatening injuries.

Genitourinary injuries commonly occur with pelvic fractures. Overall, they may be found in as many as 16% of the patients who present with pelvic fractures. Bladder injuries occur in as many as 7% of these patients. Urethral injuries occur in approximately 15% of males with pelvic fractures. If patients are stable, there is little reason not to perform a retrograde urethrogram prior to placement of a Foley catheter. The classic presentation of males with urethral injuries includes blood at the urinary meatus, a high-riding prostate or scrotal hematoma. Unfortunately, these are nonspecific. While the presence of any of these signs is strongly suggestive of urethral injury, the absence does not necessarily rule out the injury. Although urethral injury is uncommon in females, it does exist. Barach and coworkers have suggested that bilateral pubic rami fractures, significant vertical displacement of the pelvis, and symphyseal disruption are the fracture patterns most likely to be associated with urethral injuries in females. These may be very difficult to diagnose. While lacerations of the vaginal mucosa have been reported with relative frequency, the finding of blood at the urinary meatus is virtually never present. Urethral injuries in the male are typically treated with suprapubic bladder drainage. They may require acute repair in the setting of severe pelvic fractures for several reasons. Suprapubic tubes may interfere with bony fixation and early definitive repair may be associated with fewer long-term complications, such as stricture. Urethral disruptions in females typically require operative repair.

Bladder rupture also commonly accompanies pelvic fractures. It takes substantial energy to rupture an empty viscous bladder enclosed in a protective bony ring. A ruptured bladder is a good indicator of the severity of injury, particularly if the bladder was empty at the time of impact. Most patients present with gross hematuria, although in some instances hematuria may only be microscopic. The timing of diagnostics is crucial. While it is important not to delay the genitourinary evaluation; neither urethral injury nor bladder rupture is immediately life-threatening. Thus, their evaluation can be deferred until life-threatening injuries are addressed. Patients who require angiography for diagnosis and control

of pelvic blood loss should not have a cystogram performed prior to the angiogram. Extravasation of contrast into the retroperitoneum may limit the angiographer's ability to identify vascular injury. Extraperitoneal bladder rupture is the most common type of bladder rupture accompanying patients with pelvic fractures. Treatment for this is simple decompression with a Foley catheter or suprapubic tube if a concomitant urethral injury is present. Extraperitoneal bladder ruptures may require operative repair if very extensive or if anterior plating of the pelvis is to be performed, to prevent contamination of implanted hardware. Conversely, an extraperitoneal bladder rupture may be a relative indication to use external fixation as a definitive strategy to avoid the potential for contamination of the hardware.

DEEP VEIN THROMBOSIS FOLLOWING PELVIC FRACTURE

Pelvic fractures increase the risk of deep vein thrombosis (DVT). Some combination of pneumatic sequential compression devices, lower extremity elastic stockings, and low-molecular weight or low-dose unfractionated heparin is generally employed as prophylaxis for DVT. DVT may be difficult to assess on physical exam secondary to lower extremity swelling from fractures, operative fixation, or lymphedema. Duplex Doppler ultrasound screening may help to identify occult DVT. Unfortunately, thrombi may occur in the deep pelvic veins, making detection with US difficult. Patients with pelvic fractures are at particular risk for thromboembolism, because they all have some degree of pelvic venous injury and are immobilized for some time. The best treatment strategy is an aggressive program of prevention. Pharmacologic manipulations combined with early fracture fixation and mobilization is probably the best way to prevent DVT. Unfortunately, this is not always possible. Despite aggressive therapy, some patients will develop deep thrombosis.

If DVT is diagnosed, consideration must be given to whether anticoagulation is safe. Certainly, anticoagulation is contraindicated for patients who have substantial blood loss, particularly from pelvic fractures. After several days, if patients have remained stable, they may be candidates for anticoagulation. If there is any concern about the appropriateness of anticoagulation therapy, consideration should be given to placement of an inferior vena caval filter to prevent pulmonary embolism. The diagnosis of pulmonary embolism must be suspected in any patient with a pelvic fracture. Unfortunately, these patients have a multiplicity of reasons to develop hypoxia other than that caused by pulmonary emboli, such as fat embolism from long-bone fractures, atelectasis from immobilization, or pneumonia. The diagnosis of pulmonary embolism must be aggressively pursued in order to make the diagnosis in a timely manner. A combination of chest X-ray, spiral chest CT, ventilation/perfusion lung scan, and pulmonary angiography should be utilized in order to make the diagnosis.

CONCLUSION AND FUTURE DIRECTIONS

Hemodynamically unstable patients with pelvic fractures continue to represent the most frequent source of preventable death following blunt trauma. The major causes of death in these patients are early exsanguination and the late sequelae of prolonged shock and mass transfusion. It is clear that successful management of pelvic fracture bleeding is best accomplished by a multidisciplinary team approach involving a variety of specialties.

The future of pelvic fracture management will be about creating a modern synthesis of modalities to stop bleeding. The primary choice of angiography versus pelvic packing is made based on a careful assessment of hemodynamic status. Angiography and subsequent embolization can provide an effective control of ongoing hemorrhage due to arterial bleeding in patients who are hemodynamically stabilised, whereas packing should take priority over the treatment of hemodynamically unstable patients. The complementary roles of newer hemostatic adjuncts, such as recombinant factor VIIa, refinement of massive transfusion protocols, real-time monitoring of coagulopathy with routine thrombo-elastograms, and other improvements in resuscitation are critical and are in active development.

12 Thoracic Trauma

INTRODUCTION

Chest wall trauma is common and can range from an isolated rib fracture to flail chest, hemopneumothorax, cardiac injury and is found to be responsible for 25% of all deaths following road traffic accidents. Many of these deaths occur at the site of the accident following serious chest injuries such as bilateral flail chest, severe lung contusion with deep refractory hypoxia, and great vessel disruption and exsanguination.

Almost all patients who reach hospital alive can be made to survive if managed appropriately. Indeed the mortality of this group has been greatly reduced in recent years, as a result of the establishment of accident and emergency services as a distinct specialty, paramedical ambulance services and the introduction of advanced trauma life support (ATLS) training. The introduction of the ATLS program has revolutionized the management of all forms of trauma with thoracic trauma in particular. The guide lines of advanced trauma life support (airway, breathing, circulation, disability, exposure) should always be followed in the assessment of such cases.

The ATLS philosophy was developed from the airway, breathing and circulation (ABC) approach for the evaluation and treatment of injured patient. The basis of this is that life-threatening injury causes death or major morbidity within certain reproducible time limits. Therefore, the greatest threat to life must be treated first to avoid further deterioration. In all cases, a primary survey of the patient is performed in which any immediately life-threatening injury is identified and treated. Once the patient's condition is stable a secondary survey is performed to establish whether any further injury exists.

The approach to the treatment must be methodical to rule out the injuries to the underlying viscera such as lung, heart, liver, and spleen as injuries to these are often associated with chest wall trauma.

Chest injuries can be of two main groups: blunt and penetrating injury. Blunt injury may lead to fracture ribs, sternum along with pulmonary and cardiac contusion or rupture of airway, diaphragm and major vessel depending upon low impact velocity (direct blow) or high impact velocity (deceleration and crush injuries). Penetrating injury can be caused by stab, impalement or gunshot and may lead to pericardial tamponade, major vessel or intercostal hemorrhage, hemopneumothorax or at times esophageal or airway perforation. A high velocity bullet is always destructive because it creates an immense shock wave with resultant cavitation.

PATHOPHYSIOLOGY

Most patients with chest injuries can be managed by relatively simple measures (intercostal drain insertion, adequate analgesia, careful fluid management and physiotherapy) and do not require thoracotomy. If these injuries are not managed appropriately, the consequences may be fatal. Immediate threats to life are massive hemorrhage with consequent hypovolemia and low cardiac output. Hypoxia is the most common pathophysiological process in thoracic trauma and it is therefore crucial to ensure adequate oxygen delivery to viable sections of lung. Hypoxia and acidosis may occur secondary to:

- Hypovolemia caused by blood loss
- Low cardiac output as a result of tamponade
- Pulmonary contusion or collapse
- Ventilatory failure
- Displacement of mediastinal structure.

Respiratory acidosis results from inadequate ventilation, whereas metabolic acidosis is caused by tissue hypoperfusion. Untreated chest injuries may cause an increase in hypoxia and acidosis, which in turn will compound the adverse effects of other injuries.

PRIMARY SURVEY

The basic principle in resuscitation is securing the airway and restoring the circulating volume. The primary survey involves simultaneous assessment and treatment of life-threatening injuries. It follows the ABC principle of resuscitation, which may also include even emergency thoracotomy.

Airway

Patency of airway must be ensured immediately. The oropharynx must be cleared of any secretion or obstructing foreign body. Supplemental oxygen is useful in all such trauma patients. If the airway is compromised and patient is not adequately self ventilating, endotracheal intubation and ventilatory support is required (cervical spine injury should always be excluded). At times protecting or establishing the airway can be hazardous and difficult, particularly if there are severe injuries of head, neck, and upper chest causing distortion of the tissue. Inability to intubate the trachea may demand emergency tracheostomy or cricothyroidotomy with a large bore cannula.

Breathing

To assess the quality of ventilation and pattern of respiratory movement, the patient's chest must be fully exposed. A thorough inspection of chest is done to note the frequency and pattern of breathing, external evidence of trauma and structural defects of the thorax. Palpation will detect surgical emphysema, paradoxical movement (flail chest) and stove-in-chest deformity. Auscultation and percussion should reveal the existence of pneumothorax or hemothorax which may require emergency drainage.

The mechanism of breathing can be disrupted in a number of ways.
- Hemothorax, pneumothorax and pulmonary contusion reduce the volume of ventilated lung.
- Pain causes a reduction in the tidal volume because the patient protects the chest wall and uses the diaphragm as the only muscle of respiration.
- Loss of integrity of the chest wall (when it becomes flail) reduces the tidal volume.

Circulation

The initial assessment of the circulation involves
- Palpation of the pulse for its rate, quality and rhythm
- Measurement of blood pressure
- Measurement of pulse pressure
- Checking the color and temperature (indicator of peripheral circulation)
- Examination of neck veins
- ECG monitoring.

PRIORITY SITUATION

There are several immediately life-threatening conditions that must be diagnosed or excluded by clinical examination and investigation.

Pneumothorax

Any condition in which air can enter the pleural space, either through a breach in the thin and delicate visceral pleura or through an injury to the chest wall results in pneumothorax. It could be traumatic, spontaneous or iatrogenic. The term tension pneumothorax defines the condition in which the air within the pleural space is under positive pressure. On chest X-ray pneumothorax will appear black with no bronchovascular markings (Fig. 12.1).

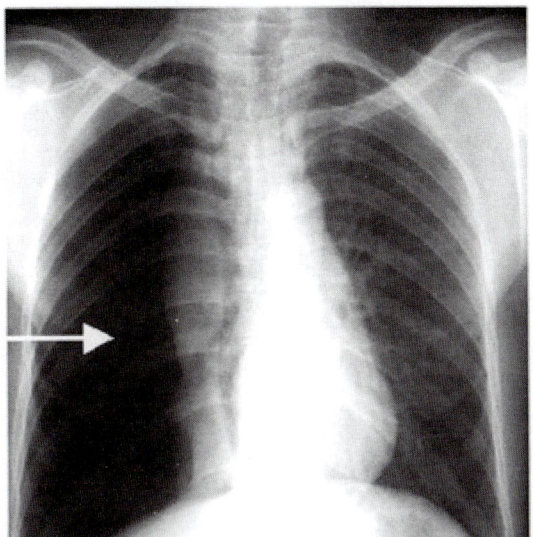

Fig. 12.1: Right side pneumothorax with collapse of right lung

Tension Pneumothorax

This occurs when air enters the pulmonary cavity during inspiration from lungs, airway, or chest wall injury that seals or closes during expiration. As the pressure rises, venous return is obstructed and the mediastinum shifts, distorting the heart and compressing the other lung. The clinical signs of tension pneumothorax are:

- Asphyxia
- Tachycardia
- Hypotension
- Tracheal deviation to the contralateral side
- Hyperresonance with loss of breath sounds on the affected side
- Engorgement of neck veins
- Cyanosis at later stage.

Tension pneumothorax should always be a clinical diagnosis, not a radiological one.

Treatment

Immediate decompression should be performed by insertion of a cannula into the second intercostal space in the mid-clavicular line which should be replaced later on with intercostal tube drain. This is a life-saving procedure and should always be done urgently.

Open Pneumothorax

This is also known as sucking chest wound, because air moves in and out through the chest wall injury with each breath. If the wound is large, air will move in and out through the wound rather than through the trachea and thus no gaseous exchange will take place and respiratory failure results. In this condition there is a chest wall defect which creates an open pneumothorax. During inspiration air passes through the wound more readily than through the bronchial tree, and the mediastinum will move towards the intact site. During expiration air exits the pleural cavity and the lung partially reexpands with air from the intact lung. This causes the mediastinum to move towards the affected side. The erect chest radiograph is the only sure way to confirm or to exclude the diagnosis of pneumothorax.

Pathophysiology

The lung contains elastic tissue and is held expanded, separated from the chest wall by a thin layer of pleural fluid. The pressure in this potential space is subatmospheric and this negative intrapleural pressure is always maintained. Therefore, whenever the air is admitted into the pleural space, the negative intrapleural pressure is lost and the lung is no longer held expanded in apposition to the chest wall and due to it own elasticity collapses to a very small volume. Subsequent result depends upon whether the source of air seals off, persists or is valve like.

a. *If communication seals off:* When communication closes, the leak in the visceral pleura usually stops as the lung collapses. Neither air nor blood enters the collapsed lung. Systemic hypoxia is not usually a feature provided the other lung has good function. The air in the space is absorbed.

b. *If communication remains open:* This is rather unusual for the communication to remain open.

This occurs when there is an injury to the chest wall, so that the air enters and exits with each respiratory movement. If resistance to flow is less than that in trachea and bronchi, air movement will occur selectively in and out of the pleural space rather than the lung leading to respiratory failure.

c. *If the communication acts as valve:* This results in a state of tension pneumothorax which is a lethal condition and at times it may pass unnoticed in anesthetized, drunk or head injury cases. In this condition, the injured patients strains, groans as he become more hypoxic. This generates positive pressure inside the airway, causing more air to pass out and get trapped in the chest cavity. As the pressure rises venous return is obstructed and the mediastinum shifts, distorting the heart and compressing the other lung. It is particularly hazardous component of multiple injuries because it may progress insidiously while other injuries attract more attention. It is also dangerous when the patient is being artificially ventilated.

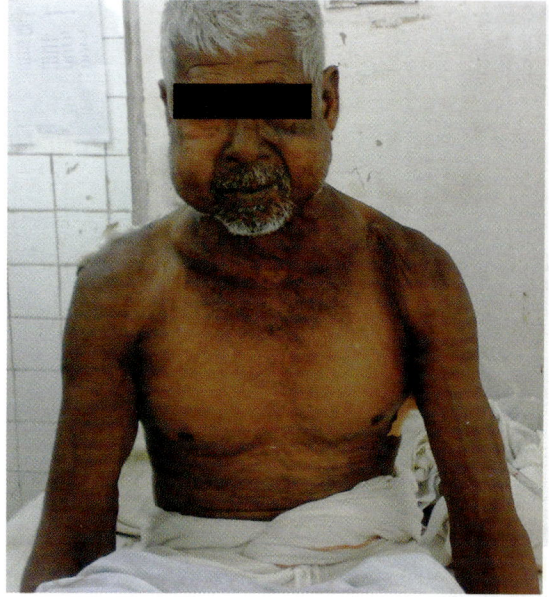

Fig. 12.2: Patient with fracture ribs and surgical emphysema in the neck, face, thorax and arms

Treatment

Initial management is closure of the defect with a sterile occlusive dressing and placement of intercostal drain should be away from the wound. Surgical closure can be undertaken when the primary and secondary survey is complete.

Traumatic Pneumothorax

Closed Pneumothorax

Pneumothorax due to trauma is usually closed. In this the chest wall is intact and the visceral pleural damage is caused by a rib fracture. It can happen after a fall against a hard edge or due to kick. At times, it can be a part of multiple injuries. This is dangerous if the patient is anesthetized, because positive pressure ventilation will lead to tension pneumothorax. Whenever the parietal pleura is torn due to rib fracture surgical emphysema may occur (Fig. 12.2). Emphysema is a characteristic physical sign and in this crepitus is felt due to the presence of air in the subcutaneous space.

Hemothorax

Massive hemothorax is defined as the loss of 1500 ml or more of blood into the chest cavity. Although it is more commonly caused by a penetrating injury, it can be associated with blunt trauma of chest wall as well.

Diagnosis

The signs are those of hypovolemic shock with absent breath sounds on the affected side. The neck veins may be full secondary to the mechanical effects of hemothorax or it may be empty in case the patient is hypovolemic.

Hemothorax is noted as a meniscus of fluid blunting the costophrenic angle when viewed on the upright chest X-ray film (Fig. 12.3). As much as 400–500 ml of blood is required to obliterate the costophrenic angle. In case of massive hemothorax the affected side of the chest will appear completely white (Fig. 12.4). In case of hemo-pnemothorax air fluid level will be present (Fig. 12.5).

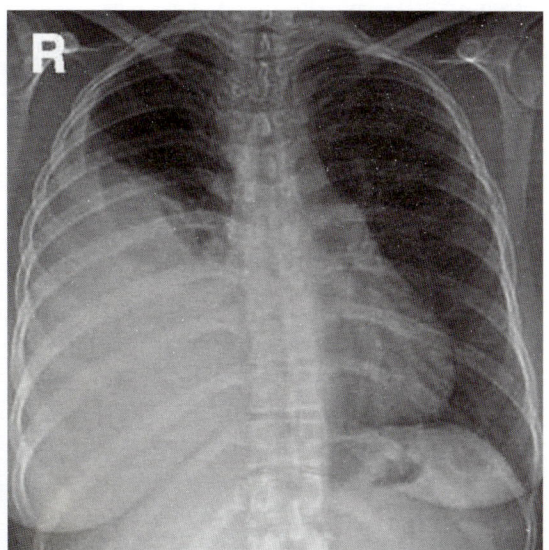

Fig. 12.3: Chest X-ray showing right sided hemothorax with blunting of costophrenic angle

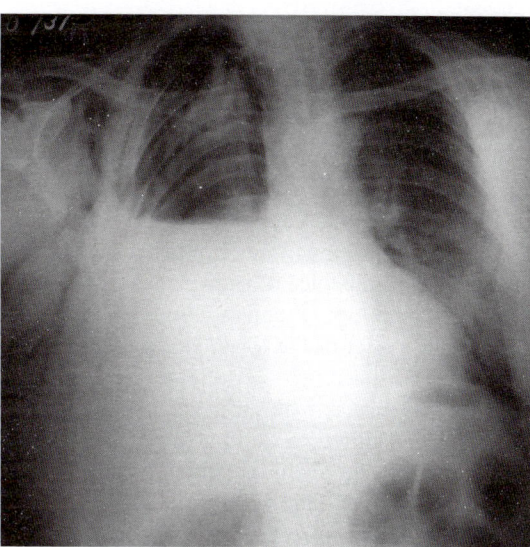

Fig. 12.5: Right side hemo-pneumothorax as suggested by air fluid level and associated ribs fracture

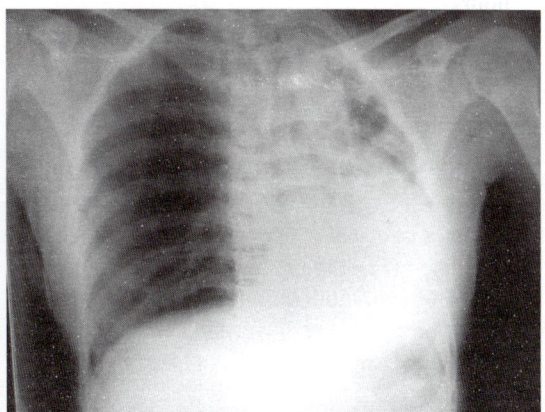

Fig. 12.4: Left side hemothorax causing white out chest

Treatment

It comprises of continued decompression of the chest and restoration of the blood volume. A large bore chest drain (32 F or larger) should be used. The rapid infusion of fluid replacement is started through large caliber venous cannula until type specific or cross-matched blood is available.

If there is continuing blood loss of more than 200 ml/hour for more than three hours, exploratory thoracotomy must be undertaken by an experienced surgeon. Any penetrating wound medial to the nipple should heighten suspicion of damage to the heart, great vessel or hilar structure.

INTERCOSTAL CHEST DRAINAGE

Underwater seal drainage successfully treats most cases of hemopneumothorax. The modern chest drains

- are made up of clear plastic
- are available in varying diameters
- have length markers
- have multiple side roles
- have radiopaque stripe to allow confirmation of tube position on radiograph.

Choosing the Site

The safest place is lateral to the anterior axillary fold, in the 4th or 5th intercostal space.

Insertions

- The skin is prepared and 10 ml of 1% lignocaine is injected (if time allows) through the skin and muscle. The pleura is penetrated and the easy aspiration of air or blood confirms that the site is well chosen.
- Bloody froth indicates that the lung has been punctured and thus one should reconsider the diagnosis and choice of site.
- Using a scalpel, 2 cm incision made on the superior aspect of the lower rib at the proposed intercostal space.
- Blunt dissection with an artery forcep is then performed down to and through the parietal pleura. The space is further enlarged to sufficient size with finger. This will have added benefit of confirming the correct location.
- Preferred chest tube is inserted into the pleura with the help of an artery forcep.
- Once the chest drain is inside the pleura, air/blood should escape. Thereafter the drain is secured firmly and immediately connected to the underwater seal drainage system.
- It is advisable to place a horizontal mattress suture around the incision to tie as it can be used later to close the hole when the drain is removed.
- The column of water should swing and bubbles should escape if the patient is asked to cough or in case of hemothorax gush of blood should come out.
- Under no circumstances should a chest drain be clamped because this could convert a simple pneumothorax to a tension pneumothorax.

A radiograph should be taken after chest tube insertion to check whether the tube is properly positioned.

Removal of Drain

The drain may be removed when radiograph shows that the
- Lung is expanded
- The tube has stopped bubbling
- There is a minimum swing in the column of fluid
- There is no further bleeding.

All these usually occurs in 3–4 days. The patient is taught to perform a valsalva maneuver at full inspiration so that on removal of the tube he can maintain positive pressure until the tube is completely removed and the mattress suture is tied (see also Chapter 5).

THORACOTOMY

Majority of chest injuries are managed conservatively by underwater seal drainage. Oxygen and physiotherapy are the mainstay in the management of blunt chest trauma. However, some patients may require thoracotomy.

Indications for Thoracotomy

- Fresh bleeding more than 1000 to 1500 ml at initial drainage
- Continued brisk bleeding >100 ml/15 min from intercostals drain
- Continued bleeding >200 ml/hr for 3 or more hours
- Rupture bronchus, aorta, esophagus or diaphragm
- Cardiac tamponade.

Preparation

- Double lumen endotracheal tube is used to intubate the patient. This allows the one lung to be collapsed while the other side is selectively ventilated (Figs 12.6A and B).
- Patient is placed in lateral position on the operating table with lower leg flexed at both the hip and the knee. A pillow is placed between the knees.
- The position is well secured with the help of strap around the hips
- Upper arm is held at 90° flexion and supported by a bracket
- The lower arm is flexed and positioned next to the head.

Incision

- The classical skin incision for a lateral thoracotomy extends from 1 to 2 cm inferoposterior to

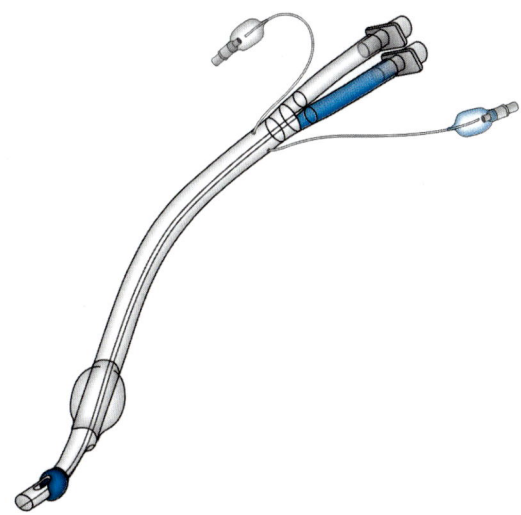

Fig. 12.6A: Double-lumen endotracheal tube

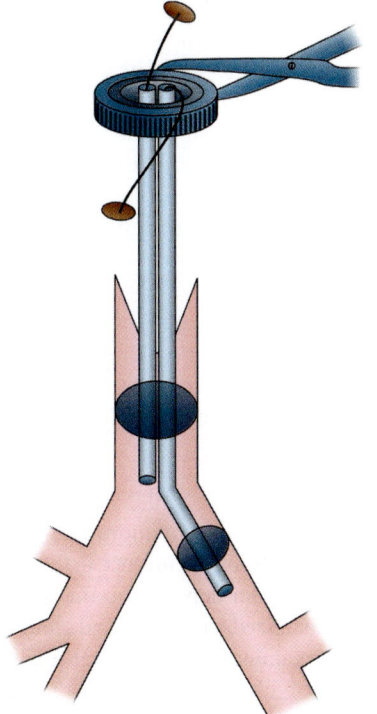

Fig. 12.6B: Left sided double-lumen endotracheal tube. Clamping the right sidewill selectively ventilate the left lung and right lung will collapse

the nipple in the male (or the submammary fold in the female) and passes to a point 1 to 2 cm below the angle of scapula. It then curves posteriorly and upward between the posterior border of the scapula and spine (Fig. 12.7A).

- The incision is further deepened into the muscle layers: The latissimus dorsi is encountered first and incised in the same line with coagulating diathermy (Fig. 12.7B).
- The plane deep to scapula and serratus anterior is identified and the ribs counted. The highest rib that can be felt is usually the second, which has a sharper surface than the lower ribs.
- A periosteum of the sixth rib is cut along a line 5 mm below and parallel to the superior edge. Periosteum is stripped from the superior aspect of the rib in the postero-anterior direction. This reveals the parietal pleura with the lung beneath (Fig. 12.7C).

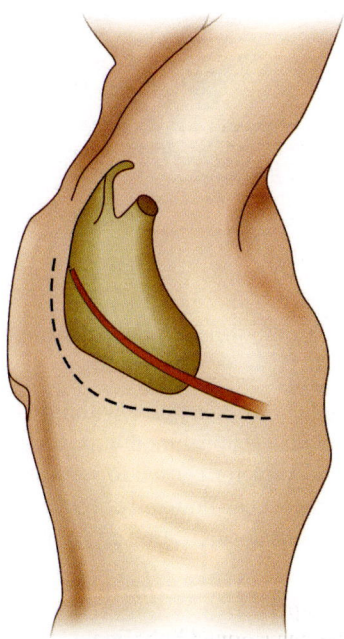

Fig. 12.7A: Dotted line shows the incision for posterolateral thoracotomy

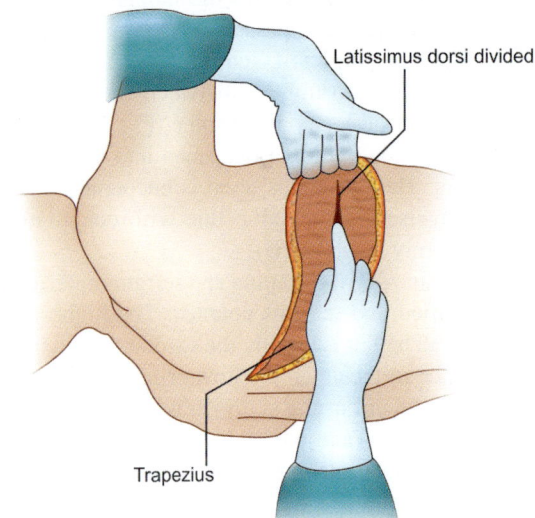

Fig. 12.7B: Latissimus is incised in the line of incision

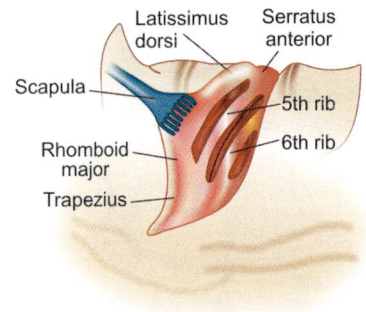

Fig. 12.7C: Incision over the sixth rib

- Parietal pleura is penetrated with instrument and the lung falls as a pneumothorax is created.
- A thoracic retractor is used to separate the ribs.
- The anesthetist can now fully deflate the exposed lung for better visualization of the hemithorax.

Closure

Two drains are usually inserted following thoracotomy; a superior one draining the apex of the hemithorax and an inferior one draining fluid from diaphragmatic surface of the hemithorax. The drain should be inserted two intercostal spaces below the incision and the muscle layer should be brought together tension during insertion to allow correct alignment. The intercostal nerves may be infiltrated with local anesthetic at the angle of the rib before closure. Anatomical alignment of the ribs is achieved by using a rib approximator. The stripped layer of periosteum and intercostal muscle are sutured to the intercostal muscle below the stripped rib using a continuous layer of absorbable suture. A non-absorbable suture may be used to maintain the closure if healing is likely to be compromised.

The muscle layer of fascia are closed in layers using absorbable sutures, skin is closed in usual manner.

Postoperative Pain

Postoperative pain can be a major problem with thoracotomy and it should be dealt effectively for normal breathing. Patient controlled analgesia is an important development, but need good supervision. Local anesthetic infiltration of the intercostal nerve above and below the incision is helpful. Sources of avoidable chronic pain include rib fracture and entrapment of intercostal nerve during wound closure.

The chest drain placed at the time of surgery is removed only when air leaks stops and lung is re-expanded. Breathing exercise and regular physiotherapy should begin early after the operation.

RIB FRACTURE

Single fracture of one or more ribs due to direct violence is a common occurrence in the chest trauma. The degree of pain depends on the number of ribs involved. Localized tenderness and crepitus are often elicited in examination. Sufficient analgesia is the treatment of choice to encourage the normal respiratory pattern. At times intercostal nerve block may be required for persistent pain.

Although the first rib is well protected and requires a considerable force for fracture, the mortality is high because of its association with injury to major vessels.

Fracture of sternum results from deceleration or seat belt injury. It generally leads to the injury of the underlying myocardium. ECG monitoring, analgesia and closed observation in intensive cardiac unit is required.

FLAIL CHEST

It occurs when several ribs are fractured at two places either on one side of the chest or on either side of the sternum. The flail segment causes severe disruption of normal chest wall function with paradoxical movement. It is usually accompanied by underlying lung contusion and the combination of the two can cause serious hypoxia.

Diagnosis

Careful observations of the respiratory movement which may be un-coordinated, and the palpation of the chest wall for fracture crepitus are required so that the diagnosis is not missed. The chest radiograph cannot always be relied onto reveal costochondral separation or rib fracture (Fig. 12.8).

Treatment

Resuscitation of a patient with flail chest involves ensuring full expansion of the lung with good oxygenation, which may require intubation and mechanical ventilation. Any hemothorax must be drained by an intracostal drain. Adequate analgesia is important because it allows the patient to self-ventilate completely as well as to clear their own airway and cope with physiotherapy.

Thoracotomy with fracture fixation is occasionally appropriate when operative procedure is required for an underlying injury.

CARDIAC TAMPONADE

In trauma patient it is usually caused by penetrating injury but disruption of the heart or great vessels with bleeding into the pericardium may also result from a blunt injury as well. The pericardium is a

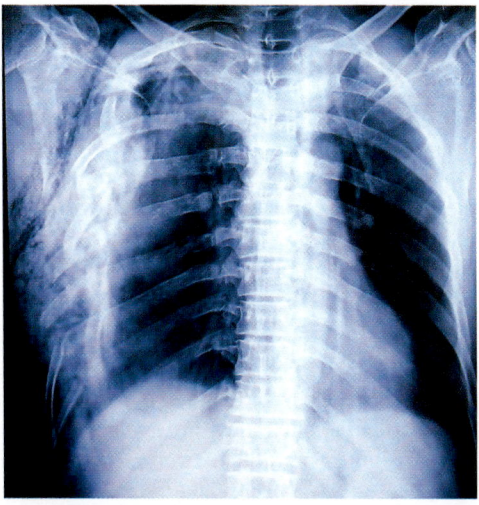

Fig. 12.8: Chest X-ray showing multiple rib fractures (3rd to 8th ribs) on the right side at two places giving rise to flail chest. Also there is right-sided surgical emphysema

fixed structure and even a small amount of blood will interfere with cardiac filling and cardiac output. Removal of as little as 20 ml of blood by pericardiocentesis can dramatically improve the cardiac function.

Diagnosis

Signs of tamponade are hypotension, muffled heart sounds and an elevated jugular venous pulse (This may be absent in the hypovolemia.).

Treatment

Immediate pericardiocentesis should be undertaken if tamponade is suspected. In 25% of patients with cardiac tamponade, clotting of blood within the pericardium will prevent aspiration. All trauma patients with positive pericardiocentesis must undergo formal surgical exploration of the heart.

Pericardiocentesis

- The patient should always be connected to ECG monitor before commencing

- Prepare drape and apply local anesthetic to the area above and below the xiphisternum, if possible
- Insert a long >15 cm large bore cannula through the skin 1–2 cm below the left xiphochondral junction. Direct the tip of the cannula towards the tip of the left scapula, maintaining an angle of 45° to the skin
- Advance the cannula while maintaining negative pressure on the syringe attached. When blood flows into the syringe, stop advancing and draw off as much blood as possible. If there are ECG disturbances or the blood is bright red (arterial) remove the cannula and start again because the tip is likely to be in the left ventricle.

SECONDARY SURVEY

The aim of the secondary survey is to identify the potential life-threatening injuries and this too should only begin when patient's condition is fully stabilized.

Essential investigations during the secondary survey are:

- ECG
- Chest radiograph
- Arterial blood gas.

POTENTIAL LIFE-THREATENING INJURIES

Pulmonary Contusion

The underlying lung often gets injured in thoracic trauma, which usually resolves but laceration with persistent air leak, features of bleeding or failure of expansion of the lung will require surgical intervention. Many of such injuries are also associated with pneumothorax or hemothorax.

Close monitoring is essential because the onset of an adult respiratory distress syndrome like condition can be insidious and intubation and ventilation may be required at any time.

Myocardial Contusion

The diagnosis of myocardial contusion is based on the ECG abnormalities or enzyme changes,

indicative of infarction. There may be arrhythmia and signs of heart failure.

Once the myocardial contusion is diagnosed, the patient should be treated as if he had sustained a myocardial infarction.

Aortic Disruption

It is usually occurs as a result of major deceleration injury. Clinical signs are interscapular pain, murmur, hoarseness, radio-femoral delay in arterial pulse. Arteriography is diagnostic and CT is of little help. If complete, it is invariably fatal at the scene, but if the bleeding is slow it needs early identification and management.

Diagnosis

The laceration is commonly in the region of ligamentum arteriosum and only advential continuity prevents sudden death. The transection of aorta must be suspected in all high speed deceleration incidents. The clinical signs may be masked by concurrent injuries.

If aortic disruption is suspected, the investigations should be undertaken urgently.

In a good quality posterolateral chest radiograph findings which suggest aortic injury are

- Widened mediastinum
- Obliterated aortic knuckle
- Fractured 1st and 2nd rib
- Depressed left main bronchus
- Elevated right main bronchus.

It should be stressed that even in the presence of normal chest radiograph, if slight suspicion exists and the diagnosis cannot be excluded then angiography should proceed urgently.

Treatment

Once the diagnosis is confirmed formal surgical repair is required and should not be delayed. Urgent exploration by left thoracotomy through 4th intercostal space is undertaken. Control above and below the transection is vital and the aorta is repaired by direct suture or interposition graft.

Diaphragmatic Rupture

At times the blunt trauma produces large radial tears which lead to herniation of abdominal viscera into the chest. This in turn may cause mediastinal compression of thoracic organs with its consequent effects. Diagnosis is often missed and contrast studies are usually required. This occurs more commonly on left because the liver prevents right sided visceral herniation. Penetrating injury of thorax may cause tear of diaphragm (Fig. 12.9).

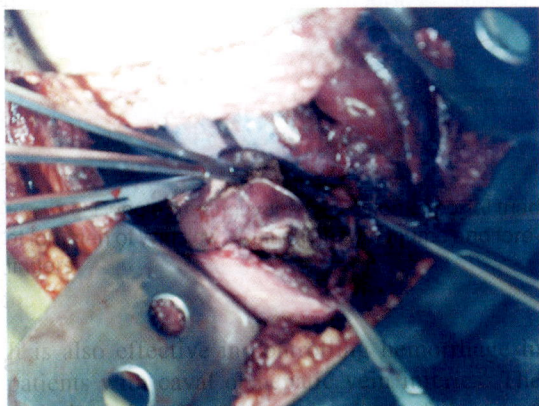

Fig. 12.9: Right side thoracotomy showing diaphragmatic tear and liver laceration caused by stab injury

Treatment

Diaphragmatic tears should be repaired with non-absorbable sutures.

Tracheal Rupture

Trachea is susceptive to blunt and penetrating trauma and the immediate concern is the patency of the airway. Stridor indicates partial obstruction which may became complete if not managed promptly.

Diagnosis and Treatment

Endoscopy and CT scanning following stabilization of the patient. Trachea if found injured should be repaired.

Esophageal rupture

It usually follows a penetrating injury. The resulting mediastinitis often causes an emphysema, if there is leakage into pleural cavity.

A radiograph is essential for diagnosis. This discloses the presence of air in the mediastinum or pleural cavity or in the neck which may easily be palpable. Left pneumothorax or hemothorax in the absence of rib fracture should raise a suspicion for esophageal rupture.

The diagnosis is confirmed by contrast studies or esophagoscopy.

Treatment is initially chest tube drainage followed by formal repair.

Role of Ultrasound and Standard CT in Thoracic Trauma

Surgeons have found ultrasound to be useful in detection of post-traumatic hemothorax. The sensitivity and specificity of ultrasound has found to be equivalent to the portable chest radiograph. The only benefit is that ultrasound examination was significantly faster.

The standard thoracic CT has been always an adjuvant to the routine chest radiograph. The spiral CT with contrast has been found to be useful in detecting blunt rupture of the thoracic aorta.

THORACOSCOPY

The use of video-assisted thoracoscopy continues to increase in major trauma centers. The indications for thoracoscopy in trauma include early evacuation of a clotted hemothorax, evaluation of left hemi-diaphragm after penetrating left thoraco-abdominal wounds and repair of pulmonary lacerations or assistance with pulmonary lobectomy.

13 Soft Tissue Injury of the Face

Soft tissue trauma to the face is a common occurrence. It has been observed from the various studies that roughly 60% of the individuals injured in automobile accidents, sustain facial injuries. The other causes of soft tissue injury of the face include gunshot wound, thermal or chemical burns, animal and human bites. One should not get distracted by the dramatic appearance of a facial wound at presentation. Always, the general condition of the patient should be assessed and underlying skeleton be examined. Status of airway, circulation and cervical spine must be determined, before focusing on the facial injuries.

COMMON SOFT TISSUE INJURIES OF THE FACE

- Abrasion
- Contusion
- Laceration
- Avulsion
- Accidental tattoos.

ASSESSMENT OF INJURY

Attending doctor must obtain a careful history, which includes the mechanism and time of injury, and any treatment if given earlier. A single laceration with a clean knife has a far better prognosis for primary healing than a grossly contaminated crush laceration. The time lapse from injury to presentation is also important. It has been a teaching that wound should not be closed primarily if presented more than six hours after the injury. Although this principle is correct, but the excellent blood supply of the face along with the use of better antibiotic cover and adequate debridement can allow primarily closure even up to 24 hours.

During the clinical examination, it is necessary to judge whether there is true tissue loss, as opposed to tissue retraction. The radiological investigations are usually undertaken to assess the skeletal injury. They can also be used to identify and localize the foreign bodies. Photography is often used to record facial injury because of the medico-legal implications.

While accessing the facial injuries it is of utmost importance to palpate with finger tips the orbital rims, bridge of the nose as well as the zygomatic prominences for any deformity, pain and tenderness. A careful ophthalmic examination is also essential to exclude both intra and extra-ocular damage. Many a time a subconjuctival hemorrhage is associated with underlying zygomatic complex fracture. Deranged facial sensation in the distribution of trigeminal nerve is indicative of bony damage and it should be assessed by using a blunt pin. The classical Battle sign (hematoma behind the pinna) also indicates skull fracture. Palpation of nasal bones and visualization of septal bone is also essential and is achieved by clearing the blood and mucus. Paresthesia of lower lip during examination suggests a significant disruption of inferior alveolar nerve running within the mandible. Limitation of the jaw function indicates significant bony damage of mandible.

In the event of chemical burn of the face, it is essential to ascertain the causative agent. Simple enquiries, such as tetanus prophylaxis, drug allergies and past medical history should be made. In case of animal bite, it is important to discover the type of animal involved (Fig. 13.1).

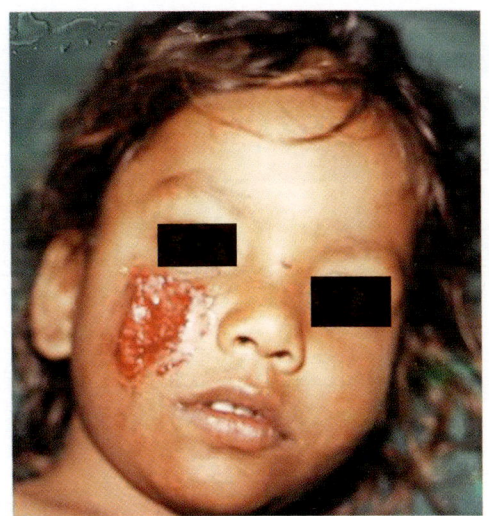

Fig. 13.1: Showing dog bite at face

Shaving of facial hairs in adult males is of utmost importance to prevent small puncture wounds being left unattended. Most soft tissue repair in adults can be performed under local anesthesia of 1% xylocaine and 1: 200000 adrenaline solution infiltrations. Knowledge of various blocks comes handy during wound repair. In children and agitated patients, general anesthesia is the best modality. While waiting for general anesthesia, bleeding is controlled and wound is properly cleansed and dressed. Repair can wait up to 24 hours without compromising the final results.

Facial abrasion must be cleansed with soap solution and examined for accidental tattoos, which may require gentle scrubbing with scrub brush and occasionally needle/scalpel are needed to scoop out deeply embedded particles. A layer of ointment is applied and wound is dressed if possible, otherwise it may be left open with regular cleaning of wound with soap solution and application of antibiotic ointment till wound heals. The new regenerated epithelium is protected from direct sunlight for 6–8 weeks to prevent hyper-pigmentation.

After the careful hemostasis, the soft tissues are repaired in layers. On the face the deep closure is usually achieved with vicryl. Suture thickness may be variable from 4/0 to 6/0 in facial injury repairs. The skin closure aims at approximation without strangulation using the minimal number of sutures. There are two viewpoints as to the best type suture for skin closure; many surgeons prefer fine 5/0 or 6/0 nylon or prolene; while those who use 6/0 silk claim better wound edge approximation and tension control. It is advisable to remove the silk sutures early in 3 to 4 days, the synthetic sutures can be left longer for up to 5 or 6 days. At times subcuticular sutures help in avoiding the suture marks on face and can be left longer (2 weeks or so). Alternative to suturing is the application of adhesive tape strips or cyanoacrylate glue especially in small superficial wounds. It is necessary to apply these with the same care as sutures, ensuring that all bleeding has been stopped and the skin is dry. Tincture Benzoin may be applied to the skin to aid adhesion.

Investigations

In all patients who have any suspicion of any bony injury radiograph must be taken in two planes. In the event of any cranial injury or complicated facial injury CT scan is mandatory. Bony detail obtained from the CT scan is of significant benefit in assessing the extent of injury and planning the treatment.

GENERAL PRINCIPLES OF WOUND MANAGEMENT

Conservation of tissue is the rule while dealing with facial trauma. Structures in the head and neck particularly face have excellent blood supply, and even the partially avulsed tissue will often survive with most tenuous attachment. The tissues of the face are unique and very difficult to replace without loss of cosmesis. Excision of wound edges and debridement should therefore be kept at minimum. All wounds should be cleansed by copious irrigation with normal saline, followed by an antiseptic solution, such as aqueous chlorhexidine gluconate (Hibitane). Saline solution is generally used to clean the oral cavity. All the wounds should be explored to find foreign bodies and the extent of damage to the structures like facial nerve or the parotid duct.

The surgical repair should take care of the anatomical landmark when structures like lip, ear, eyelid and nose margins are involved. Simple lacerations are closed in layers. Crush lacerations, where the skin had burst as a result of direct impact, often require minimal edge debridement. Contused, ragged edges must be conservatively debrided to form a single, well bleeding edge for approximation. These wounds swell significantly therefore skin should be approximated lightly. Large slicing injury or avulsion flaps on healing can be quite disfiguring due to entrapment of lymphatic and venous circulation in the "trap-door" scar. Small avulsion flaps, if possible may be excised completely and closed in layers. In case of larger flaps the thinnest, distal portion of the flap may be excised and multiple Z-plasties are incorporated in the closure to prevent trap dooring of the scar. Postoperatively, massage therapy and pressure garment is continued for several weeks to prevent lymphedema in the flap and excessive scar formation subsequently.

Occasionally close and parallel incisions can be converted to a single wound by excising the intermediate skin bridge and thus reducing the number of scar. Primary Z-plasty to change the direction of scar or to break the straight line of incision must not be attempted in haste. If required they may be performed after proper planning at the second stage during scar revision. Figure 13.2 shows poor surgical repair of facial laceration leading to wide scarring and cross hitching.

As stated earlier watching of anatomical landmarks in area such as eyebrow, eyelid margin and vermilion is essential. A preauricular wound may suggest at times the possibility of transection of facial nerve. Laceration over the cheek wound should be explored whenever there is suspicion of facial nerve injury.

Nerve stimulator is helpful in detecting the damaged nerve and preferably primary repair should be done. In case of damage to facial nerve, when injury is well outside the parotid gland and the identification of the branches is impossible, careful alignment of the soft tissue may produce satisfactory

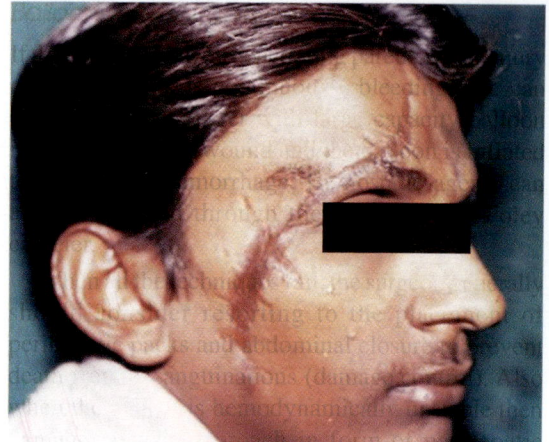

Fig. 13.2: Poor surgical repair leading to wide scar and cross hatching

result. Injury in cheek may damage not only the peripheral branches of the facial nerve and muscles of facial expression but also the parotid duct. The integrity of the parotid duct is mostly ascertained by cannulating it intraorally. If damaged, the duct should be repaired over a silicone stent, which should be retained for at least 3 weeks.

Laceration of the pinna require careful monitoring of the helical margin (Figs 13.3A and B). In crush laceration and burn of ear, careful follow-up is necessary to diagnose and treat chondritis. Pinna reconstruction is an extremely skilled job and even best reconstructive results are not at par with natural pinna. Therefore debridement must be conservative and all efforts must be made to preserve the remaining blood supply in an avulsed pinna. It is of utmost importance to avoid exposure of denuded cartilage in ragged and contused ear laceration. If this is not done, secondary infection may cause chondritis, which is difficult to treat. If the cartilage still remains exposed then the local postauricular or mastoid skin flap can be used for cover.

When pinna is totally severed, the possibility of reimplantation using microsurgical technique should be considered. Another option is to remove the skin cover and bury the cartilage framework in

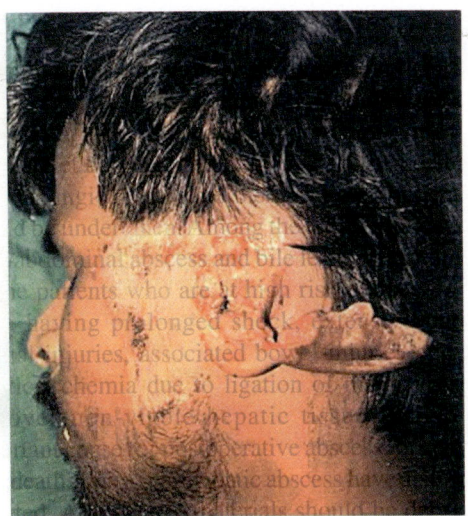

Fig. 13.3A: Laceration of pinna

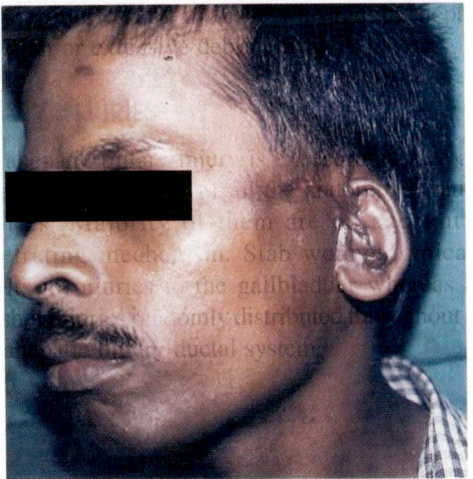

Fig. 13.3B: Photograph after repair

subcutaneous tissue over chest or abdomen, so that it can be used for future reconstruction.

The frontal impact to the nose may lead to the development of septal hematoma. Urgent drainage of this hematoma is essential in order to preserve the integrity of the septal cartilage.

Eyelid laceration: Examination of eyeball is important as the eyelid laceration may be associated with complete corneal tear. Trauma to eyeball may lead to hyphema, vitreous hemorrhage, retinal detachment, or a ruptured globe. Assessment of visual acuity is essential in all patients with evident trauma to eyelid. The correct management of eyelid injuries is important to avoid problems of epiphora and more importantly to avoid the ability to close the eye which may lead to corneal ulceration and potential loss of vision.

Eyelid laceration is repaired in layers, approximating the underlying muscles. Approximation of tarsal plate and meticulous closure of ciliary margin over "grey line" gives best result.

Human and Animal Bites

These bites present a number of problems. It carries heavy bacterial inoculum, which in the presence of inadequate drainage through punctuate wound, is likely to result in sepsis. These wounds must be cleansed, irrigated, minimally debrided and left open. Occasionally, it is possible to excise the whole wound and close it primarily.

Soft Tissue Loss

Soft tissue loss in the face varies from minor skin loss which can be treated by skin grafts or local flap. Massive injury, such as gunshot wounds require microsurgical tissue transfer. The wounds of the nose, lips and eyelids often gape alarmingly even after a single laceration giving a false impression of tissue loss. All such structures must be carefully returned to their rightful anatomical position and then sutured.

In case of definite tissue loss a thin split skin graft should be applied to the defect as a temporary measure or wound is left open with a dressing and patient is referred to a specialist service.

Nasal tip defects can usually be reconstructed with composite graft, ideally using the severed nasal part, but if necessary a graft from pinna can be harvested. If the loss is more extensive, a forehead flap reconstruction provides the best color and texture match. (Figs 13.4A to C)

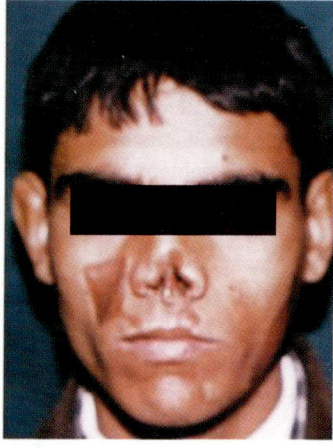

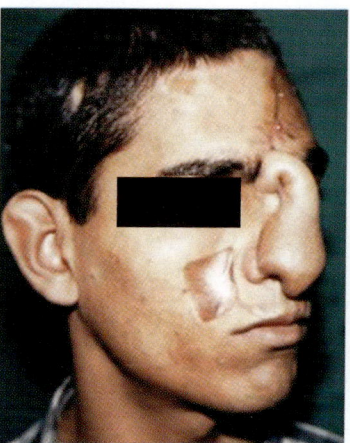

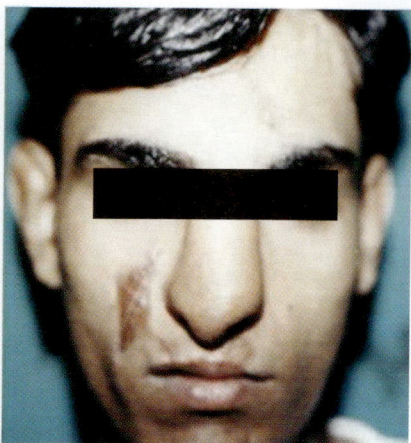

Fig. 13.4A: Soft tissue loss of nasal tip and columella

Fig. 13.4B: Reconstruction with forehead flap

Fig. 13.4C: Postoperative result

Lip defects can present challenging problems. Lacerations involving skin vermillion border require a very accurate apposition. Full thickness laceration should always be repaired in three layers—mucosa, muscle, and skin. Skin vermillion defect, which is too wide to allow for a wedge excision may be treated by re-establishing a new higher vermilion skin junction. A full thickness lip defect exceeding one third of the lip width can be repaired, using tissues of the opposite lip for reconstruction (Figs 13.5A and B).

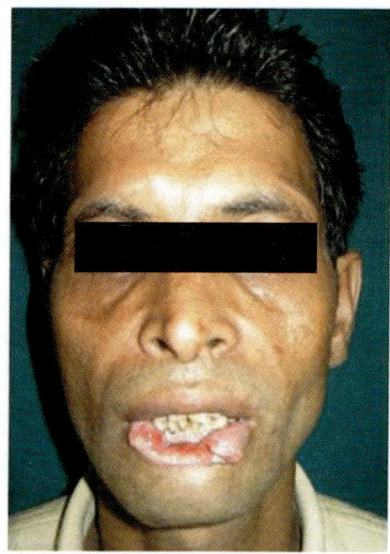

Fig. 13.5A: Human bite at lower lip

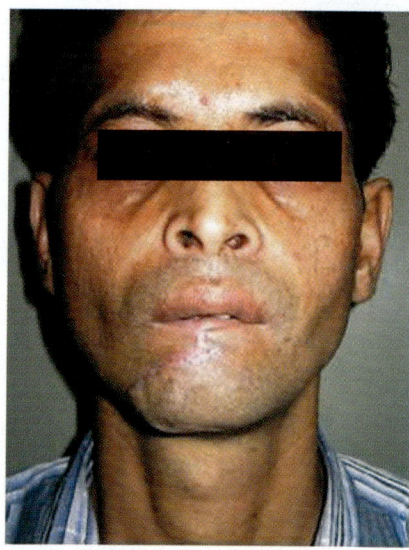

Fig. 13.5B: Reconstructed by bilateral lower lip advancement

Massive soft tissue loss of the face is often the result of gun shot wounds. In these patients early healing can be best achieved, fibrosis minimized and function maximized by using a free flap transfer.

One principle always be given priority that primary definitive repair produces the most satisfactory results; secondary correction of residual deformities are often disappointing.

Tetanus Prophylaxis

If the patient has not been previously immunized, intramuscular injection of tetanus immunoglobulin 250 units and tetanus toxoid 0.5 ml should be given in different sites. Two additional toxoid boosters at monthly intervals are necessary to complete the immunization. Previously immunized patients who received their last booster more than 10 years (or more than 5 years ago in tetanus prone wounds) should be given a single dose of tetanus toxoid.

Rabies Prophylaxis

It is always indicated following a bite from wild animal. A bite from a healthy domestic animal does not require immediate treatment, but the animal must be observed for 10 days. Bite from suspicious domestic animals requires treatment. If the patient has not been previously immunized, a single dose of human rabies immunoglobulin vaccine, 1 ml IM and five doses of human diploid cell vaccine, 1 ml IM on days 0, 3, 7, 14, 28 should be given. In addition immunoglobulin 10 units/kg is infiltrated subcutaneously at the site of bite.

Previously immunized patients who are found to have antibodies in their serum should receive a booster dose of vaccine.

Antibiotic Cover

Antibiotic cover is given in all human and animal bites, extensive injuries, associated skeletal trauma and grossly contaminated wounds.

Anesthesia

The choice of anesthesia is determined by a number of factors:

- The extent of tissue injury
- Presence or absence of associated bony injuries
- Age and general condition of the patient.

Most small lacerations can be managed by local infiltration. Regional nerve blockade (1% lignocaine with epinephrine 1:200,000) is useful in extensive injuries. General anesthesia will be necessary for extensive soft tissue injuries with associated facial fractures. Small children and un-cooperative patients are often difficult to manage under local anesthesia and require sedation or general anesthesia.

14 Head Injury

INTRODUCTION

Traumatic brain injury is the leading cause in all the traumatic deaths. Acute head injury is a progressive process. The initial and primary injury is caused by the mechanical deformation of brain tissue and blood vessel at the moment of the impact. The older terms cerebral concussion, cerebral contusion, and cerebral laceration only indicates the severity of injury of brain tissue, indicating the minor and major degree of injury. Secondary brain injury refers to delayed effects of events causing damage to neurons, axons and cerebral vasculature. The important causes of secondary injury are

- Hypoxia
- Hypotension
- Hypercarbia
- Hyperpyrexia
- Electrolyte imbalance.

Therefore the real magnitude of the head injury is determined always by total effects of primary and secondary brain injury. The injury to the brain is seen after direct penetrating trauma, acceleration or deceleration of brain within the rigid skull, or by a shearing injury.

ASSESSMENT OF INJURY

The severity of brain injury should rapidly be estimated by the level of consciousness, along with the presence or absence of lateralizing features including the pupillary changes and motor examination findings. Patients should be examined thoroughly and injuries to other organs should not be missed. The Glasgow Coma Scale (GCS) evaluates the level of consciousness based on eye opening, motor and verbal responses (Table 14.1).

Glasgow Coma Scale

GCS score is simple and objective and it can be repeated at certain intervals (Table 14.1). Even a fall of one or two indicates the deterioration and at times

Table 14.1 Elements of Glasgow Coma Scale						
	1	*2*	*3*	*4*	*5*	*6*
Eyes	Does not open eyes	Opens eyes in response to painful stimuli	Opens eyes in response to voice	Opens eyes spontaneously	N/A	N/A
Verbal	Makes no sounds	Incomprehensible sounds	Utters inappropriate words	Confused, disoriented	Oriented, converses normally	N/A
Motor	Makes no movements	Extension to painful stimuli	Abnormal flexion to painful stimuli	Flexion / Withdrawal to painful stimuli	Localizes painful stimuli	Obeys commands

warrants for neurosurgical intervention. In mild injury GCS is 12–13, whereas in moderate trauma it ranges from 9 to 12. GCS of 8 or less indicates severe head injury and coma. Along with the GCS one should also examine for the focal neurological signs and the signs of lateralization, including the pupil size and reaction, eye movements, limb movement and medullary function. While examining the pupil one must be aware that sometimes local tissue damage (globe) or drugs may affect the pupil size and reaction. Abnormal eye movement indicates depressed brain stem function, whereas abnormal limb movement indicates the local intracranial complication like hematoma causing hemiparesis or hemiplegia.

The GCS score should always be charted along with blood pressure, respiratory rate, pupillary size and pupillary response at the bed side to observe the patient's progress frequently.

RESUSCITATION

The initial evaluation is like any other injury and concerns of airway, breathing and circulation. Head injuries are at times associated with facial and cranial injury, therefore the airway must be secured. If required oral airway should be inserted. If this is inadequate, then endotracheal intubation is to be done to maintain better oxygenation and to prevent carbon dioxide retention.

While doing the initial assessment one should assess how urgent is the head injury? Are the facilities available is adequate for management of the patient or there is need to transfer to a higher center? Secondly, is patient stable to have the radiological investigation or urgent surgery is needed without having any fresh investigation. Patient should always be resuscitated and stabilized before transferring for radiological investigations, if at all required.

As for the respiratory condition, the plasma PCO_2 and PO_2 should be maintained at normal level. Abnormal PCO_2 level may cause reduction in blood flow to brain and subsequent cerebral ischemia. The circulation is judged by pulse rate, blood pressure and urine output of the patient. Isotonic fluid should

be started and initial blood loss should be corrected. All patients should undergo skull radiograph. CT scan of head if available should be done in the following conditions

- Loss of consciousness/amnesia
- Deep scalp laceration and contusion
- Palpable depressed fracture
- Patients having signs of lateralization
- Patients having seizures
- Evidence of focal neurological signs.

In case the patient needs to be transferred to specialized center one must ensure the following:
  a. Establishing the airway and respiration.
  b. Maintain cardiovascular stability
  c. Establish intravenous access
  d. Stabilize extracranial injury
  e. Ensure necessary monitoring during transit.

FURTHER MANAGEMENT

The aim is to prevent further damage of the already compromised brain. Deaths are due to prolonged hypoxia, uncontrolled raised intracranial tension (ICT) or untoward systemic events like cardio-pulmonary arrest, hypovolemia, DIC, electrolyte imbalance and renal failure. The two most important secondary phenomena that occur in progressive head injury are brain swelling with raised intracranial pressure and impaired autoregulation.

Raised ICT

Monitoring of raised ICT is very important. Generally the monitor is placed in subdural, intracerebral or intraventricular space. The ICT above 20 mm of Hg is abnormally high and above 40 mm Hg is considered to be dangerous level. Raised ICT is dealt by controlled ventilation, osmotherapy and CSF drainage if possible.

Controlled ventilation prevents hypoxic events, reduces the elevated ICT by maintaining low pCO_2 and it effectively provides adequate oxygen delivery to brain. It also helps to prevent the development of pulmonary edema. By controlled ventilation the hypoxia and hypercarbia is avoided as both lead to increased ICT.

Osmotherapy

Effective relief of raised ICT can be achieved by IV mannitol in large bolus (1–2 gm/kg 5 ml of 20% mannitol is equal to 1 gm). The effect is seen in 20 minutes and persists for four hours. Mannitol should never be used as substitute to surgical intervention. If a mass or hematoma had been excluded in CT, then mannitol can be used at regular intervals. During mannitol administration it is advisable to catheterize the patient to monitor the diuretic response of mannitol. IV furosemide 40 to 80 mg can be considered as an alternate therapy for rapid diuresis. The use of high dose of barbiturate therapy is indicated if hyperventilation, CSF drainage and osmotherapy fails and ICT is rising. The barbiturate administration may lead to fall in the mean arterial pressure to 80 mm of Hg and so the ICT. Mannitol should not be used in acute stage following injury unless the possibility of intracranial hematoma has been excluded. Also it should never be used as a diagnostic test to differentiate between hematoma and edema.

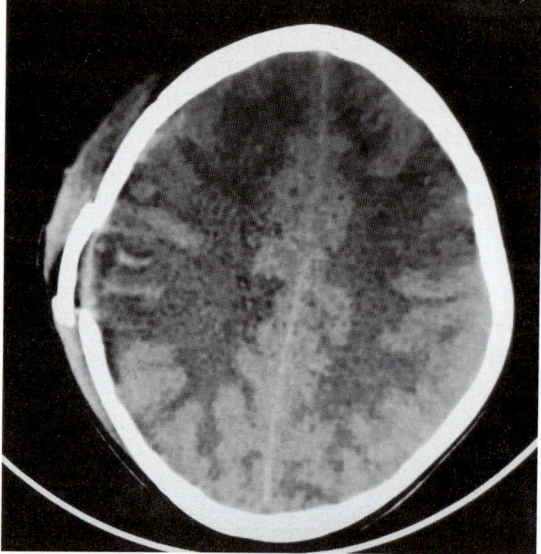

Fig. 14.1: Depressed fracture of parietal bone with contusion of brain

Autoregulation

Maintenance of normal blood pressure is mandatory because in severe injury there is always impairment of cerebral autoregulation. It is always necessary to restore the normal volume and correct the hypovolemia. Central venous pressure (CVP) is maintained at 6–8 cm of water and urine output at 30–60 ml/hr. Electrolyte imbalance should always be avoided and also the over hydration to avoid cerebral edema.

Patients of moderate to severe injury should have prophylaxis for epileptic seizures and phenytoin is the drug of choice.

FRACTURE IN HEAD INJURY

Fracture could be linear involving the entire of the skull or it can be depressed (Fig. 14.1), where at times bone fragments are driven below the inner table. These fractures may be complicated with extradural, subdural, intracerebral hematoma,

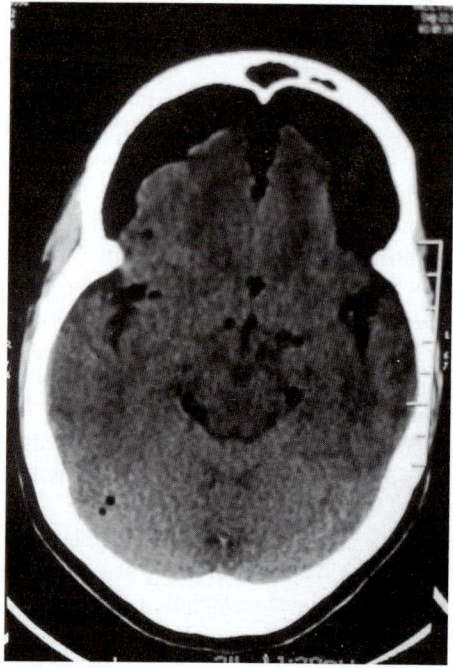

Fig. 14.2: Pneumocephalus

pneumocephalus (Fig. 14.2), seizures, infections, obstruction of major venous sinuses. Sometimes fracture at the base of the skull may lead to CSF fistula.

ACUTE EXTRADURAL HEMATOMA (EDH)

Acute extradural hematomas are generally due to injury to anterior and posterior branches of middle meningeal artery and at times due to injury to meningeal veins and dermal sinuses. Such situations are generally found when one sustains fracture at temporoparietal region of skull. The hematoma formed extradurally slowly enlarges to the size sufficient to cause rise in intracerebral pressure and causes critical distortion of midbrain at tentorial hiatus. This results in distortion of the consciousness and also dilatation of the pupil on the side of hematoma. After sometime contralateral pupil is also dilated when the stage of decerebrate rigidity settles. CT scan shows the collection of blood in the extradural space. It appears biconvex (lentiform), hyperdense, does not cross the suture line and common location is temporal fossa (Fig. 14.3). Patient may present as unconsciousness throughout or unconsciousness followed by consciousness and then unconsciousness (lucid interval).

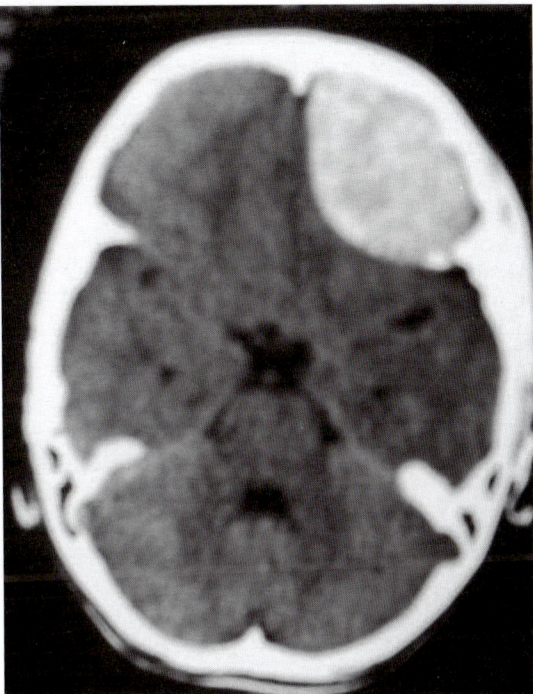
Fig. 14.3: Extradural hematoma

Treatment

If patient is asymptomatic with GCS score 14–15, on CT-scan volume of lesion is less than 25 ml and no midline shift, then a conservative approach is ideal.

If patient is symptomatic, with GCS score less than 13, patient should be subjected to burrhole evacuation of hematoma under general anesthesia.

SUBDURAL HEMATOMA (SDH)

After severe head injury there is commonly a thin layer of blood clot in the subdural layer of the brain. Tearing of bridging cortical vessels leads to the formation of subdural hematoma. There is always a severe primary brain damage so there is persisting loss of consciousness and lucid interval is very unusual. These patients deteriorate sooner than extradural hematoma. In CT scan lesion appears hyper dense, crescent shape and does not cross fax but may cross suture lines (Fig. 14.4). Mostly SDH is associated with unilateral hemisphere ischemia, cerebral edema, contusions, and intracranial hematoma and diffuse axonal injuries. If SDH is associated with laceration of underlying lobe and intracranial bleeding it is called complicated SDH. These patients present with severe degree of neurological impairment and have the potential for further deterioration; hence neuro-intensive care is needed.

Although the presentation and management of acute subdural hematoma may be similar to acute extradural hematoma, but tends to differ in certain aspects:

- Due to severe brain damage, there is persisting loss of consciousness—Lucid interval is unusual.

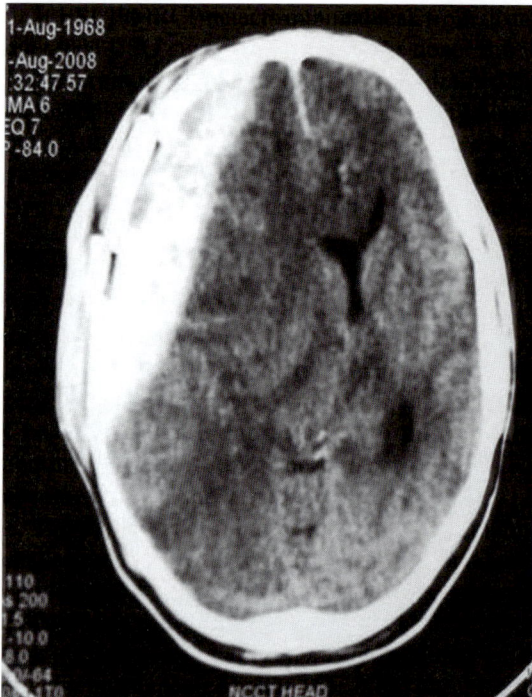

Fig. 14.4: Subdural hematoma

- Deteriation occurs sooner than extradural hematoma.
- Hematoma may be "coup" side of the blood or contrecoup, opposite side.
- Hematoma is often more extensive.

Treatment

Burr-hole surgery with craniotomy and evacuation of clot becomes necessary.

CONTUSION AND INTRACEREBRAL HEMATOMA

Pure cerebral contusions are fairly common. Their frequency has become much more apparent as the quality and number of CT scans has increased. The vast majority of contusions occur in frontal and temporal lobes. The distinction between contusions and traumatic intracerebral hematomas remains somewhat ill-defined. The classic salt and pepper lesion is clearly a contusion while a large hematoma clearly is not. However, there is a grey zone and contusions can over a period of hours or days evolve into intracerebral hematoma. Management of intracerebral hematoma is dependent on the neurological status of patient. Rapid surgical evacuation and decompression is recommended if there is a significant mass effect (i.e. midline shift greater than 5 mm).

DIFFUSE BRAIN DAMAGE

When the high velocity shearing force affects all components of brain particularly axons and the cerebral vasculature, it causes diffuse brain damage. Minor strains cause transient stretching of the axons and cerebral vasculature. The typical clinical manifestation of minor diffuse injury is momentary loss of consciousness followed by recovery (concussion injury). Axons subjected to severe strain may undergo immediate disruption. This process is termed as primary axotomy. However, some may undergo progressive swelling followed by secondary axotomy from hours to several days after injury. The injured axons can repair of its own and ultimately regain a normal appearance. Microscopic foci of axonal damage are seen in white matter of parasagittal cortex, corpus callosum, thalamus and brainstem. These changes can be seen on MRI. NCCT is not sensitive enough to detect these changes.

ROLE OF SURGICAL INTERVENTION IN HEAD INJURY

It has definite place in dealing with rapidly deteriorating patient due to increased intracranial pressure on account of extradural, subdural and intracerebral hematoma. If circumstances permits even a general surgeon may perform burrhole but ideally patients should be referred to the neurosurgical department, if facility exists. In absence of CT scan the burrhole should be done at the site of fracture in the skull or on the same side where the pupil had dilated first. Ideal placement of exploratory

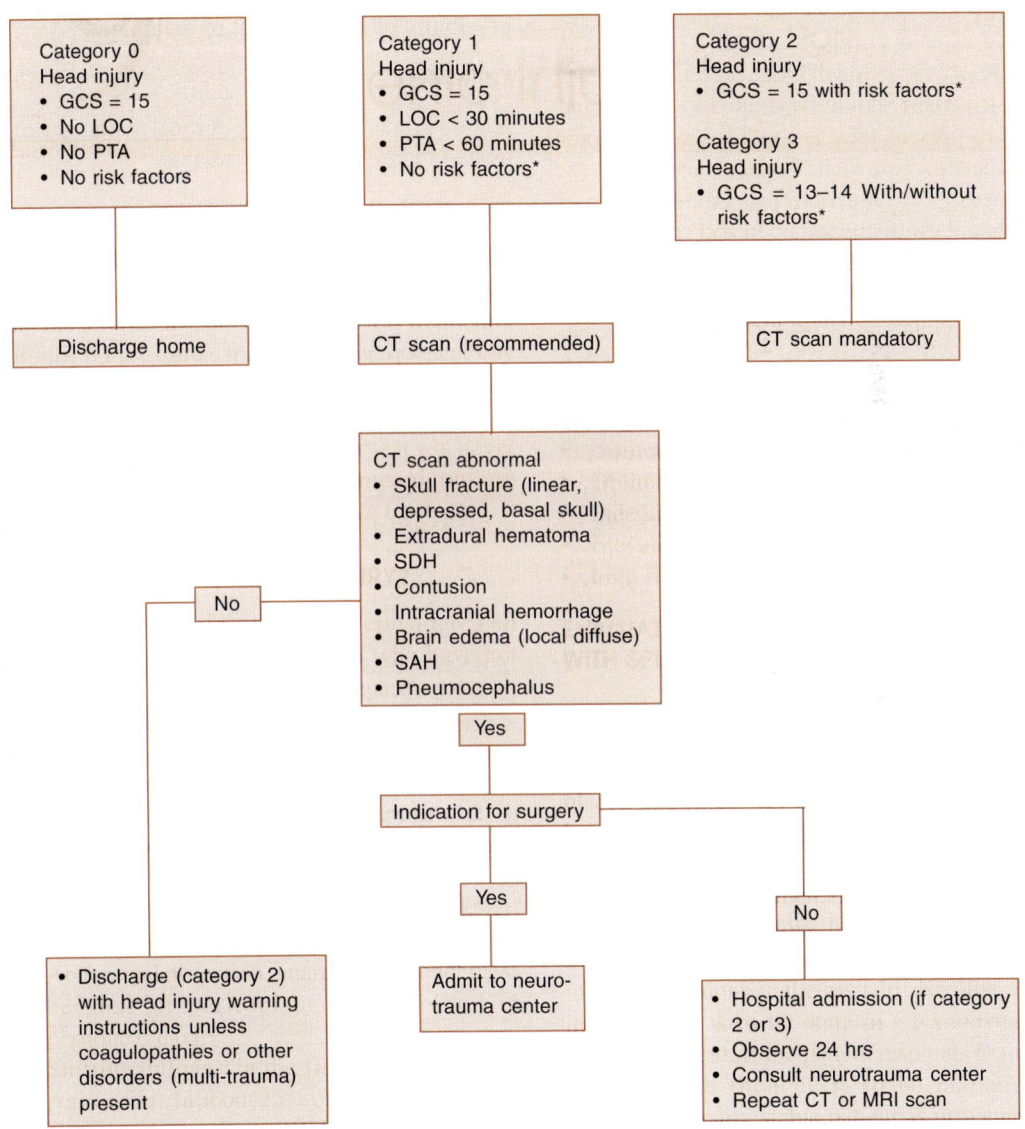

**Flow chart 14.1: Management protocol of head injury
(PTA—post-traumatic amnesis; LOC—loss of consciousness)**

Category 0
Head injury
• GCS = 15
• No LOC
• No PTA
• No risk factors

Category 1
Head injury
• GCS = 15
• LOC < 30 minutes
• PTA < 60 minutes
• No risk factors*

Category 2
Head injury
• GCS = 15 with risk factors*

Category 3
Head injury
• GCS = 13–14 With/without risk factors*

Discharge home

CT scan (recommended)

CT scan mandatory

CT scan abnormal
• Skull fracture (linear, depressed, basal skull)
• Extradural hematoma
• SDH
• Contusion
• Intracranial hemorrhage
• Brain edema (local diffuse)
• SAH
• Pneumocephalus

No

Yes

Indication for surgery

Yes

No

• Discharge (category 2) with head injury warning instructions unless coagulopathies or other disorders (multi-trauma) present

Admit to neuro-trauma center

• Hospital admission (if category 2 or 3)
• Observe 24 hrs
• Consult neurotrauma center
• Repeat CT or MRI scan

burrhole should be at temporal region. Patient is taken under general anesthesia and with help of Hudson brace or with help of electric craniotome burrhole is made. After opening the skull an overall evaluation of hematoma is done. If a significant extradural clot is present it should be evacuated with the help of fine rubber tubing. Dura in such cases are not to be opened up. Dura should be opened when there is evidence of subdural hematoma which appear as bluish collection beneath the dura, which should be evacuated after opening the dura. If burrhole is inadequate in evacuation of clot a larger craniotomy (osteoplastic flap) should be done and if bleeding vessels are present they are tackled with bipolar cautery. Bleeding from bone is stopped by bone wax. Before closing the burrhole procedure if dura is opened then it should be left open and covered with gelatin sponge. The incision is closed in two layers for the galea and for the skin. If the site of the first dilating pupil or the site of the fracture or the external trauma coincides with the hematoma then a contralateral burrhole need not be done. But if the external trauma, bruising or swelling are opposite to the first dilating pupil then compression is likely to be contrecoup. In that condition a benefit of second burrhole should to be given at the site of external injury.

Flow chart 14.1 shows the management of head injury patients.

COMPLICATIONS OF HEAD INJURY

CSF Leakage

Fracture with laceration of dura is responsible for dural tear. In the beginning CSF leak is not apparent due to edema which blocks the dural tear, but it manifests when the edema settles. Conservative management with antibiotics is done, but if it fails to stop the leakage then the dural defect should be repaired surgically.

Infection

Infection is usually seen along with CSF leakage. Suitable antibiotics should be given to avoid the possibility of development of meningitis.

Epilepsy

It is associated with severe cortical contusion and is treated by use of anti convulsants.

CHRONIC SUBDURAL HEMATOMA

Due to venous hemorrhage in the subdural space some patients present after several weeks with features of gradual deterioration in mental functions and fluctuating level of consciousness. CT and MRI detect the characteristic hematoma. Treatment is the evacuation of the clot by burrhole.

Key Points
• Through clinical examination including the bony and visceral injury to be done
• Airway clearance along with normal breathing and circulation to be maintained first
• Controlled ventilation to be done to maintain normal level of PCO_2 and PO_2
• Evaluation of GCS and focal neurological signs should be observed at regular intervals
• In deterioration of GCS and evidence of cerebral compression urgent CT should be warranted
• CT showing the evidence of clot (extradural, subdural) evacuation to be done by burhole
• In the absence of hematoma the rise in the ICT should be dealt by osmotherapy, controlled ventilation, CSF drainage and if required barbiturate

15 Neck Trauma

Many vital structures (e.g. airway, major vessels, nerve plexus and spinal cord and esophagus) are present in the neck in a very compact space. Hence, injury to the neck can cause considerable damage. Potentially lethal injuries in patients with neck trauma may not have clear symptoms and signs initially and can be easily overlooked.

Neck trauma may be caused by penetrating or blunt trauma. Most of the penetrating injuries are caused by gunshot or injuries by knife. Blunt trauma to the neck typically results from motor vehicle crashes but it also occurs with strangulation or blows from the fists or feet.

For purpose of evaluation of injuries, neck is divided into three zones (Fig. 15.1).

Zone I: It is the area of the neck between the thoracic inlet and the cricoid cartilage. Structures at risk in this zone are the great vessels (subclavian vessels, brachiocephalic veins, common carotid arteries, aortic arch, and jugular veins), trachea, esophagus, lung apices, cervical spine, spinal cord, and cervical nerve roots. Signs of a significant injury in the zone I region may be obscured and may not be clearly apparent on inspection of neck.

Zone II: It is the mid-portion of the neck, between the cricoid cartilage to the angle of the mandible. Important structures in this region include the carotid and vertebral arteries, jugular veins, pharynx, larynx, trachea, esophagus, cervical spine and spinal cord.

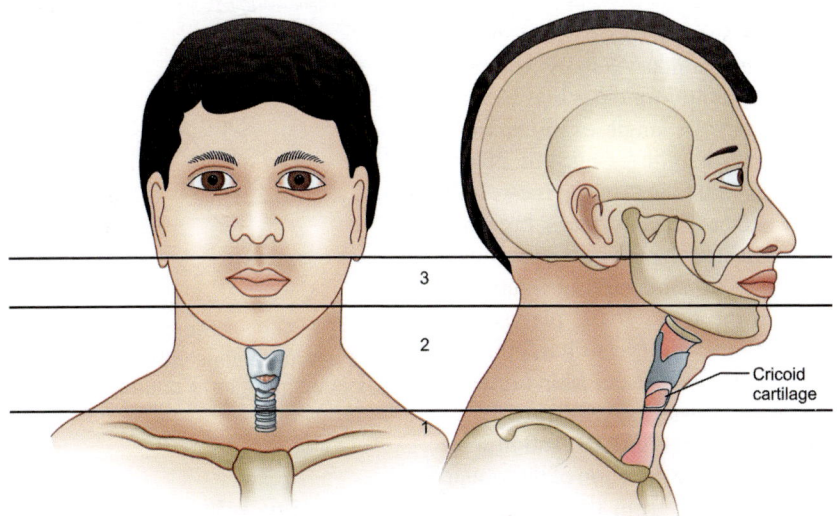

Fig. 15.1: Zones of neck injury

Zone II injuries are likely to be the most apparent on inspection and tend not to be occult.

Zone III: It characterizes the superior aspect of the neck and is bounded by the angle of the mandible and the base of the skull. Salivary and parotid glands, esophagus, trachea, vertebral bodies, carotid arteries, jugular veins, and major nerves (including cranial nerves IX-XII) are present in this zone. Injuries in zone III are difficult to access surgically.

EVALUATION OF PATIENTS WITH NECK TRAUMA

Initial management is according to the ATLS guidelines. Special points regarding neck trauma are:

History

Mechanism and time of injury is inquired from the patient and people accompanying the patient. In cases of penetrating trauma information regarding the weapon used is obtained. Symptoms relating to the aerodigestive tract (dyspnea, hoarseness, dysphonia, and dysphagia) and CNS problems (paresthesias, weakness and plegia) are asked.

Examination

It includes primary survey, resuscitation and secondary survey. On secondary survey, the neck should be examined carefully for clues that indicate damage to vital contents. A single examination is not sufficient as signs of injuries may be absent initially. Laceration or wound in the neck is carefully evaluated to see whether the platysma is breached or not (Fig. 15.2). Breach of platysma serves as a marker for presence of possible serious injuries of structures present in the neck. If the platysma is violated, location of the injury is characterized regarding whether it is present anterior (anterior triangle) or posterior (posterior triangle) to the sternocleidomastoid muscle (Fig. 15.3) and in what zone the injury is present. The direction of the wound tract (e.g. toward or away from the midline or clavicle) is determined. If the platysma is intact in

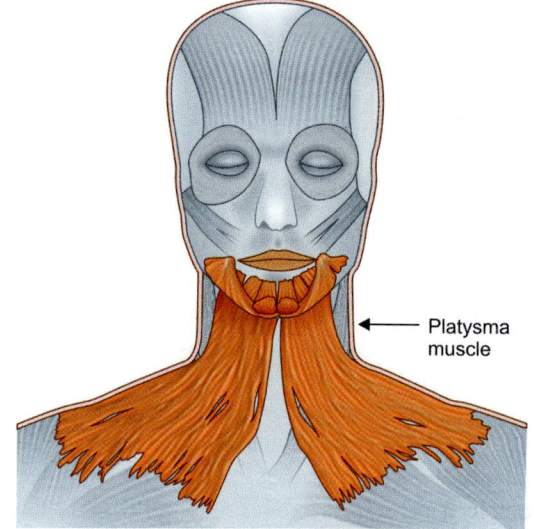

Fig. 15.2: Platysma—Intact platysma rules out significant injury in penetrating injuries

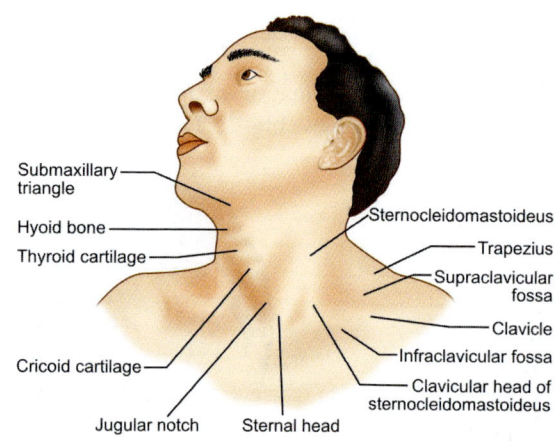

Fig. 15.3: The anterior triangles of neck lies in between the sternocleidomastoid muscles (SCM) and mandible. Posterior triangle is bounded by SCM, clavicle and trapezius muscle

penetrating injury, significant injury to the underlying structure can be safely ruled out.

Signs of Arterial Injury

Definite signs of an arterial injury include a large expanding hematoma, severe active or pulsatile bleeding, shock unresponsive to fluids, signs of cerebral infarction and diminished or absent distal pulses. It is important to remember that clinical findings are lacking initially in many patients with an arterial injury of the neck. Carotid artery injuries are associated with severe hemorrhage or hematoma and contralateral hemiparesis because of cerebral infarction.

Signs of Pharyngeal or Esophageal Injury

Signs of aerodigestive injuries include hematemesis, odynophagia, mediastinal emphysema subcutaneous emphysema, and blood in the saliva or in the aspirate of a nasogastric tube.

Signs of Larynx or Trachea Injury

Voice alteration, hemoptysis, stridor, drooling, sucking, hissing, air frothing or bubbling through the neck wound, subcutaneous emphysema and/or crepitus, hoarseness, dyspnea, and pain with tongue movement implies injury to the epiglottis, hyoid bone, or laryngeal cartilage.

Signs of Spinal Cord or Brachial Plexus Injury

Brachial plexus injuries sustained from blunt trauma generally involve the upper nerve roots (C5–C7), diminishing the capacity of the upper arm while sparing strength and sensation of the lower arm. Complete transection of the brachial plexus results in paralysis of the upper limb.

Complete transection of the spinal cord will result to quadriplegia with loss of all motor, sensory, and reflex function below the level of injury. Hemisection of the spinal cord will result in Brown-Séquard's syndrome causing ipsilateral motor paralysis with contralateral sensory deficits. Horner's syndrome (ipsilateral miosis, enophthalmos, anhidrosis) results from disturbances of the stellate ganglion. Neurogenic shock is a diagnosis of exclusion and is characterized by persistent bradycardia despite hypotension. Hypoxia and hypoventilation can follow disruption of phrenic innervation to the diaphragm.

Signs of Cranial Nerve Injuries

- Facial nerve (cranial nerve VII)—Drooping of the corner of the mouth
- Glossopharyngeal nerve (cranial nerve IX) —Altered gag reflex
- Vagus nerve (cranial nerve X, recurrent laryngeal nerve) —Hoarseness of voice
- Spinal accessory nerve (cranial nerve XI) —Inability to shrug a shoulder
- Hypoglossal nerve (cranial nerve XII) —Deviation of the tongue with protrusion.

Thoracic duct injury is asymptomatic and it is either detected incidentally during surgical exploration or manifests later as milky discharge from the neck wound.

IMAGING STUDIES

Cervical X-ray

It is done in all cases of blunt and penetrating neck trauma to evaluate for subcutaneous emphysema, fractures, displacement of the trachea, and presence of a foreign body (e.g. pallets, sharpnels).

Chest Radiography

It is done in all cases of zone I injury or in cases where thoracic injury is suspected. Chest is evaluated for hemothorax, pneumothorax, widened mediastinum, mediastinal emphysema, and foreign bodies.

Other Investigations

Additional investigations are done in stable patients if specific system injuries are suggested by the history or physical examination or initial tests. These investigations include—CT, MRI, color flow Doppler studies, contrast studies of the esophagus, interventional angiography, and endoscopic images.
- Conventional angiography or computed tomographic angiography are done to see for vascular

injury. Partial or complete occlusion, pseudo-aneurysm, dissection, and traumatic arteriovenous fistulas can be detected. Indications for angiography are (1) All stable patients with penetrating injury of the neck in zone I and III. (2) Stable patients with Zone II injury with signs of arterial injury.

- MRI is done for evaluating patients exhibiting neurological impairment with minimal or absent abnormalities on plain radiographs of the cervical spine.
- Gastrograffin study is done to see for suspected pharyngoesophageal leak. Though a normal study does not always exclude esophageal injury.
- Laryngoscopy, bronchoscopy, pharyngoscopy, and esophagoscopy is done for assessing the aerodigestive tract.

MANAGEMENT OF SPECIFIC INJURIES

Vascular Injury

Bleeding from the neck wound is temporarily stopped by external compression. Unstable patient with signs of arterial injury should be taken for immediate neck exploration after initial resuscitation. Stable patients with signs of arterial injury in zone II and all patients with zone I and III penetrating injury should undergo angiography. Angiography delineates the nature of injury and should be done prior to exploration provided that the patient is stable. There are chances of arterial injury even in absence of obvious signs in zone I and zone III penetrating injury and for this reason angiography should be done in all cases of zone I and III penetrating injury.

Carotid Artery Injury

Injury site is delineated and partial injury to the vessel is repaired with 4–O or 5–O prolene suture. If a subadventitial hematoma is noted at operation, a vertical arteriotomy is made over the area and inside of the vessel inspected for injury. If a portion of internal carotid artery is resected or there is loss of segment then saphenous vein graft is used as an interposition graft.

Exposure of high internal carotid injures can be very difficult. Additional exposure can be obtained by anterior subluxation of mandible. Other procedures that can improve the exposure are—detachment of the sternoclavicular muscle from the mastoid process, division of digastric muscle and occipital artery.

Bleeding from the distal internal carotid artery adjacent to the skull can be very difficult to manage and it can be best controlled by inserting a Fogarty balloon catheter into the distal segment and then inflating the balloon. The catheter can be left in place for several weeks until the vessel is thrombosed.

Vertebral Artery Injury

Treatment options for vertebral artery injury include surgical ligation, transcatheter embolization and simple observation. The proximal part of vertebral artery is relatively easy to expose as it takes off from the subclavian artery. However, exposure of the distal part is difficult and these are best managed by angiographic embolization.

Internal Jugular Venous Injury (IJV)

It is most frequently injured vessel in the neck. If laceration of the internal jugular vein is found during the exploration of the neck then it is repaired by 4–O or 5–O prolene suture. However, if condition of the patient is unstable and control of bleeding is required to be achieved quickly, then IJV can be ligated provided the opposite IJV is normal.

Laryngo-Tracheal Injury

The ideal way to establish airway is gentle orotracheal intubation in an awake patient. Sometimes tube cannot be negotiated through the injury site and one should be prepared to do immediate cricothyroidotomy or tracheostomy in case the orotracheal intubation fails.

Simple tracheal lacerations that do not detach a tracheal ring can be repaired without a tracheostomy (Figs 15.4A and B). More severe disruptions (gunshot wound directly to the trachea) imply more

need only observation (small laceration, shallow laceration, nondisplaced fracture) and those that require a thyrotomy or open fracture reduction and mucosal approximation. A soft laryngeal stent may be needed for badly macerated mucosa.

Injury of Pharynx and Esophagus

Pharyngeal or cervical esophageal injury is approached through an incision along the anterior border of sternocleidomastoid muscle on the side of injury. When an injury is found the tear is debrided and repaired in two layers with interrupted vicryl suture. If the mucosa is not clearly visible then a Foley catheter is inserted through the defect and withdrawn after inflating the balloon. This brings the mucosa up in the operating field. A flap of local muscle like omohyoid is used to buttress the repair. This is particularly important when there is an associated tracheal injury.

In cases of delayed diagnosis of esophageal injury, one can attempt a closure after thorough debridement if no necrosis or gross suppuration is present. If repair is not feasible then cervical esophagostomy is done.

Morbidity and mortality rates in esophageal injury are greatly increased if significant injury is missed for more than 12–24 hours.

Thoracic Duct Injury

Thoracic duct injury is rare but can occur in left sided zone I and II neck injuries. If found injured on neck exploration, it should be ligated. However, most of the times injury is missed on initial exploration and it presents as either a cervical fistula, localized swelling (chyloma), or as chylothorax.

Thoracic duct injury is confirmed by staining the drainage fluid with Sudan III dye and confirming the presence of fat globules. Patients are managed initially with adequate drainage and total parenteral nutrition, and/or modified diet contains medium chain triglycerides and little or no long chain fatty acids. If the discharge does not settle in 2–3 weeks then surgical ligation of thoracic duct is done.

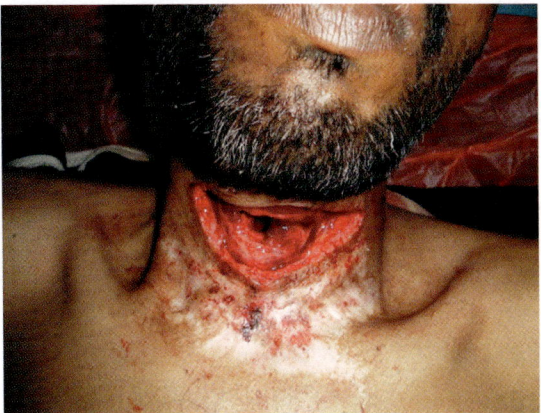

Fig. 15.4A: Cut throat injury with tracheal laceration

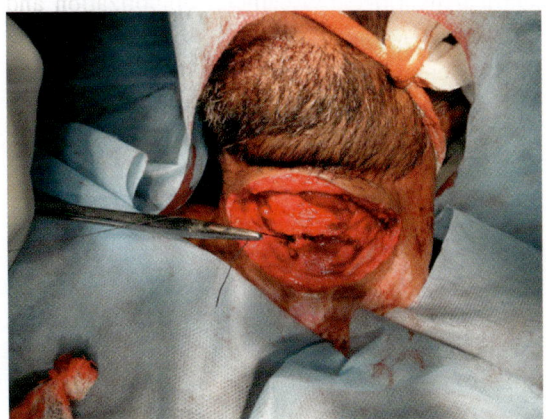

Fig. 15.4B: Repair of trachea with interrupted sutures

soft-tissue injury and a 6-week tracheostomy either below or through the tracheal injury is the safest procedure.

Laryngeal mucosal lacerations from penetrating injury should be repaired early (within 24 hours). The time elapsed before repair has an effect on both airway stenosis and on voice. Significant glottic and supraglottic lacerations and displaced cartilage fractures need surgical approximation. Endoscopy and CT will differentiate between the patients that

16 | Initial Management of Spinal Injury

INTRODUCTION

Spinal cord injuries (SCI) are among the most serious injuries resulting in a permanent loss of function and paralysis and yet retaining a keen and alert mind. The psychological, emotional and financial implications of such a catastrophe are tremendous on the patient, family and community. Incidence of spinal cord injury excluding those who die at the scene of accident is approximately 40 cases per million populations in United States. While in the absence of national spinal cord injury registry in India, the exact incidence is not known but incidence expected to be 20–40 per 100,0000 population. The most common causes of injury are motor vehicle accidents, falls, assault sports and recreational activities and work-related accidents.

Those who sustain acute spinal cord injury are not willing to accept anything but a cure for such a devastating injury. It is essential for the clinician to understand pathophysiology of acute spinal cord injury for management of the patients. Severity of the spinal cord injury and final outcome depends upon the mechanism of the injury, the severity of the force applied and the duration of the spinal cord compression. Experimental and clinical studies on spinal cord injury revealed that there was a spectrum of pathologic appearances that evolved over the initial days following injury. This led to the concept that injury process is a result of both primary and secondary insults. While the primary injury is not amenable to any pharmacological intervention, the effects of secondary insult can be mitigated if treatment is started early enough.

PRIMARY MECHANISM

Primary mechanism of cord injury can be due to four kinds of mechanical forces:

a. Impact with persisting compression, e.g. fractures, dislocations, and disk herniations.
b. Impact with no persisting compression, e.g. hyperextension injuries.
c. Distraction, e.g. hyperflexion injuries.
d. Laceration/Transection: Penetrating injuries, fracture dislocation.

SECONDARY INJURY

Mechanisms that may be involved are:

a. *Systemic shock:* Profound hypotension and bradycardia follows cord injury and may compromise an already damaged cord.
b. *Local microcirculatory damage:* This may occur due to mechanical disruption of capillaries, hemorrhage, thrombosis and loss of autoregulation.
c. *Biochemical damage:* This may occur due to excitotoxin release (glutamate), free radical production, arachidonic acid release, lipid peroxidation, eicosanoid production, cytokines and electrolyte shifts.

All these factors (along with edema) lead to loss of energy producing ability with consequent loss of impulse transmission, cell swelling, and membrane lysis and cell death.

The predictive value on the functional prognosis of the complete or incomplete status of the neurological injury is considerable. The injury is sometimes associated with "spinal shock" in the first few hours that follow the trauma, which is characterized by an abolition of all reflexes below the cord lesion. This state is transitory and disappears with the installation of cord automatism. One can assert with certainty the complete status of the injury only after resolution of the spinal shock, usually after several days.

The incomplete status of the cord injury allows classifying it among one of the different clinical syndromes which also gives an idea of the functional recovery potential. Several well defined syndromes have been described in connection with spinal cord injury

- *Central cord syndrome*: Occurs almost exclusively in the cervical region, produces a sacral sensory sparing and typically more important a motor impairment in the upper limb than the lower limb—a manifestation of damage to the central areas of the cervical cord as in whiplash injuries.
- *Syndrome of Brown-Séquard:* A unilateral lesion that produces a motor and proprioceptive impairment on the same side as the injury, and a loss of thermal and pain sensitivity on the contralateral side—a manifestation of cord hemisection.
- *Anterior cord syndrome:* An injury that produces a variable motor, thermal and pain impairment, but preserves the proprioception.
- *Conus medullaris syndrome:* Injury to the cone and lumbar roots, that produce areflexia to the bladder and lower limbs. The sacral reflexes may be preserved—a manifestation of damage to the terminal cord, common in thoraco-lumbar fracture-dislocation.
- *Cauda equina syndrome:* Lumbosacral nerve root injury, with areflexia of the bladder and lower limbs.

The goals for the emergency physician are to establish the diagnosis and initiate treatment to prevent further neurologic injury from either pathologic motion of the injured vertebrae or secondary injury from the deleterious effects of cardiovascular instability or respiratory insufficiency.

CARE OF ACUTE SPINAL CORD INJURY CAN BE DIVIDED INTO

i. Prevention
ii. First aid treatment
iii. Early management of acute spinal cord injury.

PREVENTION OF ACUTE SPINAL CORD INJURY

Since we do not have a cure for acute spinal cord injury at the moment, prevention of spinal paralysis should be aimed for at any cost. Prevention of acute spinal cord injury will require (a) education and behavior changes of high-risk-takers; (b) implementation of stricter laws by the government; (c) designing safer vehicles and use of seatbelts, airbags, etc.; (d) discouraging violence in sports; (e) implementation of strict rules regarding safety at work.

PRE-HOSPITAL MANAGEMENT

The management of the patient with a potential SCI necessitates a rigorous approach on the very place of the accident. At the site of injury resuscitation is aimed at airway maintenance, adequate oxygen saturation, restoring blood pressure to acceptable limits, preventing bradycardia, done simultaneously to prevent any ischemic damage to the already compromised cord. Recognize the need to stabilize and immobilize the spine on the basis of mechanism of injury, pain in vertebral column or neurological symptoms. Brief motor examination is to be done if feasible. Patients is transported to the hospital with a cervical hard collar on a hard backboard, if there are not available stabilize head and neck with sandbags or rolled blankets. Commercial devices are available to secure the patient to the board. The patient should be secured so that in the event of vomiting the backboard may be rapidly rotated 90 degrees while the patient remains fully immobilized in neutral position of spine. Early medical management from the pre-hospital period (role of the medical rescue units), has made great progresses in term of survival and prevention of neurological worsening. Immobilization is to be maintained during transportation.

SIGNS ASSOCIATED WITH POSSIBLE CERVICAL INJURY

• Respiratory compromise
• Physical signs of injury above clavicle
• Weakness in any or all limbs
• Neck pain and stiffness
• Abnormal head position
• Pain/tingling/numbness in arms or hands
• Priapism.

DRUG TREATMENT

Since 1990 a series of trials were done to evaluate drugs to prevent secondary neuronal damage in patients with acute spinal cord injury.

Methyl Prednisolone Sodium Succinate (MPSS)

It prevents post-traumatic lipid peroxidation, prevents destruction of neuronal and microvascular membranes and improves neurological function.

When the treatment is initiated within 3 hours of injury, MPSS is administered for 24 hours and patients who are initiated on treatment between 3 and 8 hours need 48 hours administration.

Dose

Bolus: 30–mg/kg-body weight to be given in 30 ml of water over 15 minutes.

Maintenance: 5.4 mg/kg/hour for 23 to 48 hours. This total dose of methylprednisolone is to be mixed in 100 ml of water and given at a rate of 5 ml per hour. There is no apparent beneficial effect if it is given after 8 hours, and practice of prescribing drug in dosages like 500 mg twice a day or eight hourly has nothing to commend it. In other conditions when MP is to be administered it has to be in doses of 30 mg/kg body weight given by IV infusion over a period of 30 minutes, which can be repeated 6 or 8 hourly if required. Although the National Acute Spinal Cord Injury Studies (NASCIS II and NASCIS III) have shown modest improvements in recovery of patients with SCI with high dose steroids, this therapy has only a modest functional impact in these patients. NASCIS II has found 5.1% improvement in motor score in 45.9% of patients. It is generally believed that rate of complications is not high enough to withhold the use of MP in SCI. MP is safe and reviews have not provided any support to the notion that high dose MP increases risk for mortality or major morbidity. Complication of therapy with MP include non-healing or delayed healing of wound, wound infection, GI bleeding, wound complications, pulmonary complications (pneumonia), avascular necrosis of femoral head, decubitus ulcer, urine infection, deep vein thrombosis, pulmonary embolism, hyperglycemia and sudden death.

Tirilazide Mesylate

The NASCIS III study, whose results have been published in 1997, compared the administration of methyl prednisolone for 24 and 48 hours to the administration of tirilazide mesylate 2.5 mg/ kg every 6 hours for 48 hours.

GM-1 Gangliosides

Gangliosides are purified extracts from bovine brain. Experimentally it has been shown that they favor neuronal growth after a traumatic injury or in the course of an ischemic accident. The evidence available does not support the use of gangliosides treatment to reduce death rates in SCI patients. No evidence has yet emerged that gangliosides treatment improves recovery or quality of life in SCI patients.

Calcium inhibitors, especially Nimodepin have been studied extensively in animals. Cell protecting agents and inhibitors of NMDA receptors are under evaluation.

The only medication that showed a possible positive effect in randomized clinical studies is high dose methylprednisolone.

HOSPITAL MANAGEMENT

Upon arrival at the hospital, the interaction with the medical team that has managed the initial gathering transmits information regarding the precise circumstances of the accident, timing, clinical examination data, treatment done, presence of combined initial injuries that are frequently met. The neurological examination (ASIA scoring) will be repeated at admission and during the clinical course to get an idea of evolution towards improvement or aggravation.

The American Spinal Injury Association recommends use of the following scale of findings for the assessment of motor strength in SCI

- 0 No contraction or movement
- 1 Minimal movement
- 2 Active movement but not against gravity
- 3 Active movement against gravity
- 4 Active movement against resistance
- 5 Active movement against full resistance.

RADIOLOGICAL INVESTIGATIONS

The screening examination of injured spine consists of conventional radiographs. Additional imaging modalities available include computed tomography (CT), Magnetic Resonance Imaging (MRI), Myelography either alone or combined with CT and evoked potentials.

Plain X-ray is the initial radiograph of choice and it is the foundation on which the diagnosis of spinal injury should be made. Thoracic spine is relatively fixed structure with mobile segments at either end. Therefore, fracture tends to occur at cervico-thoracic and thoraco-lumbar junction. On suspicion of neck injury it is essential to have lateral radiograph with shoulders pulled down to reveal all seven cervical vertebrae (Fig. 16.1). If the lower cervical vertebrae are not seen on the lateral film oblique views of the lower facets may be informative. Others views that may be obtained include oblique, open mouth and flexion-extension views. As high velocity injuries have a high incidence of spinal fractures at more than one level, radiographs should be taken not only of the suspected injury site but also of whole of the spine.

MRI is the procedure of choice for the diagnosis of acute injuries of the soft tissue of spine and spinal

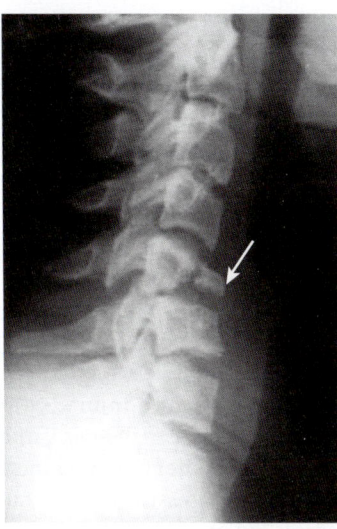

Fig. 16.1: Teardrop fracture of C5 vertebra on lateral radiograph

cord (Fig. 16.2). MR demonstrates fragment retropulsion, spinal canal compromise, spinal cord injury (edema, swelling, compression, hemorrhage), ligament rupture, vertebral mal-alignment and intervertebral disk herniation.

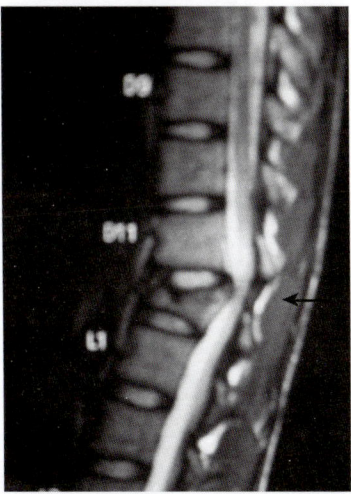

Fig. 16.2: MRI showing fracture of D12 with cord compression

CT still plays a significant role as the initial examination in acute spine injury patients. CT demonstrates bony pathology exquisitely. Posterior neural arch fracture, vertebral comminuted fracture, facet relationship and details of retropulsed fragments (intersegment fracture and rotation) are best detected by axial CT.

Most applicable evoked potential in spinal injury is somatosensory evoked potentials (SSEP). When the spinal cord is severely damaged the impulses are not conducted across the point of injury and the evoked response is absent. This then corroborates the finding of a complete cord injury. Of course, in incomplete cord injury cases there is variation in the waveform and often a delay in conduction of the evoked response. Progressive normalization of the SSEP antedates the appearance of clinical recovery and therefore the test can be of prognostic value.

MANAGEMENT OF THE INJURED SPINE

The opinion over the most appropriate method of managing spinal injuries is controversial and opinion is divided between operative and non-operative management. However, operative management results in decreased hospital stay, early mobilization of patients, decompression of neural tissue and prevention of spinal deformities.

Goals of Treatment

a. To prevent further neurological damage
b. To improve neurological function where possible
c. To restore spinal stability and alignment
d. To rehabilitate the patient to the maximal potential of his disability.

Early Management of Acute Spinal Cord Injury

This can be divided into five categories, all of which are equally important

I. General Treatment
II. Treatment of associated injuries
III. Treatment of spinal fractures with neurological deficit

IV. Prevention and treatment of complications related to spinal cord injury
V. Rehabilitation.

General Treatment

Every effort should be made to stabilize the patient by avoiding hypoxia, hypovolemia, hypotension, and hypothermia. In addition, drugs to minimize neurological deficit should be administered as soon as possible as every hour counts. Nervous tissue is exceptional in its lack of supporting fibrous network as compared to other organs. Secondly due to its lipid nature, spinal cord is susceptible to ischemia resulting into necrosis.

Treatment of Associated Injuries

High speed injuries such as motor vehicle accidents can result in multiple traumas consisting of serious head injury, chest injuries, vascular injuries, fracture of long bones, abdominal injury and peripheral nerve injuries. Some of these injuries can be life-threatening. Others will add more disability and will ultimately influence the functional outcome of spinal cord injury patients. Complex injuries in addition to prolonging patients stay in critical care unit will prevent patients from participating in active rehabilitation program.

Treatment of Spinal Injuries

Several conditions can lead to delays in the diagnosis of spinal injury. These include:
• Head injury with loss of consciousness
• Alcohol intoxication
• Associated fractures or multiple injuries.

Neurological symptoms are usually manifestation of significant instability, although some burst fractures with neurological deficits may be relatively stable. A history of progressive neurological deterioration is another indication that spine is unstable.

Most of patients following stable spinal injuries have no neurological deficits but some may develop quadriplegia or paraplegia. Spinal injuries are treated non-operatively if the fracture is relatively stable and spinal column is well aligned, i.e. < 30° kyphosis < 30° loss of vertebral heights, <10° scoliosis. The patient is kept in bed till pain is relieved. Ambulation with collar/ brace after 6–12 week is allowed. These patients require regular neurological assessment and radiographic studies. Patients with progressive neurological deterioration or radiological evidence of progressive disruption of spinal column must be managed surgically. If late deformity develops fusion is carried out.

Diagnosis of Instability
- A history of violent forces affecting the spinal column with associated neurological symptoms or progressive neurological deficit.
- Physical findings indicative of rotational forces as well as local features in the spine representing posterior element disruption.
- Presence of neurologic signs.
- Radiographic evidence of anterior, middle and posterior spinal column disruption as evident by fracture patterns and displacement (angular and translational).
- Presence of two or more adjoining fractures.

Management of Unstable Spinal Injuries: Surgical stabilization is the mainstay of treatment.

There are generally two indications for early surgery:
- Progressive neurological deficit is the absolute indication of surgery and requires emergency decompression of neural tissue.
- A neurologically incomplete patient with deterioration of neurological injury and demonstrable compression of spinal cord on MRI, should be decompressed with removal of all bone and disk fragments to provide an optimum environment for spinal cord recovery.

Other Indications of Surgical Intervention
- *Dural laceration:* Dural lacerations should be identified and repaired. In dorsolumbar injuries, portion of cauda equina may herniate through dural defect and following the process of healing and scarring, chronic pain syndrome may occur.
- *Fracture-dislocation:* Unstable spine that can not be reduced closely and is causing compromise of neurological tissue should be stabilized.

- *Open Spinal injuries.*

Surgical approach depends on anterior or posterior compression. Surgical management focuses on the specific injury encountered, which can be classified as involving:

1. Anterior column or vertebral body primarily;
2. Posterior column with pedicle, facet or lamina injury; or
3. Both columns. Spinal realignment generally is emphasized.

This begins with application of cervical tongs and serially increasing traction until normal spinal alignment is achieved and bony compression is reduced.

In cervical spine injury, if injury primarily involves the anterior column, a standard anterior approach is used to allow anterior decompression and reconstruction with either allograft or autograft and stabilization with locking plates. Posterior approach is indicated when the pathoanatomy involves posterior elements and is basic midline approach with muscle retraction to the lateral aspect of facets bilaterally. Occasionally a dual approach is necessary to remove offending anterior compression prior to reduction followed by posterior stabilization. These global injuries are quite unstable and patient benefits from both anterior and posterior reconstruction.

In dorsolumbar region, burst fracture involves anterior and middle columns. Pedicle screws and anterolateral plates stabilization by posterior approach is simple and helps in decompression of the cord and corrects kyphosis effectively. Posterior approach is also important in cases of dural laceration. Anterior surgery achieves more complete and reliable decompression with interbody strut graft fusion which is important in the biomechanics of the spinal functioning. Anterior surgery has better advantage of canal clearance than posterior pedicle and plates systems. Anterior surgery alongwith posterior pedicle screw stabilization gives patients rigid stabilization, effective canal decompression, allows early rehabilitation with shorter hospital stay and early return to work.

Prevention of Complications Related to SCI

Acute spinal cord injury results into alteration of many body functions. Every effort should be made to prevent complications that could result in serious morbidity or even death.

a. Respiratory complications
b. Thrombo-embolic complications
c. Genitourinary complications
d. GI complications
e. Autonomic dysfunctions
f. Pressure sores
g. Spasticity and contractures
h. Pain
i. Psychological and behavior disorders.

Respiratory Complications

Due to paralysis of intercostal and abdominal muscles, occurrence of bronchitis, pneumonia leading to respiratory failure is not uncommon with cervical cord injury. Similarly respiratory complications can arise in high level paraplegics and other spinal cord injured patients who sustain trauma to chest. Treatment of respiratory complications requires vigorous chest physiotherapy, suctioning and appropriate antibiotics. Ventilatory support and tracheostomy become necessary for those spinal cord injured patients who need prolonged respiratory support and intubation.

Thrombo-embolic Complications

Spinal cord injury patients are at high risk of developing deep vein thrombosis and pulmonary emboli which could lead to death. Prevention of deep venous thrombosis requires use of antiembolic stockings and early mobilization. In absence of any contraindication anticoagulation therapy with low molecular weight heparin should be implemented.

Genitourinary Complications

Cystitis and pyelonephritis are common in acute spinal cord injury patients. Prevention of GU complications require adequate fluid intake, avoidance of urinary retention and periodic examination of urine for bacterial growth. In addition urological review to assess the status and function of kidneys and lower urinary tract must be undertaken on a regular basis. Emptying of bladder on a regular basis with intermittent catheterization is an acceptable method of management of neurogenic bladder in most spinal cord centers around the world.

Autonomic Dysfunctions

Postural hypotension: Fainting due to drop in both systolic and diastolic blood pressure can occur in acute phase. This can be prevented by gradual mobilization to the upright position, using pressure gradient stockings and abdominal binder.

Autonomic dysreflexia: This is a syndrome characterized by elevated blood pressure, pounding headache, flushing, excessive sweating and piloerection followed by bradycardia. It is seen in patients with spinal cord paralysis at D6 or above. It can be triggered by distended bladder, fecal impaction, infection, pressure sores or tight clothing. Elevated blood pressure needs immediate attention. Management of autonomic dysreflexia consists of elevating patient's head and treatment of precipitating cause. In addition, administration of drugs such as nitroglycerin, nifedipine, beta blockers become necessary. Failure to receive appropriate treatment for the autonomic dysreflexia could lead to serious complications like ventricular fibrillation, cardiac arrest or cerebral hemorrhage.

Pressure Sores

Prevention of pressure sores requires daily inspection, maintaining clean and dry skin and lubrication of skin over the bony prominences. A patient with spinal cord injury must be turned every 2–3 hours when in bed. Common sites for pressure sores are coccyx, ischial tuberosity and greater trochanter. Treatment of pressure sore depends on grading of ulcer. Superficial and clean ulcer will heal with conservative treatment. Deep and infected ulcers will need debridement and surgery.

Spasticity and Contractures

Contractures can be prevented by daily range of movement exercises as well as by proper positioning. Moderate to severe spasticity can interfere with patients functions and cause skin breakdown. Lioresal, Dantrium or Tizandine alone or in combination have proven to be useful. In addition hydrotherapy and use of equipment such as standing frame becomes necessary.

Pain

Almost all patients with spinal cord injury experience pain in acute phase. Nociceptive pain can be controlled by use of analgesics, narcotics and physical modalities. For neurogenic and deafferentation pain, use of antidepressants or anticonvulsant medications becomes necessary. Other methods of pain management such as relaxation technique, hypnosis, acupuncture, use of cordotron or TENS machine can be implemented.

Psychological and Behavior Disorders

Acute spinal cord injury resulting into permanent loss of function can lead to depression, anger, frustrations and feeling of hopelessness. Lack of physical, psychological and financial support can lead to isolation and dependence on drugs and alcohol. Death due to suicide is more common in spinal cord injured patients as compared to general population. Prevention of suicide will need collective effort from healthcare providers, psychotherapists, vocational counselors and use of antidepressant medications.

Every spinal cord injury patient must find a reason to live and get out of bed every morning.

17 Burn: Initial Management

Burn injuries are one of the most devastating kinds of trauma worldwide, affecting all age groups. Although advances in modern medicine has helped immensely in improving the mortality in severe burns and the post-burn quality of life but its catastrophic influence on human life is still a challenge for medical/paramedical staff and the patient who has to come to terms with psychological as well as physical scars and chronic disability for his entire life. The management of burn is a multidisciplinary approach including burn surgeon, physician, nurses, physiotherapist, nutritionist, and psychological support staff. This chapter addresses the emergency room management of acute burns along with general understanding of burns and its management.

ETIOLOGY OF BURN

- Thermal Burn
  - Flame
  - Scald
    - Liquid
      - Spill
      - Immersion
    - Grease
    - Steam
  - Contact
- Electrical Burn
  - Contact
  - Flash
- Chemical
  - Acid
  - Alkali.

BURN PREVENTION

More than two million burn injuries occur each year in India and the fact that 90% of these injuries are preventable, effective social, educational and legislative efforts can hugely impact the incidence of burn which is almost endemic in Indian subcontinent. In India, burn is mainly a problem of low socio-economic strata with clustered living, illiteracy and poverty being its major determinant. Few safety measures that can be taken to prevent burns are as follows

- Do not ignite if there is smell of gas leakage
- Safety certification of gas stoves and kerosene stove
- Avoid cooking on floor
- Avoid wearing loose clothing in kitchen
- Plugging electric sockets when not in use to prevent children from electrocution
- Burn safety programs directed at school aged children
- Legislative measures
- Strict punishment norms for products non complying to safety standards
- Severe punishment for culprits involved with homicidal acid attack.

PATHOPHYSIOLOGY OF BURNS

Cutaneous burn is caused by application of heat to the skin. Severity of burn injury is related to the rate at which heat is transferred from the heating agent to the skin. This depends upon specific heat of the agent, duration of contact and conductivity of the local tissue.

Methods of Heat Transfer

- *Conduction:* Hot, Solid object in direct contact with skin
- *Convection:* Hot spills/Steam (Scald)
- *Radiation:* Sun burn.

The Physiologic Response to Burn Injury

Burn injury results in both local and systemic response.

Local Response

Skin being a barrier to the transfer of heat energy from the source to the underlying tissues, suffers most of the damage. Burn causes coagulative necrosis of the epidermis, dermis and the underlying tissues. This is the main mechanism of cellular damage due to flame, scald and contact burns (thermal burns). Chemical and electrical burns in addition to it also cause direct injury to the cellular membrane.

Jackson in 1947 described three zones of cutaneous injury due to burns, which are three dimensional in nature.

Zone of Coagulation This is the central zone corresponding to the area of maximum damage. In this zone there is irreversible tissue loss due to coagulative necrosis of the constituent proteins.

Zone of Stasis The area surrounding the necrotic central zone is characterized by decreased tissue perfusion. It is a potentially salvageable area associated with vascular damage and vessel leakage. The main aim of burn resuscitation is to increase tissue perfusion in this zone and prevent any damage becoming irreversible. Adverse wound environment such as infection or edema and hypotension can convert this to zone of coagulative necrosis.

Zone of Hyperemia Outermost zone is characterized by vasodilatation due to inflammatory response to injury. This zone of tissue invariably survives unless there is severe infection or prolonged hypotension.

Systemic Response

The body response to major burn is profound involving all major body systems. It manifests as Systemic inflammatory response syndrome (SIRS) involving metabolic, cardiovascular, neuro-endocrine, respiratory, gastrointestinal and renal system. This along with infection setting in 48–72 hrs after injury is the major cause of mortality and morbidity in burn patients.

Cardiovascular System

The inflammatory response to burn results in release of local and systemic mediators (histamine, serotonin, PGs, thromboxane) which disrupt vascular endothelial integrity, causing increase in vascular permeability. This leads to leakage of intravascular proteins and fluid to the interstitial space. The increase of interstitial oncotic pressure further drives fluid from intravascular compartment to the interstitial compartment. Hence plasma volume is severely depleted (**hypovolemia/burn Shock**) while there is marked increase in interstitial fluid (**tissue edema**). The edema formation is generalized involving local as well as distant organs. The endothelial permeability starts getting restored within 8–12 hours after burn injury and is completely restored by 24 hours. This is the rationale behind using maximum fluid resuscitation in first 8 hours after injury. **Decreased cardiac output** owing to depressed myocardial contractility, systemic hypotension and peripheral/splanchnic vasoconstriction is completely restored with resuscitation.

Respiratory System

Inflammatory mediators cause pulmonary **hypertension** and **edema** along with **bronchoconstriction** and in severe case **adult respiratory distress syndrome** can occur.

Neuroendocrine System

Hypermetabolism follows severe burn injury. This is in response to the release of catabolic hormones, namely catecholamines, glucagon and glucocorticoids. The basal metabolic rate increases up to three times the resting rate. Glyconeogenesis, glycogenolysis and lipolysis cause hyperglycemia leading to "diabetes of the burn". Proteolysis is increased with accelerated breakdown of muscle protein during the catabolic phase. Therefore recommended protein intake is 2 g/kg/day for patient with severe thermal injury.

Other Systemic Effects

- Suppression of cellular immunity
- Impairment of neutrophil function
- Systemic clotting disorder
- Early destruction of RBCs
- Decreased renal blood flow
- Oliguria, ATN, renal failure
- Gastrointestinal mucosal atrophy
- Decreased blood flow to gut, gastric mucosal ulcers, increased permeability to bacteria.

AN UNDERSTANDING OF BURN DEPTH AND BURN WOUND HEALING

A proper assessment of burn depth is the cornerstone of burn management and the standard technique till date is clinical assessment of the burn wound. The subjectivity of the observer and the dynamic nature of burn wound (an initial superficial burn may become deep due to hypovolemia, infection or poor dressing technique) limits the accuracy of clinical assessment to 50–70% in various studies. As modern management of acute burn has evolved from non-operative, conservative management to surgical excision of deep burns, accurate assessment of burn depth is essential before subjecting the patient to excisional surgery. Various techniques: Biopsy, thermography, MRI have been reported to accurately quantify burn depth but laser Doppler is one of the most promising and is gaining popularity amongst burn surgeons.

Assessment of burn depth is also important at places where non-operative treatment is the mainstay of burn management. Excisional surgery in burns require a state-of-the-art burn center with dedicated support from anesthetist, blood bank, ICU which is lacking in most developing countries including India.

A fair understanding of burn depth helps in understanding the natural progression of the injury process and the functional outcome. Burns are classified according to the increasing depth of the injury. Skin consists of epidermis and dermis along with epithelium-lined skin appendages: sweat gland, hair follicles and sebaceous gland (Fig. 17.1).

In cases of first-degree burn (epidermal burn) the dead epidermis desquamates and is replaced by a new layer within few days without any scarring. As the depth of burn increases, the superficial layer of dermis (papillary dermis) also gets involved leading to second-degree superficial burn.

In Second-degree superficial burn upon shedding of dead dermal tissue, the epithelial cell from the skin appendages namely hair follicle, sweat gland and sebaceous gland proliferate and cover the thinned out dermis. As most of the appendages are located in deeper layer of dermis, they are relatively unharmed in Second-degree superficial burn and therefore the proliferation is faster and the wound heal in two weeks. Scarring is minimal except sometimes altered pigmentation of the regenerated skin.

Second-degree deep burn extends into the deeper layer of dermis, i.e. reticular dermis. As most of the epithelial appendages are also burned, healing is slow, from few remaining skin appendages. The remaining dermis is even thinner and there is more of scarring. The wound heals in three to six weeks with scarring, hypertrophy and depigmented patches. Thus at centers, where excisional surgery is the norm, deep burns with projected healing time of more than three weeks are routinely excised and grafted.

Third-degree burn involves whole of the dermis, and thus there is no chance of epithelial regeneration from skin appendages. This requires excision and grafting but if managed conservatively will heal by epithelialization from the margin and contraction of the wound bed leading to contractures and non-healing ulcers.

Fourth-degree burn involves not only skin but also underlying subcutaneous tissue and deeper

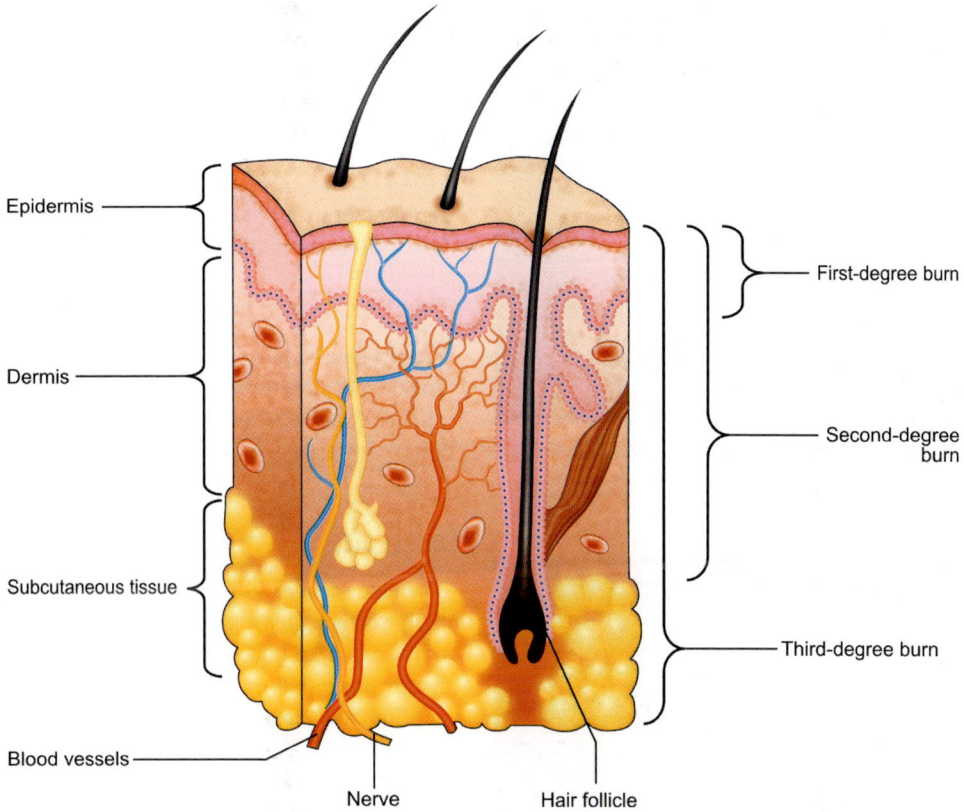

Epidermis

Dermis

Subcutaneous tissue

Blood vessels

Nerve

Hair follicle

First-degree burn

Second-degree burn

Third-degree burn

Fig. 17.1: Layers of skin

structures. If managed conservatively, it will heal with contractures and deformities.

First-degree Burn

As mentioned previously, these burns involve only the epidermis. They are painful, erythematous and blanch to the touch. Example includes periphery of second-degree burn, sunburn or minor scald burn. These burns heal within 3 to 5 days with no scarring.

Second-degree Superficial Burn

Second-degree superficial burns include epidermis and papillary dermis. They are painful, moist pink in appearance, blanch to touch form blister (Fig. 17.2) and heals in 10 to 14 days without scarring.

Second-degree Deep Burn

Deep dermal burns are pale, dry, do not blanch to touch, painful to pin prick and may or may not form blister (Fig. 17.3). If not excised and grafted, the wound heal in 3 to 7 weeks with scarring and hypertrophy. Long-term measures such as pressure garment, physiotherapy and massage is required.

Third-degree Burn

Third degree or full thickness burn involves all layers of the dermis. They are characterized by white or

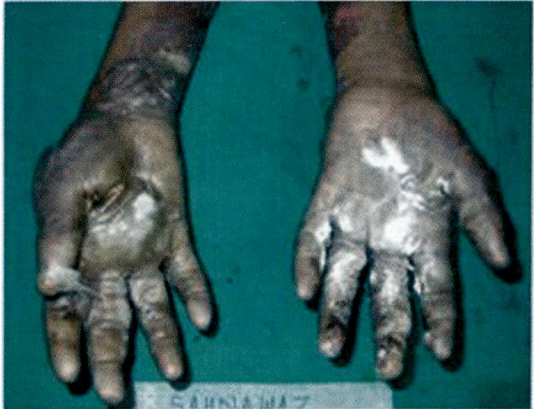

Fig. 17.2: Second-degree superficial burn

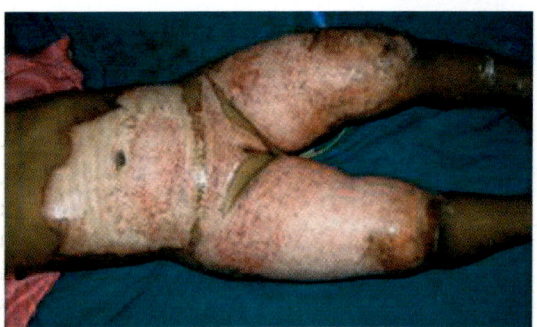

Fig. 17.3: Second-degree deep burn

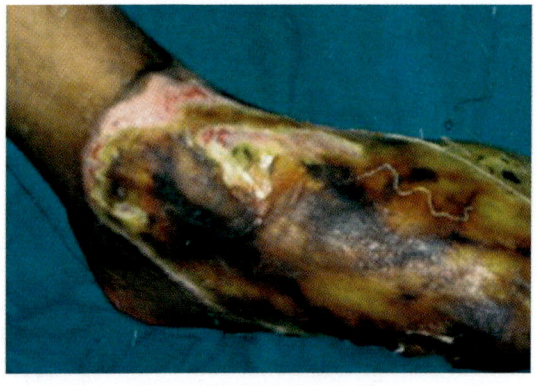

Fig. 17.4: Third-degree burn

black, firm, leathery eschar which is painless, dry and has visible thrombosed veins (Fig. 17.4). The eschar is nothing but coagulated, denatured dermis which if not surgically excised and grafted, separates from underlying viable tissue by subeschar abscess. After eschar separation, underlying viable tissue requires grafting or else wound will heal by epithelialization and contractures.

Fourth-degree Burn

Fourth-degree burn involves skin, subcutaneous fat and deeper structures. The burns almost always have charred appearance, many a time requiring amputation of the involved extremity. The most common example is high voltage electrical burn.

BURN SIZE

The size of burn in proportion to the patient's total body surface area is the most important determinant of the extent of injury. It is the single, most important factor in predicting burn related mortality, complications and the prognosis of the patient. All fluid resuscitation formulae and subsequent nutritional requirement calculation is directly related to the size of burn.

There are numerous formulae mentioned in literature to calculate the size of burns but the most common and simplest one is the Wallace's Rule of Nines (Fig. 17.5). Although this gives a fairly accurate estimation of burn size, more accurate charts—Lund and Browder, Berkow's are more precise in burn estimation especially in children where proportion of head, limbs and trunk is different from that of adults (Fig. 17.6).

FLUID RESUSCITATION IN BURNS

Fluid resuscitation is started while primary/secondary assessment is being carried out in all patients having critical or moderate burns. Resuscitation is started with Ringer's lactate at 1 lit/ hr in adults and 20 ml/kg/hr in children. This rate should be continued until a formal calculation of the resuscitation need is done. There is no ideal

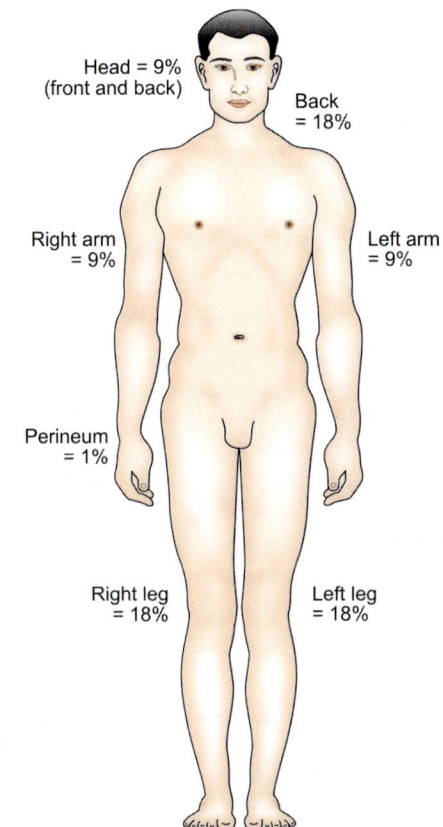

Head = 9%
(front and back)

Back
= 18%

Right arm
= 9%

Left arm
= 9%

Perineum
= 1%

Right leg
= 18%

Left leg
= 18%

Fig. 17.5: Wallace's Rule of Nines for calculating size of burn

8–12 hours after injury. The rate of fluid infusion has to be critically balanced, too little fluid will cause hypoperfusion and whereas too much will help only in increasing the edema due to increased capillary permeability. The increased capillary permeability is the result of inflammatory response to burn injury and starts getting restored 6–8 hrs after injury and returns to near normal by 24 hours. The composition of the interstitial edema fluid is similar to plasma, i.e. the capillary permeability is increased both for water and proteins. If colloid resuscitation is done during these initial hours, most of it will be lost to the interstitial space and will help only in aggravating the edema. This is the reason behind most resuscitation formulae advising colloid resuscitation only after 24 hrs.

The most commonly used formula for fluid resuscitation is the Parkland formula. This is a pure crystalloid resuscitation and recommends 4 ml/kg/% TBSA of Ringer's lactate over the first 24 hrs, with one half of this amount administered in first 8 hrs and the remaining half in next 16 hrs. As mentioned previously, formula is only a guide for fluid resuscitation. The protocol has to be modified in cases of electrical burns, burn shock, elderly patients and inhalation injury. There are numerous other formulas for fluid resuscitation. However, discussing all of them is beyond the scope of this chapter.

MANAGEMENT OF BURN

First Aid

The management of burn starts right at the scene of the event. The aim is to stop the burning process, shift the patient to open space, cool the burn, cover and promptly shift the patient to hospital.

Extinguish the Fire

Removal of heat source is primary. Flame should be doused with water or by covering with blanket or rolling the patient on ground. Care must be taken to avoid further injury to the patient and to avoid rescuer from getting burnt. Burnt clothing should be removed at the earliest but adherent clothing

resuscitation regimen and many are in use. All fluid resuscitation formulae are only guidelines and volume and rate of infusion has to be altered according to various physiological parameters being monitored, most importantly, urine output. All patients having critical and moderate burns must be catheterized and hourly urine output must be monitored and charted. The goal of fluid resuscitation must be a urine output of 1 ml/kg/hr in children and 0.5 ml/kg/hr in adults.

The aim of fluid resuscitation is to prevent systemic hypotension caused by general shift of fluid from intravascular compartment to the interstitial space. This shift is most pronounced during first

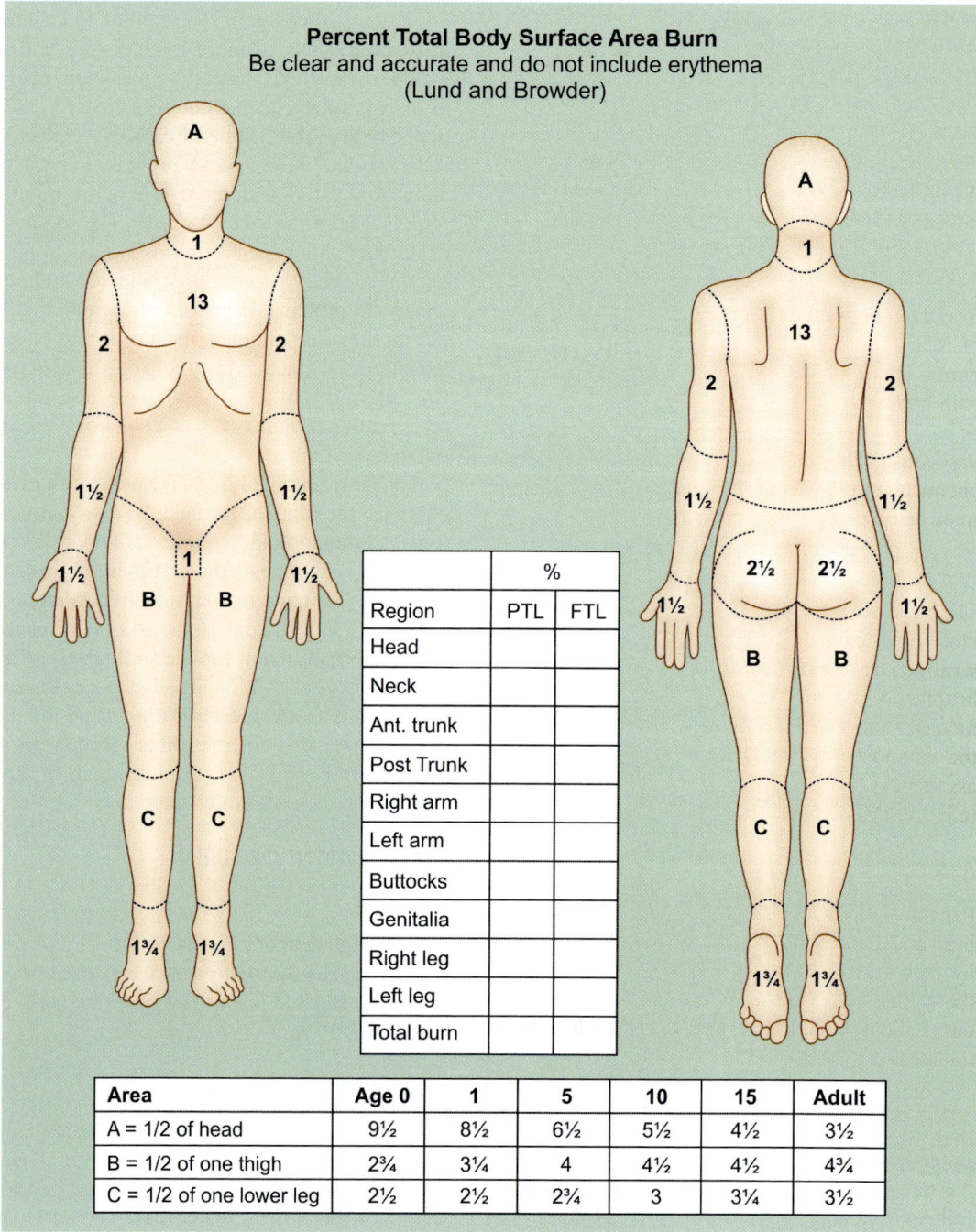

Percent Total Body Surface Area Burn
Be clear and accurate and do not include erythema
(Lund and Browder)

	%	
Region	PTL	FTL
Head		
Neck		
Ant. trunk		
Post Trunk		
Right arm		
Left arm		
Buttocks		
Genitalia		
Right leg		
Left leg		
Total burn		

Area	Age 0	1	5	10	15	Adult
A = 1/2 of head	9½	8½	6½	5½	4½	3½
B = 1/2 of one thigh	2¾	3¼	4	4½	4½	4¾
C = 1/2 of one lower leg	2½	2½	2¾	3	3¼	3½

Fig. 17.6: Lund and Browder chart for estimation of burn size

material, e.g. nylon must not be peeled but left to be taken care at the hospital. In case of electrical burn, victim must be disconnected from the source of electricity before starting first aid management. In cases of flame burn in an enclosed space, the patient must be immediately shifted to an open area. All metallic items, e.g. ring, jewelry, watch must be removed before edema sets in.

Cooling the Burnt Area

Room temperature water poured within 15 minutes of injury removes heat and prevents deepening of burns. This also removes noxious agents, decreases pain, reduces edema and cleanses the wound. Iced or cold water is not recommended as it may lead to vasoconstriction and deepening of burn. In case of chemical injury, copious irrigation with water/saline must be carried out for 15–20 minutes.

Covering the Burnt Area

The burnt area must be covered with a piece of clean cloth or in case of major burn the patient may be wrapped in clean sheet/blanket and shifted to hospital. It is advised not to apply locally available medicament on the wound as it may be harmful to the wound (e.g. tooth paste) or may hamper the assessment of wound size or depth at the hospital (e.g. methylene blue) (Fig. 17.7).

Shift to Hospital

Patients with major burns must be shifted to hospital in an ambulance with administration of 100% oxygen by face mask. Neck and spine must be supported during transport and shifting till spinal injury is ruled out. Patient should be kept nil orally while being transferred to the hospital.

Hospital Management

Emergency room management of burn starts with basic rules of trauma management. ABC protocol is followed and once other life-threatening injuries are ruled out, only then attention is directed to the burn injury.

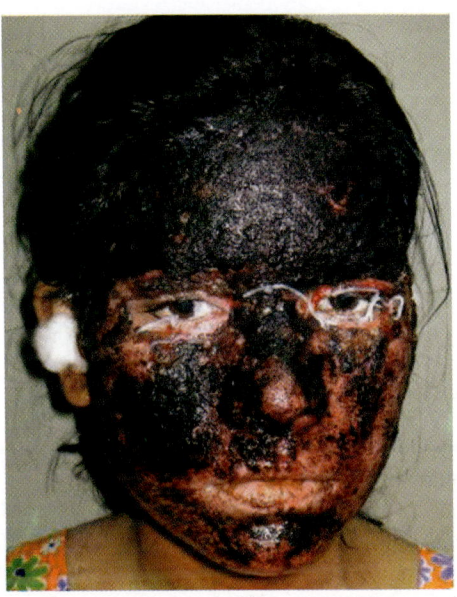

Fig. 17.7: Topical application of 'Ratanjyot'

Steps of Management of burn
• Primary assessment
• Secondary assessment
• Definitive assessment
  – Critical burn
  – Moderate burn
  – Minor burn
Critical and moderate burn: Referral to burn unit and admission
Minor burn: OPD management.

Primary Assessment

Primary assessment in burns is like any other trauma patient. It is a rapid, systematic approach to identify and treat life-threatening conditions. ABC protocol must be strictly followed, emergencies identified and treated.

Airway injury and compromised breathing status should always be suspected in patients with inhalation injury. This topic will be covered later in the chapter. However suspicion of airway injury and its quick management during primary assessment will help in saving many lives and complications.

- Establish clean airway
- Expose chest to assess ventilatory exchange
- Monitor respiratory status
- Assess pulse and blood pressure
- Actions
  - Endotracheal intubation if compromised respiratory status
  - IV line and fluids to restore circulation (1 lit/hr in adults and 20 ml/kg/hr in children)
  - Tracheostomy (Rare): In case of severe laryngeal edema and difficult intubation.

Secondary Assessment

Secondary assessment, like Primary assessment should be carried on in all patients of burn irrespective of the etiology and the percentage of burn. It's a more thorough head to toe evaluation to rule out other co-existing injuries, co-morbid conditions and proper action is taken accordingly.
- Rule out other concomitant injuries
- Neurological evaluation including GCS
- History taking, past medical history, drug allergies, medication
- Actions
  - 100% oxygen by mask
  - Cervical collar, splints if injuries suspected
  - Reference to other specialties if required, e.g. Ophthalmology, Orthopedics, etc.
  - Catheterization
  - Information to Burn Specialist.

Definitive Assessment

Definitive assessment is directed more towards burn and its management. It includes the primary and secondary assessment, and a final diagnosis and establishment of treatment plan.
- Primary assessment
- Secondary assessment
- History taking
- Complete physical examination
- Severity of burn assessment
  - Size of burn
  - Depth of burn

- Classify burn accordingly to Critical, moderate and minor burn
- Critical and moderate burns: Admission
- Minor burns: Discharge and OPD management
- Perform escharotomies in constricting/circumferential deep burn
- Monitor urine output
- Dress the patient
- Base line blood investigations.

History taking in Burns

- Mode of injury: Flame/scald/chemical/electrical
- Accidental/suicidal/homicidal
- Concomitant injuries: Fall from height or explosion
- Loss of consciousness
- Time elapsed since burn
- First aid/fluid resuscitation given prior to reaching hospital
- History of other co-morbid conditions (Diabetes, Hypertension, tuberculosis, Neurological problems, seizures)
- Past-medical history
- History of drug allergy
- Menstrual history
- History of drugs, alcoholism.

Flame Burns
- Cause of injury
- History of inhalation injury (especially flame burn in enclosed space)
- Type of clothing worn (Cotton/synthetic/mixed)

Scald Burns
- Nature of fluid (Oil/grease scalds are deeper than water scalds)
- Immersion scalds are deeper than spill scalds
- Deliberate scalds: Child abuse
- Steam burn: More severe than scald.

Electrical Burn
- Whether Contact/flash/arching
- Voltage: Low (< 1000 V) or High (>1000 V)
- Duration of contact
- Loss of consciousness/concomitant injuries
- Entry and exit wound.

Chemical Burn

- Acid/Alkali (Acid burns more self limiting than alkali burns)
- Duration of contact
- First aid given (irrigation with copious amount of water done or not)
- Ophthalmologic work up in case of facial burns.

Critical Burn (needs admission)

- Partial thickness: >25% in adults, >15% in children and > 5% in infants
- Full thickness: > 10% in adults and 3% in children
- Inhalation burn
- Burns involving hand, face and genitalia
- Burns complicated by other concomitant injuries
- Electrical burn
- Chemical burn.

Moderate Burn (needs admission)

- Partial thickness: 15–25% in adults, 10–15% in children, and 2–5% in infants
- Full thickness: 3–10% in adults and 1–3% in children.

Minor Burns (managed as outpatients)

- Partial thickness burn < 15% in adults, < 10% in children, and < 2% in infants
- Full thickness burn < 2% in adults.

Escharotomy

A circumferential deep dermal or full thickness burn is inelastic and unyielding in nature. Edema collection underneath the eschar especially after fluid resuscitation blocks venous return in extremities leading to circulatory failure. The resulting ischemia, if untreated may lead to distal gangrene and/or neuromuscular deficit. Similarly deep, circumferential and inelastic burn around the thorax may lead to ventilatory compromise and respiratory distress. Both these conditions require escharotomy i.e. the release of burn eschar longitudinally along its length and down through the full thickness of eschar to the viable subcutaneous tissue.

Escharotomy is best done in an operation theater with an electrocautery unit but can be done bedside if the need arises (Fig. 17.8). Incision for various areas is shown in Figs 17.9A and B. Following escharotomy, the wound is dressed and the limb is elevated to further improve the venous return.

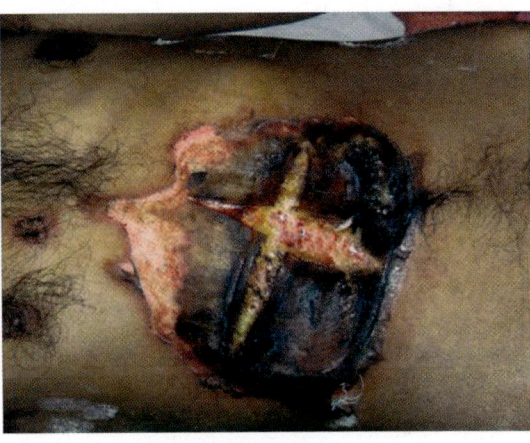

Fig. 17.8: Escharotomy

Sign and symptoms of ischemia
- Cyanosis
- Numbness/tingling/deep tissue pain
- Sensation of cold extremity
- Progressive weakness or loss of function
- Progressive paresthesia
- Progressive decrease or absence of pulses.

Assess on hourly basis
- Nail bed capillary refill
- Pin prick oozing from finger tip
- Skin color and temperature
- Sensation.

Investigations
- Ultrasonic Doppler for assessing arterial blood flow
- Tissue pressure > 40 mm Hg.

Fasciotomy

Release of the deep fascia (fasciotomy) in limbs to decompress various muscle compartments is done

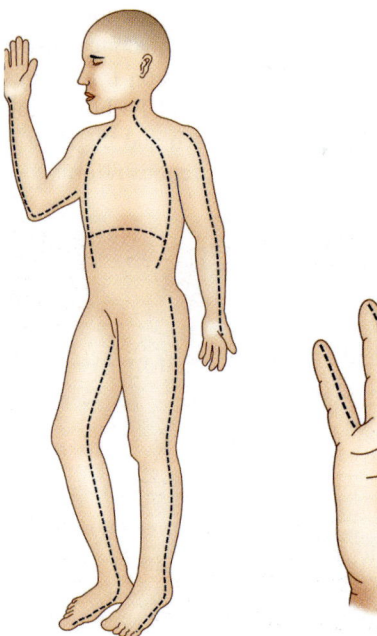

Fig. 17.9A: Escharotomy incisions for the chest, neck, and limbs

Fig. 17.9B: Escharotomy incisions for the digits

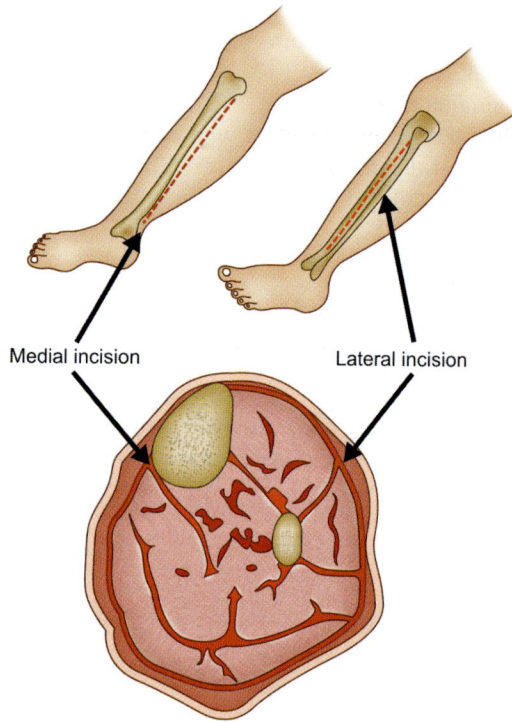

Medial incision   Lateral incision

Fig. 17.10A: Incision for fasciotomy at leg

in compartment syndrome. This is most commonly required in major electrical burns and best done in operation theater. Incisions for fasciotomy at forearm and leg are shown in (Figs 17.10A to C).

Burn Wound Management

Modern techniques of burn wound management along with latest antibiotics are the two most important factors which have considerably reduced burn morbidity and mortality at the present time. Superficial burns heal by epithelialization within 2 weeks and are thus managed conservatively with dressings. However, early surgical excision of deep second degree and third degree burns, has drastically changed the picture of burn wound management. Earlier, the treatment was conservative for all type of burns, whether superficial or deep. It involved frequent baths and daily dressing of wounds.

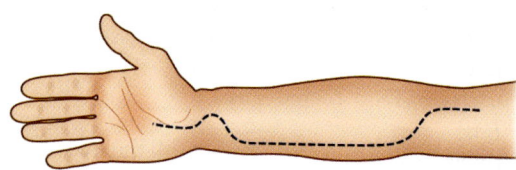

Fig. 17.10B: Volar incision for forearm fasciotomy

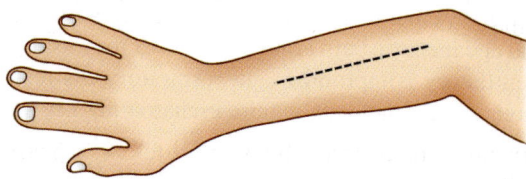

Fig. 17.10C: Dorsal incision for forearm fasciotomy

Burn Wound Excision

Dead eschar tissues in deep burns serve as a nidus for bacterial proliferation and infection subsequently leading to septicemia and mortality. Early excision of the dead tissue to viable bleeding bed and split skin grafting is the standard procedure today. The excision is performed preferably within a week of burn as soon as the patient is hemodynamically stable. The viable bed after excision is grafted with thin, autograft. If the donar autograft is limited in area, it can be meshed and expanded up to 1: 8 to cover the freshly excised bed. However, mesh > 4:1 leaves significant raw areas between the meshes leading to infection and graft loss. Excisional surgery in major burn should be attempted only at a burn center with following facilities

- Well equipped blood bank
- Dedicated burn anesthesia teams
- Well equipped ICU
- Skin bank (for supply of allograft)
- Availability of skin substitute.

Types of burn wound excision

a. *Tangential excision*

   Excision of dead tissue till viable dermal bed is reached in second degree deep burns.

b. *Sequential excision*

   Excision of dead tissue till viable subcutaneous tissue, in third degree burns.

c. *Fascial excision*

   Excision of tissues up to deep fascia irrespective of the thickness of the burn. This is performed with an electrocautery (different from sequential and tangential excision which is performed with dermatome/skin grafting knife). It has limited application as the cosmetic result is poor. It is mainly indicated in life-threatening, full thickness burn which requires minimal blood loss and faster surgery.

   Following excision of burn wound, the resultant raw area is covered by split thickness graft (for large areas) or full thickness graft (for small areas).

Wound Coverage

a. *Full thickness graft (FTG)*: FTG includes epidermis and full thickness of dermis. The graft is harvested with a scalpel and the donor area is closed primarily. In spite of the better cosmetic and functional result due to more relative thickness of dermis in comparison to split thickness skin graft (STSG), the role of full thickness graft is limited in acute burn wound management. This is owing to its limited availability and poor 'take'.

b. *Split thickness skin graft (STSG)*: STSG includes epidermis and variable thickness of dermis, depending upon which it is classified as thin, intermediate and thick. The graft is harvested with a dermatome or skin grafting knife (Humby, Watson) and the donor area heals by epithelialization within 2 weeks depending upon the thickness of the graft harvested. Serial skin grafts can be harvested from the same donor site after healing is complete.

c. *Skin substitutes:* When the area of burn exceeds 30–40%, it becomes increasingly difficult to cover the excised wound with patient's skin graft (*autograft*) due to limitation of donor areas. There comes the role of skin substitutes, which can be temporary or permanent (Fig. 17.11). The classical temporary skin substitute is cadaveric skin (*allograft*), stored in skin banks. The availability of allograft has changed the course of modern burn treatment for these massive wounds. The substitute is applied over the excised burn wound that could not be covered by meshed autograft. Allograft prevents the wound from getting infected and prepares it for subsequent autografting, once the donor sites have healed. However, allograft is a temporary wound cover. As soon as the graft is vascularized by the recipient blood vessels, the immunological reaction to the donor cells present in allograft sets in, leading to rejection of the graft. Removal of epidermis and treatment of the remaining dermis makes cadaveric skin free of any cellular antigen

Permanent skin substitute
- Dermal substitute
  - Alloderm
  - Dermagraft
  - Integra
- Epidermal substitute
  - Apligraft
  - Cultured epithelial autograft (CEA)

Temporary skin substitutes
- Collagen
- Allograft (Cadaveric skin)
- Xenograft (Other species)
- Amniotic membrane

Fig. 17.11: Skin substitute

and is thus not rejected by the immune reaction. This principle is used to prepare allodermis which is a permanent skin substitute (*Alloderm*). Alloderm is applied over freshly excised wound bed and covered with thin STSG.

Integra was developed by Burke and Yannas and is gradually becoming a popular dermal substitute. It is bilaminate structure, consisting of a dermal analogue covered with a thin silicone layer. The silicone layer acts like a temporary epidermis. As the dermal analogue gets vascularized in two weeks, the silicone layer is peeled off and is replaced by thin STSG or a layer of cultured epithelial autograft

d. *Skin culture*: Cultured epithelial autograft (CEA) is a sheet of keratinocytes cultured from patient's skin, obtained as full thickness skin biopsy. The technology is promising, but the present disadvantages are the main limiting factor in its popularity.

Limitation of CEA
- Long time to culture (3 weeks)
- Poor 'take' rate
- Poor durability due to absence of dermis
- Poor cosmetic result
- Expensive.

Inhalation Injury

Inhalation injury consists of three different aspects of inhaling hot smoke in the process of burn injury.

Although the pathophysiology of each component of inhalation burn is different, the treatment is concomitant. The presence of inhalation injury increases risk of mortality in a burn patient by two to three times.

Components of inhalation injury are:
- Carbon monoxide poisoning
- Thermal injury to upper airway
- Smoke inhalation.

Carbon Monoxide Poisoning

CO toxicity is one of the most frequent immediate causes of death following smoke induced inhalation injury. It must be suspected in every flame burn patient and treated promptly. When inhaled and absorbed, CO binds with hemoglobin to form carboxyhemoglobin (COHb) which interferes with the oxygen delivery to the tissue. Measurement of blood level of carboxyhemoglobin is diagnostic.

Treatment is by administration of 100% oxygen, which displaces CO from proteins 4 times faster. Patients having COHb > 20% must be intubated and ventilated with 100% oxygen (Table 17.1).

COHb levels (%)	Symptoms
0–10	None
11–30	Headache, dilatation of cutaneous blood vessels
31–50	Dizziness, nausea, vomiting, collapse
50–70	Convulsions, increased pulse and respiratory rate, coma
> 70	Death with hours to minutes

Table 17.1: Symptoms of inhalational injury according to the level of COHb

Thermal Injury

Thermal injury to the respiratory tract is usually limited to the upper airway. The heat dissipation in upper airway prevents heat injury to the lower tracheobronchial tree. The pathophysiology is similar to cutaneous burns and manifests as mucosal edema, erythema, hemorrhage and ulceration which is diagnosed by direct visualization of mouth and pharynx, and upper airway through fiberoptic bronchoscope. The edema gets more severe following fluid resuscitation and may lead to upper airway obstruction and difficult intubation.

Smoke Inhalation

The toxic compounds are carried with the smoke to the distal tracheobronchial tree. These compounds dissolve in the mucous and form various chemical causing acute inflammatory responses akin to chemical burn.

Inhalation injury is suspected in the presence of the following:

- Injury occurring in enclosed space
- Burn around mouth and nose
- Singed nasal hairs
- Intra-oral burns, tongue burn
- Dyspnea, hoarseness of voice
- Pharyngeal edema
- Inspiratory stridor
- Laryngeal edema
- Carbonaceous sputum
- Anxiety, disorientation
- Coma.

Investigations Done in Inhalational Injury

- Blood gas analysis
  - COHb: CO poisoning
  - P:F ratio: Decreased suggesting compromised pulmonary function
  - Hypoxemia.
- X-ray chest.
- Serial fiberoptic bronchoscopy.
  Most reliable method. Pharyngeal/laryngeal edema, mucosal erythema/ulceration, carbonaceous particles, exudative casts can be easily visualized.
- Xenon ventilation scanning: Area of lung retaining isotope 90 sec after IV injection, suggests airway obstruction.

Treatment of Inhalational Injury

Aim of treatment is to maintain a patent airway and maximization of gaseous exchange

a. *Oxygen by mask*: A conscious, actively coughing patient who can clear the secretions effectively must be managed on mask and oxygen.

b. *Intubation and hyperventilation with 100% oxygen:*
   Indications
   - COHb > 20%
   - Unconsciousness, altered sensorium
   - Increasing respiratory tract edema
   - Hoarseness of voice
   - Respiratory/ventilatory failure
   - $PaO_2 < 60$ mm Hg
   - $PCO_2 > 50$ mm Hg
   - PaO_2/FiO_2 ratio < 200

c. *Chest physiotherapy*
   - Cough, deep breathing exercises every 2 hours
   - Turn patient from one side to other every 2 hours

d. *Nebulization*
   - 3 ml N-acetylcystine 20% solution every 4 hr for 7 days
   - 5000 units of heparin with 3 ml of normal saline every 4 hr for 7 days

e. Frequent nasotracheal suctioning

f. Sputum culture

g. *Early ambulation and mobilization:* Helps in secretion removal, prevents atelectasis and pneumonia, and improves oxygenation

h. *Hyperbaric oxygen (HBO)*: The use of HBO therapy for patients with COHb poisoning is controversial as well as impractical.

MANAGEMENT OF MINOR BURN

Minor burns are treated on an out patient basis.

Cleaning of Wound

The wound is thoroughly washed with normal saline to remove dust and foreign bodies.

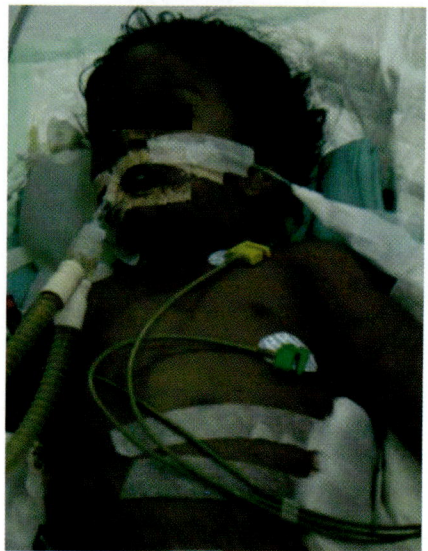

Fig. 17.12: Intubated child with inhalational injury

Debridement of Blisters

Small blisters are punctured and the overlying epithelium is left intact to act as biological dressing. Large blisters especially over hands hamper active and passive movement, they are debrided and the exudate is drained.

Dressing

Wound is covered with paraffin embedded gauze dressing (Jelonet) and topical antibiotic cream (Framycetin, Mupirocin, Povidone-iodine, Bacitracin, Polymyxin-B, Silver nitrate, Chlorhexidine) is applied over it. Cotton pads are applied and the dressing is secured with crepe bandage or elastoplast. Dressing is changed every 48–72 hrs depending upon soakage. If the paraffin gauze is firmly adherent to the wound, it is left intact as removing it will peel off regenerating epithelium and delay wound healing.

Facial burn is usually left open. The face is cleansed thrice a day with chlorhexidine solution and topical antibiotic ointment is applied. Burns over pinna must be dressed with cotton fluffs as contour dressing to prevent chondritis.

Hand burns after dressing must be elevated to prevent edema and swelling.

Splintage and Range of Motion Exercises

In hand burns, splintage in functional position may be required initially. During dressing change, active and passive range of motion (ROM) exercises must be encouraged to prevent stiffness.

Analgesia

Analgesics and mild sedatives (in children) must be administered before dressing to alley pain and anxiety.

Electrical Burn

Electrical injury can be classified as low voltage (<1000 V) or high voltage (>1000 V) burn. It can be in form of true electrical injury due to current flow through the tissue or an arc injury, when the current jumps from one part of the body to another, sparing the intermediate tissues example cubital fossa or axilla. Flash injury occurs when surface burn is caused by sparking and the cloth catching fire. It is similar to the flame burns.

Clinical features may include entry and exit wounds, tetanic contractions, fractures and dislocations (Fig. 17.13). Compartment syndrome especially of upper limb is fairly common feature of high voltage electrical injury. Passage of electric current through cardiac tissues may cause abnormal ECG, ventricular fibrillation or asystole. Myoglobinuria is caused by heat injury to the muscle fibers through which the electric current has passed.

The general principle of burn management also applies to electrical burns. Primary, secondary and definitive assessment is performed and the patient is admitted for hospital management. Even patients with seemingly minor burn must be admitted for observation and discharged only after normal ECG and no complains of myoglobinuria. Fluid

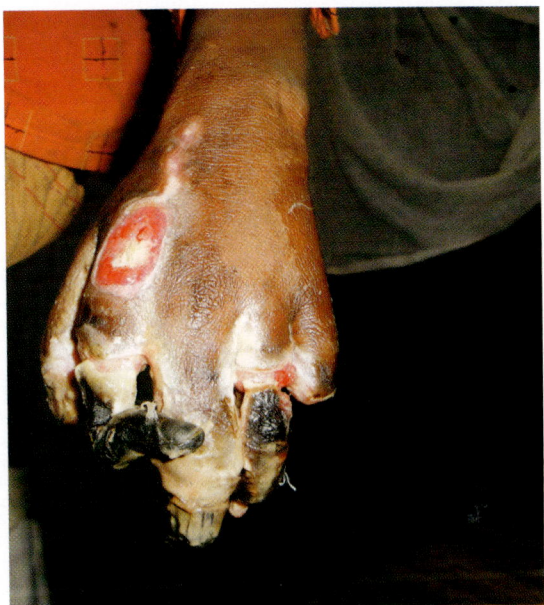

Fig. 17.13: Electrical burn of hand

resuscitation with Ringer lactate solution is started to maintain urine output of 2 ml/kg/hr. Injury to muscles with loss of pigments lead to acidic urine. 5% sodium bicarbonate infusion is added to maintain alkaline urine. Mannitol infusion @ 25 g 6 hourly must be given to flush out cellular debris and pigments from the renal system. Early compartment decompression by fasciotomy and carpal tunnel release may be required in high voltage injury.

Chemical Burns

Chemical burns are caused by an acid or alkali. Industrial accidents are the common cause of chemical burns. Homicidal injury caused by throwing acid over face of young girls is not uncommon in Indian subcontinent. These are usually deep second-degree or third-degree burns, although the depth of burn is directly related to the concentration of the chemical agent and the nature of the chemical. Alkali cause deeper injury due to the process of saponification. In a victim of chemical injury, all the clothing must be removed to prevent further injury and the involved area is irrigated with water for 15–20 minutes. Neutralizing agents must not be used as they can cause more harm by producing heat of neutralization. Incidence of ophthalmic injury is high and expert opinion must be taken even for the most trivial injury to the eye. All chemical burns must be admitted and routine management protocol is followed. The depth of injury is assessed on regular basis and usually the burn appears deeper in the following days. The treatment is conservative for superficial burns and excisional surgery for the deep burns.

18 Abdominal Compartment Syndrome

INTRODUCTION

Abdominal compartment syndrome (ACS) is defined as complex of adverse physiological consequences that occur as a result of acute rise in intra-abdominal pressure usually more than 20 mm Hg. This condition is seen in patients who have massive abdominal trauma, have an operation for multiple intra-abdominal infections or in those who have undergone prolong abdominal surgery like necrotizing pancreatitis and intestinal obstruction. In all such cases due to associated intestinal edema, congestion and accumulation of blood, the closure may lead to intra-abdominal hypertension causing ACS.

The normal intra-abdominal pressure is 0–5 mm Hg only. ACS is manifested when the intraabdominal pressure rises to 25 mm/Hg and characterized by distended tense abdomen, hypoxia with respiratory compromise and poor renal perfusion with oliguria. If it remains untreated patient develops renal failure, respiratory failure, acidosis and finally goes into shock. This is a surgical emergency and patients should be taken to operating room for removal of fascial closure of the abdominal wound. After a week when the edema resolves and the patient's general condition improves, formal abdominal closure is done.

COMMON CAUSE OF INCREASED INTRA-ABDOMINAL PRESSURE

1. Abdominal trauma
   - Use of abdominal packs
   - Post-resuscitation visceral edema
   - Pelvic or retroperitoneal hematoma
   - Intraperitoneal bleeding
   - Burn of the abdominal wall (eschar).
2. Tense ascites
3. Acute necrotizing pancreatitis
4. Sepsis
5. Secondary to mesenteric vascular infarction
6. Paralytic ileus
7. Intestinal obstruction
8. Rupture abdominal aortic aueurysm
9. Laparoscopic (tension pneumoperitoneum).

MEASUREMENT OF INTRA-ABDOMINAL PRESSURE

Intra-abdominal pressure is traditionally should be measured in surgical ICU, but as the ACS may develop in other situation as well, a high index of suspicion must be maintained even in a non-ICU set up. There is no characteristic clinical sign indicative of abdominal compartment syndrome. The measurement of abdominal girth is a poor indicator of raised intra-abdominal pressure. In accordance with the Pascal's law, pressure within the abdominal organ reflects as intra-abdominal pressure. The widely accepted method of measurement of intra-abdominal pressure is the transvesical pressure, which is inexpensive and simple to perform.

Procedure

100 ml of saline is introduced through a Foley urethral catheter in the urinary bladder and the draining tubing is clamped thus producing a

continuous column of fluid in catheter. Using the symphysis pubis as zero point, a water manometer (preferably a pressure transducer) is attached to the catheter which gives an accurate reading of intra-abdominal pressure. In case of bladder trauma the intra-abdominal pressure measurement can be done by transgastric pressure by a nasogastric tube.

This procedure allows repeated estimation of intra-abdominal pressure without any risk of introduction of infection. In general intra-abdominal pressure measurement of 20 mm Hg (27 cm of saline) or higher define significant intra-abdominal hypertension.

Grading of Increase Intra-abdominal Pressure

Grade	Intra-abdominal pressure (mm Hg)
I	12–15
II	16–20
III	21–25
IV	>25

PATHOPHYSIOLOGY

Since the contents of the abdomen are relatively non compressible and contained within a confined space of the abdominal cavity, an increase in the volume of retroperitoneum or abdominal contents will lead to rise in intra-abdominal pressure. According to many studies the highest incidence of intra-abdominal hypertension (IAH) is observed in patients who have undergone laparotomy for abdominal trauma and massive fluid resuscitation is the major contributory factor. The IAH leads to significant dysfunction to almost all the organ system. Such physiological derangements become more pronounced and clinically significant when IAH is more than 20 mm Hg.

Abdominal wall compliance allows compensation of chronic or subtle increase in intra-abdominal pressure. A critical intra-abdominal pressure is reached where viability of the other tissue is threatened if abdominal wall compliance is reduced

(e.g. peritonitis, burns) or there is a rapid increase in intra-abdominal volume (hemorrhage, after trauma). It is in these circumstances the multi-organ effects of the abdominal compartment syndrome develop.

Abdominal compartment syndrome can be primary which is always due to trauma of abdominal and pelvic organ. The secondary abdominal compartment syndrome is seen in patients with sepsis, burn and having massive fluid resuscitation, whereas tertiary ACS develops following an attempt of temporary abdominal closure.

EFFECTS OF IAH ON DIFFERENT SYSTEMS

Cardiovascular System

Intra-abdominal pressure (IAP) more than 20 mm Hg has a profound influence on cardiovascular system. The hemodynamic compromise is due to complex alteration in pre-load, after load and intra-thoracic pressure. The raised IAP reduces the cardiac output; compression of IVC diminishes the venous return of the heart (pre-load) which is further compounded by pooling of blood in the retroperitoneum and extremities. Such venous pooling and stasis in the lower extremity may predispose to venous thromboembolic phenomenon. Appropriate mechanical and pharmacological measures must be taken in such situation to decrease the incidence of pulmonary embolism. The increase after load is because of raised vascular resistance and raised intrathoracic pressure. In accordance to the Starling's law, stroke volume decreases, reducing cardiac output. This effect is compounded by hypovolemia. Acidosis reduces the myocardial contractility and the elevated diaphragm distorts the shape of ventricle resulting in reduced ventricular compliance. Volume resuscitation leads to improvement in cardiac output and stroke volume.

Respiratory System

The raised IAP leads to respiratory failure. Upward displacement of diaphragm is responsible for declining lung and chest wall compliances, reducing the intrathoracic volume, increasing the intra-thoracic pressure and compressing the lung parenchyma—a situation similar to restrictive lung disease. Hypoxia may result consequent to hypoventilation and abnormal ventilation perfusion matching. The compromised elimination of carbon dioxide results respiratory acidosis. The associated rise in the vetriculo-perfusion mismatch and pulmonary dead space lead to hypoxia and hyper-carbia which need mechanical ventilation, otherwise these effects may further impedes the venous return and exacerbate the co-existing lung disease.

Renal

In raised intra-abdominal pressure there is fall in the glomerular filtration rate. The increased pressure also leads to decrease in renal flow and increase in renal vascular resistance. Compression on renal parenchyma and rise in inferior vena cava pressure along with decreased arterial pressure together leads to oliguric renal failure. Oliguria is observed at intra-abdominal pressure between 15 and 20 mm Hg. It may further progress to a stage of anuria when pressure exceeds 30 mm Hg. Decompression of the abdomen becomes necessary to treat such oliguria. Effects of raised intra-abdominal pressure are shown in Fig. 18.1.

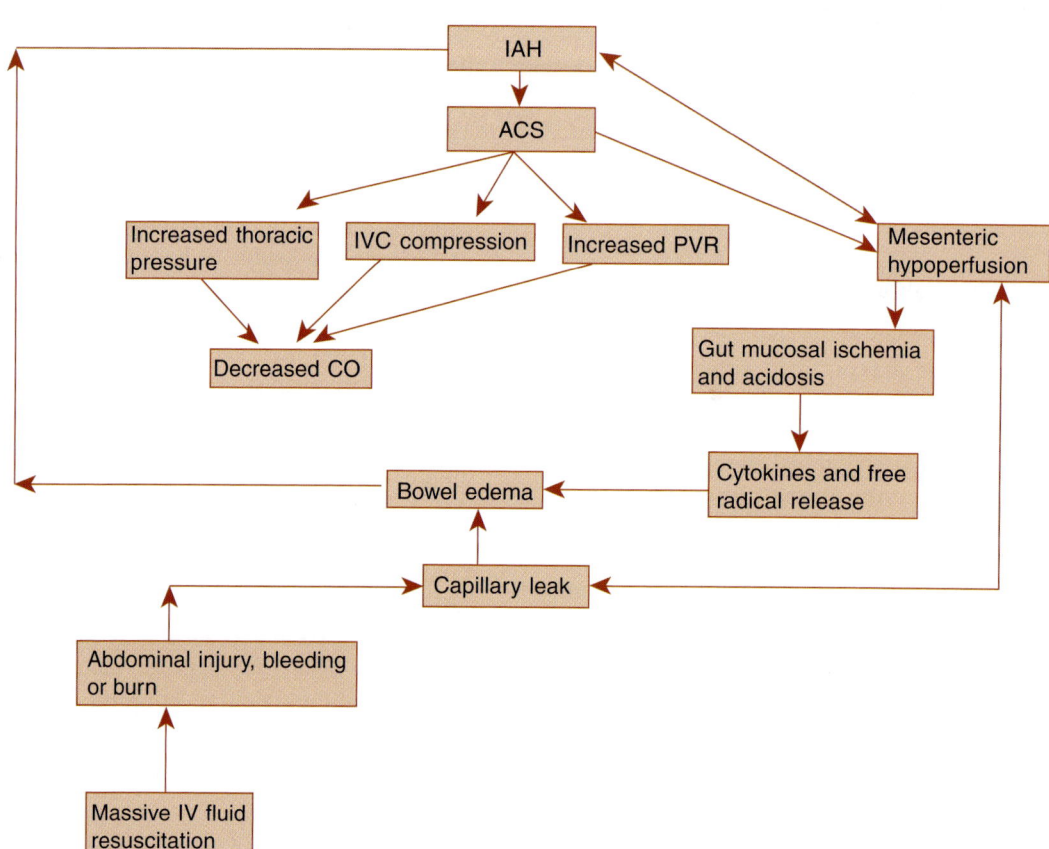

Fig. 18.1: Effects of raised intra-abdominal pressure (PVR—Peripheral vascular resistance; CO—Cardiac output; IAH—Intra-abdominal hypertension; ACS—Abdominal compartment syndrome)

The only effective treatment of ACS is to decompress the abdomen simply by reopening the abdominal sutures. Where the patients have no abdominal incision a long vertical midline incision would be appropriate. The intravenous fluid resuscitation is recommended along with the use of mannitol. After achieving adequate decompression by opening the abdomen the area is covered by plastic "Bogotá bag" fitted to the edges of the fascia preferably by interrupted sutures. A small perforation in the bag is done for the fluid to escape.

Another technique for the closure to the open area is by large sheet of absorbable woven mesh which is also to be sewn to the fascia with a placement of suction drain. It is important that polypropylene mesh should not be used in this situation because of its potential danger caused by the mesh adherence to the intestine. Vacuum-assisted wound closure (VAWC) has become a routine technique in the management for all kinds of open abdominal wound (abdominal wound dehiscence/ burst abdomen). The VAWC dressing can be held in place by interrupted stay sutures placed in fascia in each side and tied over the VAWC dressing. Once the patients' general condition improves and intestinal edema subsides the fascial defects should be repaired. In cases the approximation of the fascia is difficult the wound can be again covered with absorbable woven mesh. Ultimate closure of the open abdominal wound may take several weeks or months.

19

Abdominal Wound Dehiscence

ABDOMINAL WOUND DEHISCENCE

Abdominal wound dehiscence is a serious postoperative complication that concerns every surgeon. The incidence of this complication varies from 1 to 5%. Efforts have been made to overcome this complication with various innovations in the technique of closure of laparotomy incisions and use of different types of suture material.

DEFINITION

Abdominal wound dehiscence is also known as burst abdomen, wound failure, wound disruption, evisceration, and eventration. It is defined as partial or complete postoperative separation of an abdominal wound closure with protrusion or evisceration of the abdominal contents. Wound dehiscence and incisional hernia are part of the same wound failure process; it is the timing and healing of the overlying skin that distinguishes the two. The full healing of the skin incision is used to make a convenient distinction between wound dehiscence and incisional hernia. Dehiscence of the wound occurs before cutaneous healing, while incisional hernias lie under a well-healed skin incision.

PRESENTATION

Wound dehiscence commonly presents a week after surgery. It has been observed that dehiscence is preceded by serosanguinous discharge. The extent of dehiscence can be superficial or deep. In superficial dehiscence there is breakdown of skin and subcutaneous tissue, whereas in complete dehis-cence there is opening up of fascial layer resulting in exposure of abdominal viscera (Fig. 19.1). Bowel loops can prolapse out of the wound in deep dehiscence (Fig. 19.2). Patients often tell that some

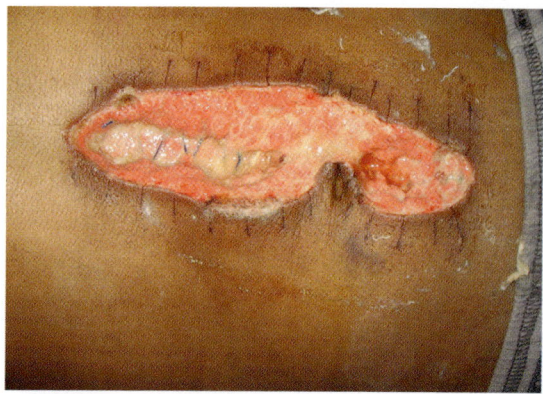

Fig. 19.1: Deep dehiscence with bowel exposed

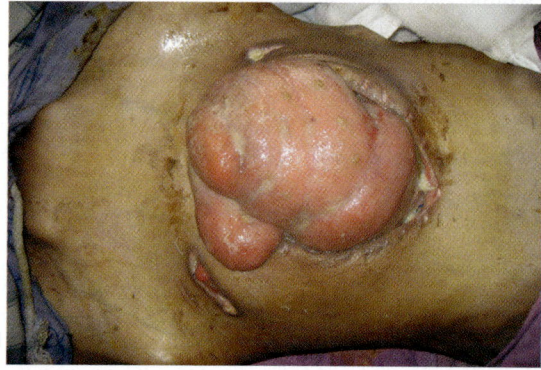

Fig. 19.2: Wound dehiscence with prolapsed bowel loops

thing had given away. Such dehiscence is the commonest cause of incisional hernia.

PREOPERATIVE RISK FACTORS

These risk factors of surgical wound complication which can be broadly categorized in to local and systemic causes.

Systemic causes

- Malnutrition (vitamin C and zinc deficiency, anemia and hypoproteinemia)
- Chronic disease (cirrhosis of liver, uremia)
- Pharmacological agent (prolonged steroid therapy)
- Shock
- Age (advance age)
- Increased intra-abdominal pressure (postoperative paralytic ileus, persistent cough, i.e. COPD patients, vomiting and obstructive uropathy).

Local Causes

- Contamination
- Trauma
- Tissue hypoperfusion
- Irradiation
- Neoplasm.

Contamination

A clean operative field minimizes contamination of wound with bacteria. The bacterial organisms that normally colonize skin surface are predominantly gram-positive *Staphylococcus* and *Streptococcus* species. Following clean operations, wound infection, is found to be 1–3%, e.g. breast biopsy and inguinal hernia repair. Clean contaminated wounds are those where the organ that is colonized with high number of potentially pathogenic bacteria is breached like in colorectal surgery. Wound infection rate in such cases is around 10%. In contaminated wound there is an uncontrolled bacterial contamination, e.g. repair of gunshot injury of colon and rectum. Wound infection in such setting is found to be around 30–60%. Necrotic tissue always exacerbates defective wound healing. Bacterial invasion use the debris as a source of nutrition causing further invasive wound infection. The necrotic debris is also responsible for acting as a mechanical barrier to the healing cells like fibroblast.

Tissue Hypoperfusion

Hypoperfusion due to hypotension and acidosis in shock increases wound infection and dehiscence rate by many fold. Tissue perfusion gets impaired also in peripheral vascular disease, hypothermia, vasospastic disease and venous hypertension. Previously irradiated tissue is also highly susceptible to wound dehiscence due to reduced capillary blood supply as a result of microangiopathy. Reduced perfusion leads to low tissue oxygen tension which further get associated with collagen defect and increased wound infection rate.

Malnutrition

Malnutrition plays an important part for non healing of the wound as it limits the collagen synthesis, fibroblast proliferation and neovascularization. Serum albumin of <3 gm/dl is seen to increase the risk of wound dehiscence and incisional hernia. Serum albumin level has been found to be the single most predictable factor in predicting the surgical morbidity and acute wound failure. Abundant amino acid is necessary for protein synthesis and cell division at the wound sites to sustain the repair. Cancer cachexia is found to delay wound repair. Nutrients like vitamin A, vitamin C, vitamin K are helpful in better healing of the wound.

Chronic Diseases

Uncontrolled diabetes mellitus is well known for wound failure due to wound infection because of impaired nutrophil chemotaxis and phagocytosis. Increasing age of the patients, atherosclerosis, immunodeficiency state, long-standing jaundice, malignancy and acute or chronic liver diseases is found to be associated with delay in wound healing and associated wound dehiscence.

Pharmacological Agents

Long continued use of steroids has been shown to inhibit fibroblast function in vitro. Cytotoxic agents are known to induce profound delay in wound repair by inhibiting the cell proliferation, DNA and protein synthesis. Chemotherapeutic drugs might suppress the normal wound inflammatory response as well as fibroblast proliferation and collagen deposition.

Poor Surgical Technique

Poor surgical technique is equally responsible for wound infection that may lead to acute dehiscence. Acute dehiscence is the commonest cause of incisional hernia. All the above risk factors (as stated above) are also associated with poor wound healing, dehiscence and incisional hernia. A sound surgical technique with appropriate suture material, good bites of tissue, properly laid knots and avoidance of excessive tension are important factors to avoid the wound dehiscence and incisional hernia. Restoration of normal anatomy during closure of abdominal wound should always be attempted, i.e.in the midline incision it is the apposition of linea alba and in lateral or horizontal incision it is the closure of tendinous, aponeurotic and fascial structures in layers.

There has been a growing interest in transverse incision in laparotomy as this approach also gives surgeon a good access to see most of the intraabdominal structures. The rate of dehiscence is higher in midline incisions than in transverse incisions. Midline incision is non-anatomic. It cuts across the aponeurotic fibers, as opposed to the transverse incision which cuts parallel to the fibers. Contraction of the abdominal wall causes laterally directed tension on the closure. In the midline incisions, this may cause the suture material to cut through by separation of the transversely orientated fibers. Conversely, in the transverse incision, the fibers are apposed on contraction. This incision is also associated with less pain and reduced incidence of wound dehiscence and incisional hernia. Mass closure or layered closure, continuous or interrupted and closure of peritoneum do not make any difference in the incidence of burst abdomen. A continuous suture ensures that the tension is distributed evenly along the length of the wound.

Minimising Infection Risk for the Surgical Wound

- **Avoid skin shaving:** Hairs to be clipped in atraumatic fashion immediately prior to the surgery. Alternatively removing no hair at all appears acceptable.
- **Adequate skin preparation:** Skin should be free from gross contamination prior to initiation of skin preparation. Antiseptic solution to be applied in a concentric circle beginning at the area of proposed incision and working out to the periphery of the field. The area should be wide with a provision to extend the incision. The antiseptic agents generally used are povidone-iodine, chlorhexidine and alcohol containing products.
- **Appropriate use of prophylactic antibiotic for high risk patient:** Antibiotic prophylaxis is best delivered just prior to the operative incision. The therapeutic levels of the antibiotics in the tissue at the surgical site during incision reduce the incidence of wound infection. The selection of antimicrobial agents can be guided by the likely infections that can occur with the operative procedure.
- **Minimal dissection of tissue**
- **Good hemostasis**

All these factors in surgical technique are important in reducing the incidence of wound dehiscence and formation of incisional hernia.

Management of Surgical Wound Dehiscence

In majority, patients with **superficial wound dehiscence**, can easily be managed conservatively with frequent dressing of wound and good drainage. If the sutures or the clips are preventing the drainage, those should be removed. Pus swab for culture and sensitivity should be sent and appropriate antibiotics should be continued to control the ongoing infection. Frequent dressing is always helpful in better healing of the wound. The ideal wound dressing should protect a wound against desiccation (hydrophobic dressing). In addition dressing should keep a wound clean, absorb exudates and minimize the wound pain. In case of larger wound dehiscence, the parts which are not viable should always be debrided and dressing should continue regularly. Supportive measures like improving the hemoglobin status, serum protein, use of vitamins should be advocated.

When patient's wound condition improves, a delayed primary closure can be undertaken to produce a better cosmetic outcome.

A **complete dehiscence of the wound** also known as burst abdomen is due to disruption of fascial layer with exposure of viscera in the main wound. A complete dehiscence is an emergency situation requiring surgery. If the general condition of the patient is good for surgery, all earlier sutures should be removed and closure to be done by application of retention sutures. It has been observed that such retention sutures at times may lead to abdominal compartment syndrome. Therefore many believe to leave the patient with laparostomy and have a second look for the surgery. In cases where the wound is infected with necrotic tissues, proper debridement should be done. Necrotic tissue should be excised back to healthy bearing soft tissue with obvious blood supply.

Wound Closure

A marked reduction in the incidence of burst abdomen can be achieved by utilizing a proper suture material and by employing a correct technique of abdominal closure. A suture material to be labeled as near-ideal for abdominal closure should have the following properties

- It should have excellent handling and knotting properties.
- It should slide through the tissues readily.
- It should be non-irritant and should not provide nidus for infection.

- It should neither disappear nor lose its tensile strength until the wound has regained near normal tensile strength.
- It should not cause discomfort to the patient.

The choice of suture material varied with the different surgeons operating on adult patients. In children, vicryl is used in all cases. For midline incisions, closure of the linea alba with continuous nylon/prolene suture is the standard practice. In transverse incisions, the transversalis muscle is included in the closure of the peritoneum, the internal oblique and the external oblique were closed separately. Tension sutures were used at the discretion of the surgeon in patients who were deemed to run a high risk of wound dehiscence.

Retention Sutures

There are a number of techniques, but the basic principles are: use heavy non-absorbable suture, e.g. No 1 monofilament nylon/prolene. It is advisable to take wide interrupted bites of at least 3 cm from the wound edge and a stitch interval of 3 cm or less should be kept. Either external (incorporating all layers-peritoneum through to skin) or internal (all layers except skin) may be used. Internal retention sutures avoid producing an unsightly ladder-pattern scar, however, they are unable to be removed subsequently (increased infection risk). A buttress device is used to prevent suture erosion into the skin, e.g. thread each suture through a short length (5–6 cm) of plastic or rubber tubing (Fig. 19.3). Do not tie too tightly. External retention sutures are usually left in for at least 3 weeks.

Size of Tissue Bite and Suture Length-to-Wound Length Ratio

Suture length-to-wound length ratio (SL:WL) influences the rate of wound dehiscence. Most studies support the use of an SL:WL of greater than 4:1 for continuous mass closure. This is achieved if both the stitch interval and the tissue bite are 1 cm. Increasing the bite to 2 cm produces a ratio of 8:1. An SL:WL of less than 4:1 is associated with an

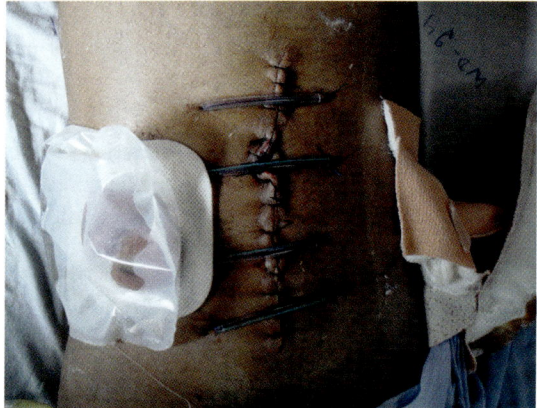

Fig. 19.3: Retention sutures

increased risk of abdominal dehiscence and the later development of incisional hernia.

The Uncloseable Abdomen

In a small number of patients it is inappropriate, technically unsafe, or even impossible to close the abdominal wall primarily.

Conditions which may predispose to an uncloseable abdomen include:
– Major abdominal trauma
– Gross abdominal sepsis
– Retroperitoneal hematoma
– Loss of abdominal wall tissue, e.g. necrotizing fasciitis.

Attempted closure may lead to sustained elevation of intra-abdominal pressure and subsequent abdominal compartment syndrome. In certain cases (e.g. if the cause is likely to resolve rapidly) it may be possible to temporarily close the abdomen by packing the wound and taking a further look after 24–48 hours. Clinicians today have also accepted the concept, that the prevention and treatment of intra-abdominal hypertension is always beneficial.

In laparostomy the friable dilated bowel wall does not tolerate the trauma of exposure and repeated dressing changes. Therefore, the temporary abdominal closure (TAC) devises to cover the laparostomy wound are highly recommended. The preferred method of TAC could be use of "Bogota bag", made of large sterile intravenous fluid bag or urobag. It is better to suture the TAC device to the fascial edges because just placing "on top" will result in huge abdominal wall defect. During the second look surgery abdominal reentry through the TAC device is simple as it can be divided in its center and if required can be resutured again. Whenever the defect is small it may be possible to close it completely. If healthy surrounding skin comes nicely together then close the skin over the defect and forget the fascia. Laterally placed relaxation incisions occasionally help to bring the midline together. The ensuing certain hernia is of minor importance at this stage. In cases of larger defect the use of absorbable mesh is of great help.

Complications do occur with laparostomy, the most morbid being spontaneous enteric fistula.

MANAGEMENT OF INCISIONAL HERNIA

Almost all the patients of burst abdomen invariably progress to incisional hernia. Some remain asymptomatic but other does have symptoms like
• Restriction of movement
• Embarrassment on account of disfigurement
• Discomfort or pain
• Obstruction/ischemia of bowel.

On examination the edges of the defect can easily be palpated. Size of the defect (Fig. 19.4) and reducibility of the hernia should always be assessed before surgery. In long-standing cases of incisional hernia contents of the abdomen lie outside the abdominal cavity and attempt to reduce the content into the peritoneal cavity at times may lead to abdominal compartment syndrome.

Repair of Incisional Hernia

Smaller hernia is suitable for anatomical repair. But most of the larger incisional hernias need repair with mesh. Polypropylene and polyethylene are commonly used which are flexible and can easily cut to size. Drawbacks of these mesh are that they become adherent to the abdominal contents. Therefore the other meshes like polytetrafluoroethylene

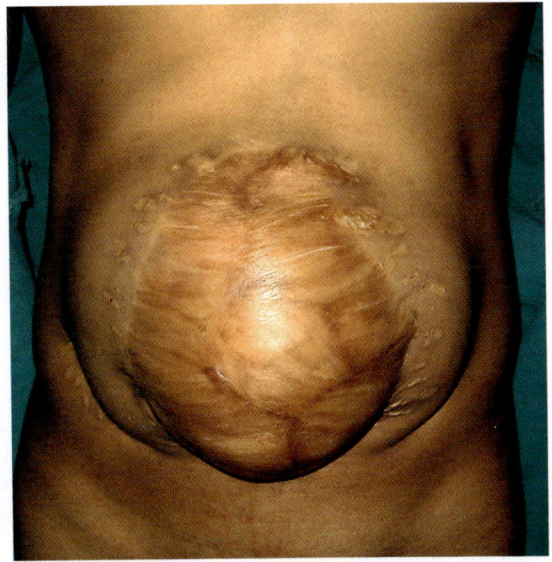

Fig. 19.4: Incisional hernia following burst abdomen

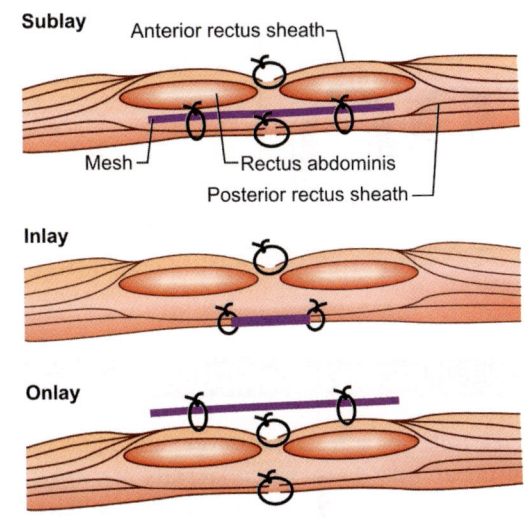

Fig. 19.5: Position of mesh in sublay, inlay and onlay repairs

and Dacron has been used successfully without causing any adhesion or erosion of the bowel. There are three general techniques for using the mesh in incisional hernia—onlay, inlay, and sublay. During surgery the old scar and redundant skin should be always excised and the underlying hernial sac is defined by careful dissection. Hernial sac preferably to be opened. Adhesion between the contents and the sac should be divided.

Onlay: During dissection the fascial edges are sutured by non-absorbable monofilament sutures preferably applying 1 cm bite at 1 cm interval. There after the mesh is placed over the suture line flat with no folds and no tension. Mesh should be secured by non-absorbable suture to the underlying fascia. Suction drain may be used and kept beneath the skin flaps (Fig. 19.5).

Inlay: This technique involves suturing the mesh to the fascial edge without closing the defect. It is important to use the correct mesh in this situation because of its contact with the underlying viscera (Fig. 19.5). Dacron mesh results are excellent. This technique should only be done when there is a substantial defect that cannot be bridged.

Sublay: In this technique the posterior rectus sheath and peritoneum is closed and the mesh is placed above this. Rectus muscles are allowed to cover the mesh and the anterior rectus sheath is closed (Fig. 19.5). This procedure is useful only in the midline.

In the present scenario laparoscopic repair of incisional hernia is also a promising technique. The postoperative complication rate is found to be 10% and recurrence rate around 3–4%.

20 Vascular Emergency

Acute ischemia affects the lower limb more than the upper limb because collaterals are usually adequate in arms in contrast to legs where collaterals are not present, unless a preexisting arterial disease has created enough collaterals. Sudden occlusion of artery occur commonly either due to embolus or thrombus. The outcome depends on the location of occlusion and the degree of collateral flow. In a sudden block of blood flow irreversible muscle damage may occur in few hours. Therefore, early diagnosis and treatment of acute limb ischemia is vital.

ETIOLOGY

Acute arterial occlusion could be intrinsic like embolic or thrombotic occlusion or extrinsic resulting from trauma. Embolism is the most common cause of acute limb ischemia. The common source of emboli is from left atrium in atrial fibrillation. Other sources of emboli are from mural thrombus after myocardial infraction, from aneurysm or from atherosclerotic vessels.

The upper extremities and cerebral vascular tree receive 20% of the peripheral emboli in cases of myocardial infarction. The terminal aorta and iliac system receive about 30% of the emboli. Carotid emboli are often multiple and have high mortality. Additional sources of cardiac emboli results from cardiomyopathy and congestive heart failure.

Patients with long bone fractures can have vessel disruption, angulation contusion or laceration. Arteries so affected are prone to thrombosis. Common sites are supracondylar dislocations or fracture of humerus or femur. The brachial and popliteal vessels are particularly at risk. Tibial plateau fracture affects distal popliteal integrity. Massive soft tissue swelling can also produce acute arterial occlusion. The lower extremity in the infrapopliteal region with its rigid fascial sheath can produce increase fascial compartment pressure.

Foreign bodies, tumor emboli, infection, ergotism are rare causes along with venous obstruction producing arterial occlusion.

Acute thrombus is generally seen in vessels which have been affected by atherosclerosis. In these cases, the ischemia is not that severe like embolic occlusion because of presence of some degree of collateral vessels. Most commonly affected vessel is superficial femoral artery which is often affected by atherosclerosis. Second most common vessel involved is popliteal artery where thrombus formation in popliteal aneurysm may lead to limb ischemia. Acute thrombus is also reported in previous arterial bypass causing recurrent ischemia.

PATHOPHYSIOLOGY

Site and degree of blockage, condition of distal arterial bed, pre-existing collateral circulation and overall metabolic condition of patient are important factors for the outcome of acute limb ischemia. In total blockage of major vessels the outcome is poor than the small vessel occlusion. Emboli generally tend to lodge at the bifurcation of arteries, most commonly the femoral bifurcation. Other uncommon sites are popliteal, iliac and aortic bifurcation. Whenever the arterial thrombosis is accompanied with venous thrombosis, the outcome is poorer because of the high risk of pulmonary embolism.

The blockage occurring in major vessel lead to proportionate increase in the metabolic demand of the tissue with a greater stress on the body as a whole. Total aortic blockage has more serious consequences than blockage of paired vessels in the distal extremity of leg or arm. Due to increase collateral pathways, small vessel occlusions are better tolerated.

CLINICAL MANIFESTATION AND EVALUATION

The hallmark of acute limb ischemia are 5 Ps.
- Pain
- Pallor
- Pulselessness
- Paresthesia
- Paralysis

Pain

Pain is the most common presentation and is present in more than three-fourths of the patients. The degree of pain depends on the severity of ischemia which is further determined by the level of obstruction and pre-existing collateral circulation. Sudden onset of pain in a previously asymptomatic patient clearly suggests the possibility of embolic phenomenon. In thrombosis, it is less sudden, and all such patients might have earlier features of claudication. In embolic occlusion foot will often be white in color with no capillary return, whereas in thrombotic occlusion when ischemia is less severe, foot may simply be paler with delayed capillary returns. Patients with embolic occlusion will generally be having atrial fibrillation or recent myocardial infarction, whereas in thrombotic occlusion there will be no such history.

Pallor

Pallor results from peripheral vasoconstriction associated with arterial spasm and decreased blood flow. Peripheral nerves are highly susceptible to hypoxia in such condition. Patients who have anesthetic paralytic ischemic limb are the poorest candidate for revascularization because of advanced tissue ischemia and hypoxemia. Sensory loss is an important sign of acute limb ischemia and dictates the need for acute intervention. Degree of nerve dysfunction is directly proportionate to the degree of ischemia. In such patients, paresthesia is characterized by numbness of the toes, and decrease in sensation compared to the other site for light touch and pin prick sensation. Weakness of limb is another important sign of limb ischemia.

Pulselessness

Absence of peripheral pulses may be acute or chronic. Contralateral palpable pulse with ipsilateral absence of pulse may suggest an embolic phenomenon. The character of peripheral pulse proximal to block may indicate the level of emboli. Bounding pulse of water hammer nature is suggestive of occlusive site. This situation may be helpful in surgical approach. A hand held Doppler examination plays an important role in evaluation of patients of acute limb ischemia.

Diagnostic Evaluation

- Careful history and physical examination
- Patients having embolic phenomenon have the risk factors like atrial fibrillation, recent acute MI and prosthetic heart valves.
- More sudden onset, no past history of claudication, unilateral edema and contralateral palpable pulse favors embolic occlusion.
- Routine blood examination, X-ray chest and ECG should be obtained.
- Whenever the diagnosis of embolism is doubtful and the site of arteriotomy is not clear, arteriogram should be done to define the anatomy which is helpful in operative procedures of revascularization.
- The patient having atrial fibrillation and signs of arterial occlusion suggest the diagnosis of arterial emboli. Such patients need not go for invasive

procedures like arteriography and immediate embolectomy should be undertaken. Whereas, in absence of atrial fibrillation acute arterial thrombosis is the most likely diagnosis.

- A non-invasive evaluation by Doppler USG is very useful. A Doppler probe confirms the presence of normal arterial signal. Recently the USG has revolutionized the vessel imaging. With added color coding it gives the detail of velocity profile and the change in the direction of blood flow which can be used to grade the severity of obstructive lesion.

- Aortic and lower limb arteriography generally performed by needle puncture of femoral artery followed by guide wire insertion and catheter insertion by Seldinger technique. After visualizing the catheter fluoroscopically, radiopaque contrast is injected and images are obtained. The catheter and puncture related hazards like hematoma, local thrombosis and arteriovenous fistula should be kept in mind. Post processing of digital images allows subtraction of overlying bones and other enhancement to facilitate visualization of the vessel and its lesion (Digital subtraction angiography).

DIFFERENTIAL DIAGNOSIS

The diagnosis most easily confused with acute arterial occlusion is deep vein thrombosis (DVT). Swelling is not an early component in cases of acute ischemia, whereas in DVT it is often the hallmark. DVT often presents with superficial venous fullness and non collapsed superficial veins. In cases of phlegmasia cerulea dolens there is a massive edema and skin necrosis in more than 50% of cases.

TREATMENT

Early recognition of acute ischemia and treatment is vital to save the limb. Lower limb is placed in the dependent position protected from the environment. There is no role of vasodilatation in cases of acute ischemic limb. The anticoagulation therapy and early embolectomy are the widely accepted treatment of acute embolic arterial occlusion. The anticoagulation

measures should be substituted immediately to prevent the propagation of thrombus and further embolization. Heparin infusion in a loading dose of 5000 IU should be given intravenously and maintained by infusion sufficient to prolong the PTT to 2.0–2.5 times of the control level. A high dose of heparin is advised as the sole therapy for patients who are unfit for surgery. Relief of pain with narcotics and management of systemic disease may at time prove to be the most important treatment for the debilitated patient. Primary amputation is the most beneficial therapeutic regimen in selected patients. One should always consider the entire patient when weighing the value the immediate surgical therapy versus the conservative non-operative therapy. The absence of both sensation and motor activity with flabby muscle mass do contraindicate the procedure of embolectomy.

Surgical Procedure— Embolectomy/Thrombectomy

It is always advisable that the operating table should be equipped with fluoroscopy. In urgent situations, this procedure can be undertaken under local anesthesia but it is safe to have the anesthetist available for monitoring of the patient and if required to give general anesthesia.

Adequate surgical exposure should be obtained for all vessels while attempting embolectomy.

- In the lower limb transfemoral embolectomy is the operation of choice by exposing the common femoral artery and its bifurcation by a vertical incision.

- Choice of arteriotomy may be tangential, vertical or horizontal depending upon the atherosclerotic pattern of the particular vessel. In relatively normal vessel transverse arteriotomy is justified above the orifices of superficial and profunda femoris artery. Transverse arteriotomy is easier to close without narrowing the vessel. Longitudinal arteriotomy is advantageous if arterial reconstruction becomes necessary.

- After opening the artery, Fogarty balloon embolectomy catheter is inserted to extract the thrombus from the proximal vessels (Fig. 20.1).

- Routinely distal embolectomy is preferred to extract thrombus from superficial femoral artery and profunda femoris artery.
- Passing of the Fogarty catheter should be done repeatedly until no further embolus is withdrawn.
- During the procedure of balloon inflation and traction of catheter one has to be careful not to damage the artery.
- After all clots have been extracted and good flow of blood has been established, distal heparinization is done with saline flushing. On removing the clamp, extremity should become pink with return of pulses. Thereafter arteriotomy is closed.
- In case, the clot cannot be removed from above, retrograde embolectomy is carried out by cut down over posterior tibial and anterior tibial vessel over the ankle.
- If the catheter has failed to pass distally or the result of embolectomy is not satisfactory, on table arteriography should be done. Intraoperative Doppler ultrasound may also be helpful in determining the vessel patency. In such situations

bypass grafting may be undertaken if required. The determinant whether a successful embolectomy has been performed is dependent on the feel of the catheter as it is withdrawn through narrowing. Over inflation of balloon may cause balloon or arterial rupture.

COMPLICATIONS

During the entire procedure of embolectomy the greatest single hazard is mismatch of catheter and vessel size. Although the catheters are specifically designed for flexibility and excellent pliability, vessel perforation, subintimal dissection and vessel damage can occur.

POSTOPERATIVE CARE

- Repeated examination of extremity for vasculariztion
- Repeat Doppler for patency of vessel
- Patient should have treatment of underlying disease.
  Overall mortality still remains at around 20–30% following the peripheral artery occlusion. Morbidity associated with the loss of lower limb is associated with multiple emboli.

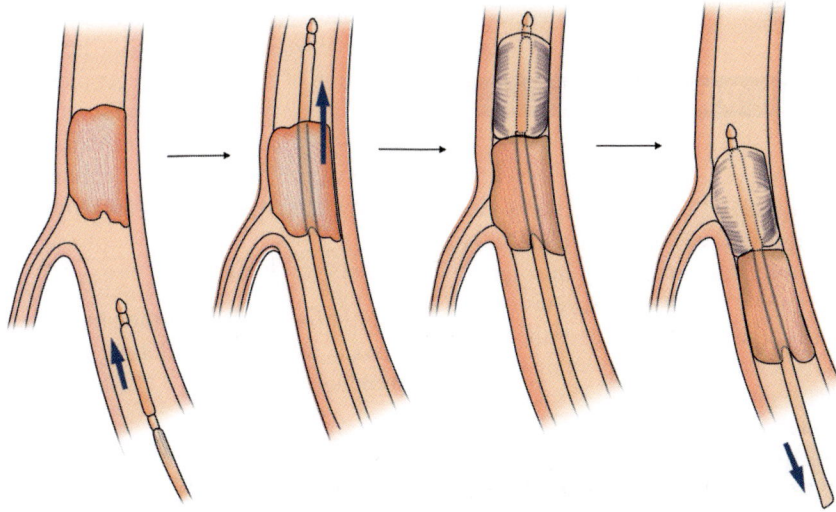

Fig. 20.1: Steps of embolectomy by Fogarty catheter with catheter insertion in the distal vessel

ROLE OF FIBRINOLYSIS

Embolectomy remains the gold standard for acute arterial occlusion. In certain cases intra-arterial dissolution of thrombus by streptokinase and urokinase can be used. These agents convert plasminogen to plasmin, which degrades the fibrin. After fibrinolysis, heparin infusion is administered to prevent further formation of clots. In case clots could not be removed with embolectomy, intra-arterial catheter is left in place for postoperative thrombolytic infusion.

ROLE OF ANTICOAGULATION

Heparin infusion is given after embolectomy for preventing further formation of thrombus. Patient is later maintained on warfarin. Warfarin is continued till the primary cause of embolism is corrected.

Management of acute arterial occlusion remains ever challenging in the surgical discipline. The balloon embolectomy catheter has significantly reduced the morbidity and mortality in these cases. One must remember that the patients with acute arterial occlusion always have significant underlying pathology and that leads to poor long-term prognosis.

DEEP VEIN THROMBOSIS

INTRODUCTION

Deep vein thrombosis (DVT) is an important acute condition involving the lower extremity and is a major cause of morbidity and mortality in surgical patients. DVT commonly affects the leg veins (such as the femoral vein or the popliteal vein) or the deep veins of the pelvis. Occasionally the veins of the arm are affected (if spontaneous, this is known as Paget–Schrötter disease). DVT can occur without symptoms or may results in pulmonary embolism. But in majority of the cases, the affected extremity will be painful, swollen, red and warm with engorged superficial veins.

ETIOLOGY

Virchow's triad is a group of three factors known to affect clot formation:
- Rate of flow (decreased flow rate of the blood)
- The viscosity of the blood (an increased tendency of the blood to clot)
- Quality of the vessel wall (damage to the blood vessel wall).

The triad of Virchow's still holds true in causing DVT in surgical patients.

Stasis

Diminished flow occurs during and after surgery. It has been documented that in supine position. Blood flow in soleal vessels or sinuses is extremely sluggish and thrombus formation is seen in patients predisposed for formation of thrombus.

Hypercoagulability

The important anticoagulant mechanisms responsible for restricting the formation of thrombus formation are antithrombin, protein C, protein S, tissue factor inhibitor and fibrinolytic systems. Deficiency in any of these mechanisms can cause a prothrombotic state. In patients with high risk like malignancy, obesity, prolonged immobilization, long pelvic surgery, congestive heart failure, etc. formation of thrombus can get precipitated. During major surgery, large amount of tissue factor is released into circulation from damaged tissues along with rise of platelet and decreased fibrinolytic activity, thereby causing a prothrombotic state.

Vessel Wall Injury

Endothelial damage either by direct trauma or hypoxia, activates the clotting factors and initiates thrombus formation.

COMMON RISK FACTORS

- Recent surgery of long duration or hospitalization
- Advanced age
- Obesity

- Infection
- Immobilization
- Use of combined (estrogen-containing) forms of hormonal contraception
- Pregnancy.

SYMPTOMS

Patient may present with the following symptoms.

- Pain
- Swelling
- Redness of the leg
- Tenderness along the thigh or calf
- Muscle induration and mild pyrexia.

Many patients however will have no appreciable symptom or sign in the affected limb. Unilateral pitting edema to the affected limb may indicate underlying thrombosis in DVT.

PHYSICAL EXAMINATION

1. *Homans' test:* Dorsiflexion of foot elicits pain in posterior calf. However, it must be noted that it is of little diagnostic value and is theoretically dangerous because of the possibility of dislodgement of loose clot.
2. *Pratt's sign:* Squeezing of posterior calf elicits pain.

However, these medical signs neither confirm the diagnosis nor quantify the severity of the disease process. Physical examination is unreliable for excluding the diagnosis of deep vein thrombosis.

Phlegmasia Alba Dolens

In this condition the leg is pale and cold with diminished arterial pulse due to spasm. It usually results from acute occlusion of the iliac and femoral veins due to DVT. The pallor is probably a result of capillary compression in the skin by the edema. This condition is also known as white leg syndrome.

Phlegmasia Cerulea Dolens

With further progression of the disease and involvement of whole iliac venous system produces a more dramatic edema causing arterial insufficiency with sever pain and cyanosis known as Phlegmasia Cerulea Dolens (Figs 20.2A and 2B). At times areas of patchy skin gangrene may also develop in the affected limb. This venous gangrene can be differentiated from the arterial by the marked edema and cyanosis in the skin in contradiction to the pallor and absence of swelling which is typical of arterial occlusion.

Differential Diagnosis

Conditions which may mimic like DVT are ruptured Backers cyst, calf muscle hematoma, superficial

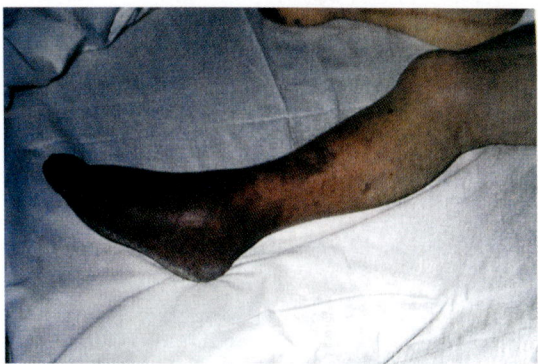

Fig. 20.2A: Phlegmasia cerulea dolens in a patient of DVT

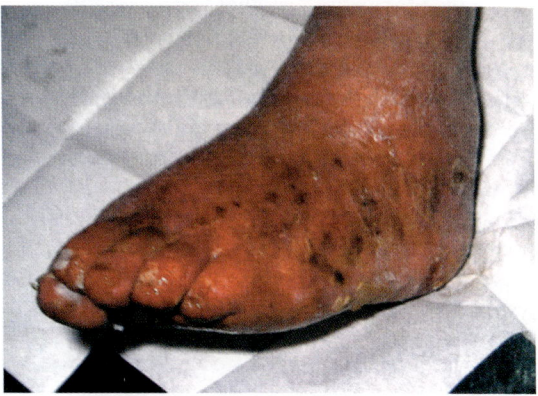

Fig. 20.2B: Same patients after treament

thrombophlebitis, ruptured plantaris tendon and cellulitis. Duplex scanning will confirm the diagnosis in most of the patients.

DIAGNOSIS

Doppler Ultrasonography

This is a simple noninvasive test for diagnosing DVT. Absence of flow signal over the femoral vein, loss of phasicity (absence of change in audible signal on deep inspiration) and failure of augmentation of signal on squeezing the calf are some of the important signs of DVT on Doppler ultrasonography.

Duplex Ultrasonography

This test involves both B-mode ultrasound and Doppler flow analysis (Fig. 20.3). The ability of high resolution to actually visualize the deep vein, their flow, location and nature of thrombus make this investigation an ideal modality for diagnosing DVT.

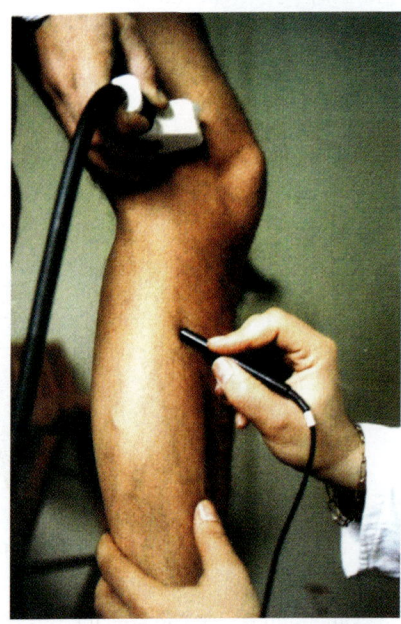

Fig. 20.3: Duplex USG in a patient of suspected DVT

Intravenous Venography

It remains the gold standard in the diagnosis of DVT. In this contrast is injected in foot vein after the superficial veins are occluded with tourniquet. Because of its invasiveness and risk associated with contrast injection, this test is rarely performed. The indications are
- High clinical suspicion but not confirmed by the noninvasive tests.
- Prior to iliofemoral thrombectomy and placement of IVC filter.

D-dimer

It measures the degradation of intravascular fibrin. D- dimer is usually elevated after surgery, therefore positive D- dimer test in postoperative patient is of little use. However, negative D- dimer very credibly excludes the possibility of DVT.

Impedance Plethysmography

It measures the change in venous capacitance and rate of emptying of volume of veins. It has an overall sensitivity of 80% when DVT involves major veins but sensitivity is poor for small veins.

Spiral CT and CT pulmonary angiography are the first line investigation for the diagnosis of pulmonary embolization.

COMPLICATION

The greatest complication of DVT is that the clot can dislodge and travel to the lungs, which is called a pulmonary embolism (PE). A late complication of DVT is the post-phlebitic syndrome, which can manifest itself as edema, pain or discomfort and skin problems.

MANAGEMENT

The aim of treatment of stable patient with DVT should be
1. Stop the propagation of the clot
2. Prevent the risk of pulmonary embolism
3. Resolution of thrombus by fibrinolysis.

Anticoagulation

Anticoagulation with heparin and warfarin are the mainstay of treatment and prevention of venous thromboembolism. It dose not lyse the thrombi but prevents the propagation and embolization. Proximal lower limb thrombosis requires anticoagulation to prevent the embolization. Calf DVT seldom emobilize but if left untreated may extend above the knee in 10% of the cases. Repeat imaging should be done to detect this phenomenon.

Heparin

Standard regimen is to give 100–200 IU per kg of unfractionated heparin as a bolus dose followed by 18 IU per kg hourly infusion to achieve APTT (activated partial thromboplastin time) 1.5– 2.5 times of the normal value. Warfarin is started simultaneously along with heparin (10 mg on first day and 5 mg later on) and is continued until the International normalized ratio (INR) is 2.0–2.5 for two consecutive days. Regular monitoring by measurement of INR is essential. Anticoagulation with warfarin is continued for three to six months.

Problems with Heparin

- *Bleeding:* The risk of major bleeding is low at prophylactic doses but increases to 2.5% with therapeutic doses of unfractionated heparin compared with 1.5% with low molecular weight heparin (LMWH). The concurrent illness, age and use of aspirin increases the risk of major bleeding.
- *Thrombocytopenia:* Reduction in platelet count is occasionally seen with heparin therapy. This result from platelet aggregation and does not occur with LMWH.
- *Osteoporosis:* It can develop after several months of heparin treatment. Fracture may occur. It is rare with LMWH.

Warfarin Therapy

Warfarin acts by interfering with the production of vitamin K dependent factors like II, VII, IX, X in addition to protein C and S. As mentioned earlier, warfarin is monitored by INR. High loading dose of warfarin results in rapid reduction of the anticoagulant protein C and S which can cause thrombosis of subcutaneous vessel and necrosis. To prevent this, heparin is always given before starting warfarin in patients of venous thrombo-embolic disease and is continued until the INR is more than two at least for two days. Warfarin is well absorbed from the gut and is mainly bound to albumin and has a circulating half-life of 36 to 40 hrs.

Problems with Warfarin Therapy

There are various factors which affect the warfarin requirement like congestive heart failure, liver failure and alcohol intake.

- *Drug interaction:* Patients on warfarin should avoid all preparations containing aspirin.
- *Bleeding:* The risk of bleeding increases whenever the INR is more than five. Warfarin should always be reduced or withheld until the bleeding is controlled by the help of prothrombin complex concentrate, fresh frozen plasma (FFP) and vitamin K.
- *Pregnancy:* Warfarin crosses the placenta and can cause adverse effect in the fetus. Exposure to warfarin during organogenesis is associated with chondrodysplasia and severe fetal deformity. The risk of fetal damage must be weighted against the problems and risk of converting to heparin in mother. Heparin does not cross the placenta but can cause adverse effects in mother. Therefore, LMWH is safe and effective in prophylaxis and treatment of venous thrombosis in pregnancy.

Low Molecular Weight Heparin (LMWH)

LMWH is as effective as unfractionated heparin in the treatment of DVT. They differ from heparin in following ways

- The bioavailability is >90% after subcutaneous injection compared to 20% with heparin

- Prolonged half-life with predictable linear clearing, so it can be given as once or twice daily dose.
- Predictable therapeutic response, so no monitoring is required and can be used as out patient basis
- Little effect on platelet and vascular permeability, so there is less chance of bleeding

For these reasons LMWH is found to be safe, efficacious, with lower risk of bleeding compared to heparin.

Thrombolysis

Thrombolysis by streptokinase and urokinase has got a role in extensive iliofemoral clot and pulmonary embolism. However, thrombolysis is also associated with increased chance of bleeding. Venous thrombectomy can be done alternatively.

Inferior Vena Cava Filter

Inferior vena cava filter reduces pulmonary embolism and is an option for patients with an absolute contraindication to anticoagulant treatment (e.g. cerebral hemorrhage) and in patients with objectively documented recurrent pulmonary embolism while on anticoagulation. IVC filters are temporizing measure for preventing life-threatening pulmonary embolism and these should be removed after 4–6 weeks.

Prophylaxis of Venous Thromboembolism

LMWH in conjunction with mechanical methods like compression stocking reduces the thrombo-embolic phenomenon associated with orthopedic and other high-risk surgery. Graduated compression stockings are a simple, safe, and moderately effective form of thromboprophylaxis. These stockings work by increasing the velocity of venous blood flow. Combination of LMWH and mechanical methods particularly compression stockings have shown superior efficacy in DVT prevention in several studies. Low intensity warfarin (target INR 1.5) is used in some patients with long-term indwelling venous catheter.

PULMONARY EMBOLISM

It is a spectrum of disease between insignificant microembolization of pulmonary vessel to a massive fatal pulmonary embolization affecting both the pulmonary arteries. Thrombus generally develops in the deep veins of the lower limbs especially in stasis and hypercoagulable states. At times the clot propagates and dislodges and embolizes to the pulmonary vessel thus depriving a segment of lung from their arterial supply. This further leads to pulmonary edema and hinders blood gas exchange. As the alveolar dead space is increased, gaseous exchange is further impaired. There is increase in right ventricular load, leading to right sided heart failure.

Pulmonary embolism accounts for 3% of all surgical deaths. The risk factor for Pulmonary Embolism (PE) includes

- High body mass index (obesity)
- Cigarette smoking
- Hypertension
- Prolonged surgery like orthopedic surgery to lower limb and extensive pelvic surgery
- Factor V laiden deficiency
- Hypercystinemia.

CLINICAL PICTURE

It is commonly not diagnosed prior to patient's death because of its few clinical manifestation. The common presentations suggestive of PE includes

Symptoms

- Dyspnea on mild to moderate exertion
- Dyspnea at rest
- Pleuritic chest pain
- Hemoptysis
- Central chest pain and syncope in cases of massive embolism.

Signs

- Tachypnea usually RR>20/min
- Abnormal physical findings on chest examination

- Elevated jugular venous pressure
- Pleuritic friction rub
- Central cyanosis
- Left parasternal heave
- Loud second heart sound.

INVESTIGATIONS

Urgent investigations required in such situation includes—Arterial blood gas, ECG and X-ray chest.

ECG shows right axis shift, right bundle branch block, tachycardia and T-wave inversion in anterior chest lead (V1–V4).

X-ray chest is frequently normal. Westermark's sign (decrease pulmonary vascular marking in peripheral lung field) or Pall's sign (enlarged right descending pulmonary artery) may be seen.

In cases where there is a less possibility of pulmonary embolism, the D-dimer enzyme linked immunosorbent assay and the Doppler ultrasound of the lower extremity is performed. Negative D-dimer shows that pulmonary embolism is very unlikely.

Other tests which are helpful are—ventilation perfusion lung scan, echocardiography, high resolution spiral CT and the pulmonary angiography.

Ventilation Perfusion lung scan

The use of ventilation perfusion lung scan as a diagnostic test for PE is based on the assumption that ventilation is preserved in the areas of reduced perfusion due to PE and that ventilation is abnormal when perfusion defects are due to the primary lung disease. But this assumption is known to be incorrect as ventilation perfusion matching may occur in early PE. In cases of decreased perfusion with normal ventilation there is a high probability of pulmonary embolism. Helical CT is helpful in defining the thrombosis in the pulmonary artery.

MANAGEMENT

Prevention

As most of the patients die with minimal symptoms, preventive measure is more important than therapeutic measure. There are two approaches for prevention of pulmonary embolism.

- Primary prophylaxis using drugs or physical methods which are effective against deep vein thrombosis.
- Early detection of subclinical venous thrombosis by screening high risk patients (postoperative scanning with iodine-125 fibrinogen) which provides the opportunity for treating silent thromboses early, before they embolize.

Primary prophylaxis is probably the more effective and less expensive approach. The main focus of thromboprophylaxis has been in the surgical disciplines, but there is a similarly strong need for the prophylaxis in non-surgical patients as well. Several recently completed trials in medical patients suggest that the use of LMWH is recommended in all the high-risk patients particularly those with heart failure and stroke.

Treatment

Anticoagulation, oxygen and analgesic are mainstay of the management. Heparin is the main component of the management. It enhances the anti-thrombotic activity and prevents the further propagation of the thrombus. Bolus dose of 5000–10000 IU is given IV followed by continuous infusion of heparin in dose 18 IU/kg/ hr not exceeding more than 1600 IU/ hr to achieve APTT level to a range of 1.5 to 2.0 times the normal. Oral anticoagulation with warfarin is started simultaneously in a dose of 5 mg OD and the dose is adjusted till INR is 2.5. Heparin is stopped when the INR level of 2.5 is achieved and warfarin is continued for minimum of 3 months. Patients who are at a high-risk for anti-coagulation therapy, placement of IVC filter should be considered. Efficacy of IVC filter is 95%. Thrombolytic therapy with streptokinase or urokinase is given in patients with massive thromboembolism. If thrombolytic therapy is unsuccessful then catheter suction embolectomy or open embolectomy is done.

21 Urogenital Emergency

HEMATURIA

Hematuria is an alarming situation indicating the presence of blood in the urine. Even a single episode of hematuria needs thorough investigation. Early intervention is important as delay may make curative treatment difficult. Hematuria may present as painless hematuria, painful hematuria, incidental finding of microscopic hematuria or positive dipstick hematuria.

TYPES OF HEMATURIA

Macroscopic or Gross Hematuria

Presence of frank blood causing red urine is the most common presentation of transitional cell carcinoma and papillary tumors of urinary bladder. It is often found in cases of renal cell carcinoma as well. Pseudo-hematuria may result from ingestion of foods like beetroot and blackberries. Use of certain drugs like rifampicin, phenothiazides may also turn the urine red in color.

Microscopic Hematuria

Presence of 5–10 RBC/ HPF in urine is considered as microscopic hematuria. All positive dipstick tests should be confirmed by microscopic examination of urine to label them as microscopic hematuria. All such patients warrant full investigation to find out any underlying disease even when the patient appears to be asymptomatic.

Dipstick Hematuria

It detects the hemoglobin in RBC by using the reagent strips in urine. Positive dipstick for blood in urine indicates hematuria, hemoglobinuria, or myoglobinuria. This chemical detection of blood in normal urine is based on the peroxidase like activity of hemoglobin. The degree of change in the color is directly proportionate to the presence of hemoglobin found in the urine specimen. The sensitivity of dipstick test is over 90% but there could be false positive dipstick reading due to contamination of urine specimen with the menstrual blood. False results can also be seen in cases of dehydration due to increased concentration of erythrocyte and hemoglobin. The efficacy of hematuria screening by dipstick test to find out the underlying urological pathology is very controversial as it has very low rate in detecting significant diseased pathology.

Important Causes of Hematuria of Surgical Importance (Fig. 21.1)

- *Renal*
  1. Tumors (Renal cell carcinoma or Hyper-nephroma and TCC of Renal Pelvis)
  2. Infection /inflammation
  3. Trauma
  4. Renal cyst
  5. Arteriovenous fistula
  6. Nephrological (Glomerulonephritis)
  7. Stones.

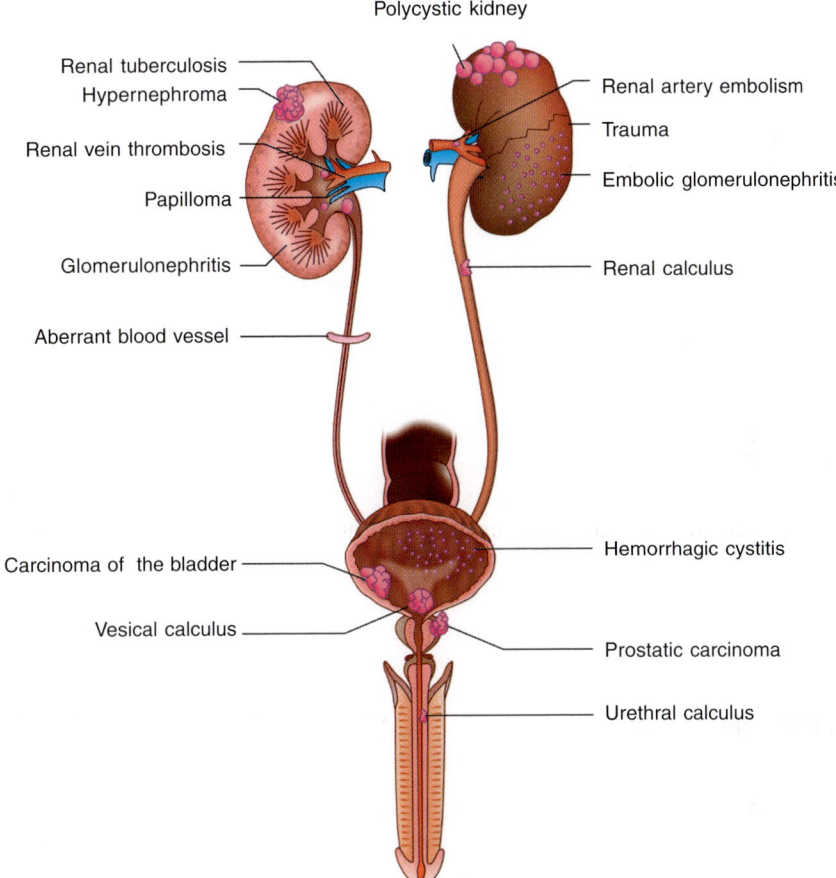

Polycystic kidney

Renal tuberculosis
Hypernephroma

Renal vein thrombosis

Papilloma

Glomerulonephritis

Aberrant blood vessel

Renal artery embolism

Trauma

Embolic glomerulonephritis

Renal calculus

Carcinoma of the bladder

Vesical calculus

Hemorrhagic cystitis

Prostatic carcinoma

Urethral calculus

Fig. 21.1: Important causes of hematuria

- *Ureter*
  1. Tumors (Transitional cell carcinoma-TCC)
  2. Stone
- *Bladder*
  1. Tumor (TCC) or papillary tumor
  2. Infection/inflammation
  3. Stone
- *Prostate*
  1. Tumors (Adenocarcinoma)
  2. BPH/post-TURP and Prostatis
- *Urethra*
  1. Infection/inflammation (urethritis).
  2. Stone and Trauma

CLINICAL FEATURES

Presentation

Hematuria when appears in the beginning of urinary stream (initial hematuria) indicates that the lesion is in the urethra or prostate. Total hematuria arises from bladder and upper urinary tract (kidney and ureter) on account of stone, trauma, tumor or inflammation due to bacterial or interstitial cystitis. The ribbon like threads or clots usually suggests bleeding from ureter. These clots occasionally are responsible for urinary retention. The terminal hematuria is seen at the end of micturition after passing the normal clear urine. This condition reflects the pathology lying in the urinary bladder at trigone or bladder neck. Terminal hematuria can also be seen in vesical calculus and hypervascular prostate in cases of BPH. Bleeding is also seen after TURP (transurethral resection of prostate) in postoperative period. Painless gross hematuria is mostly associated with urinary tract tumors like transitional cell carcinoma, renal cell carcinoma, and bladder papilloma. The painful hematuria indicates underlying inflammatory pathology either in the urethra or in the bladder.

Symptoms Associated with Hematuria

- Renal pain—caused by renal tumor, calculi, renal obstruction and infection
- Bladder pain—tumor, stone and infection.
- Dysuria—urinary infection, bladder and urethral tumor or calculi
- Ureteric colic—tumor, stone and ureteric calculus
- Frequency—urinary tract infection, ureteric calculus, bladder tumor or calculus, BPH or carcinoma prostate
- Strangury—urinary infection, tumor or stone
- Retention—due to clots retained in the bladder, BPH or urethral stone

Clinical Examination and Evaluation

Before proceeding to clinical evaluation one should elicit the past history of tuberculosis, drug intake like anticoagulants and family history of bleeding disorders. The examination should focus on the examination of genitourinary system. Abdominal examination should be done to look for any renal, abdominal or pelvic mass. External genitalia should also be examined. Digital rectal examination and per vaginal should not be missed. In elderly male prostate examination is mandatory.

INVESTIGATIONS

Urine Analysis

Routine urine examination for pus cells, RBC and proteinuria should be done. Further microscopy of the

urinary sediments obtained from the centrifuging the fresh samples of the urine should also be done. Urinary casts on microscopic examination suggests renal disease and crystals suggests calculus disease. The urinary cytology is also important to find out the presence of malignant cells which get shed from the tumor in the urine. Simple culture may reveal the infection.

Blood Test

The full blood count and serum creatinine and blood urea as well as electrolyte are important base line investigations. They reflect the degree of renal impairment.

Evaluation of Lower Urinary Tract

Cystourethroscopy

It is mandatory to subject all the patients of hematuria for cystourethroscopy with an end viewing telescope (0/30 degree). It should be performed in both men and women to exclude bladder carcinoma, papilliferous growth of bladder and urethral lesions (Fig. 21.2). All suspicious area during cystoscopy should be biopsied for histopathological examination.

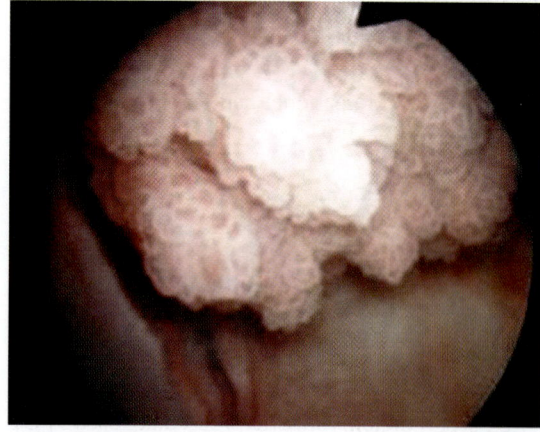

Fig. 21.2: Cystoscopy showing papilliferous bladder growth

Ureteroscopy

With the recent development, rigid or flexible ureteroscopy can be performed to evaluate the ureters and to take biopsy, brush cytology and selective ureteric urine sampling for cytology.

Evaluation of Upper Urinary Tract

On account of varieties of possible pathology causing hematuria no single imaging modality can be considered as gold standard.

Ultrasonography (USG)

USG of abdomen and pelvis is good for the diagnosis of renal tumors, stone and calcification as well as bladder growth, stone and prostate enlargement. It is also good for detecting the hydronephrosis and hydroureters. The transrectal USG is considered as a good imaging modality for the investigation of prostatic enlargement and malignancy. USG for urinary tract is safe and noninvasive investigation.

Intravenous Urogram (IVU)

All patient subjected to IVU should be prepared with dulcolax and charcoal, which helps to remove the bowel gas and feces. An initial plain supine abdominal radiograph should be performed to see the soft tissue mass and calculi. Before injecting the contrast (urograffin), a sensitivity test should always be done. It is helpful in detecting renal tumor, stone, cyst and ureteric TCC and functional status of both the kidney. However, small urothelial tumors may be missed in urography.

CT Scan

CT is not a first line investigation of hematuria but is helpful to evaluate mass lesions of kidney, retroperitoneum and bladder and helpful in planning the treatment (Fig. 21.3). Tumor infiltration into surrounding tissue or renal vein in RCC is well demonstrated by CT scan. Angiomyolipoma is best diagnosed by CT scan because of differential shadows produced by the constituents of this uncommon benign tumor.

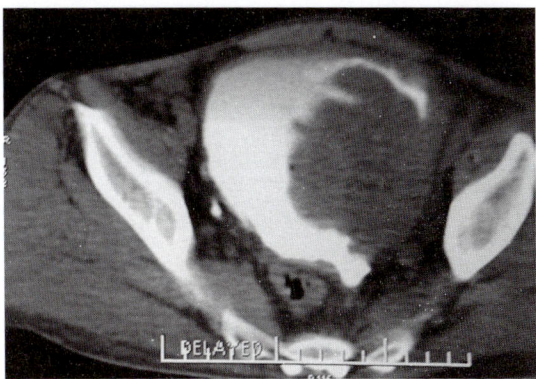

Fig. 21.3: CECT abdomen showing mass in the urinary bladder

MRI

It is a useful method of investigation for urinary tract abnormalities. It helps to supplement CT scan for evaluation of renal mass. In recent era it is turned out to be a good imaging for internal anatomy of prostate.

Arteriography

Arteriography has a role in selective embolization of tumor vessel when uncontrolled bleeding occurs in a frail patient.

MANAGEMENT

In patients presenting in the emergency with acute hematuria, resuscitation is done with intravenous fluids, blood is sent for hemoglobin estimation and blood is transfused if required. Three-way Foley catheter is inserted and bladder irrigation is started (Figs 21.4A and 4B). Sometimes cystoscopy is required for evacuation of bladder clots. Coagulation abnormality if present is to be corrected. In almost all cases hematuria settles on its own.

Further management of hematuria depends on the cause found. Clear diagnosis is possible in 70% of cases only. If cause is not found in gross hematuria, there could be a possibility of enlarged prostate or engorged bladder neck and it can be detected by cystoscopy. In women cystitis is a common cause of hematuria which

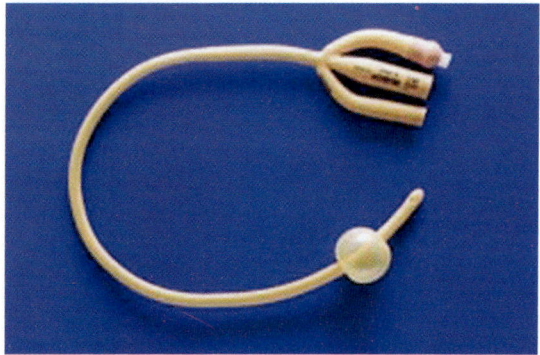

Fig. 21.4A: Three-way Foley catheter

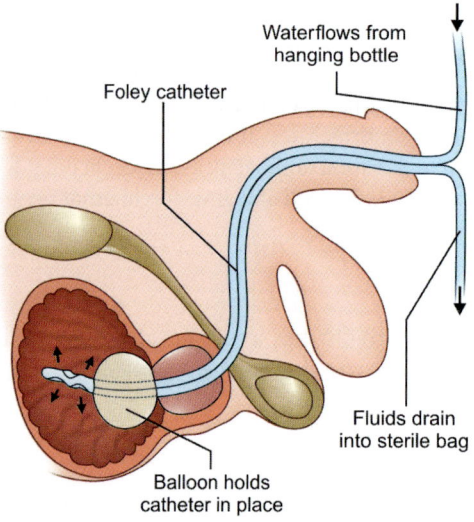

Waterflows from
hanging bottle

Foley catheter

Fluids drain
into sterile bag

Balloon holds
catheter in place

Fig. 21.4B: Bladder irrigation

is always associated with dysuria and frequency. Microscopic hematuria is seldom due to malignant disease but it is important to exclude malignancy as a potential cause and patient should be followed closely with imaging study and urine cytology.

RETENTION OF URINE

Urinary retention may be acute or chronic, painful or painless, complete or overflow incontinence. In acute condition it is always painful and complete, whereas in chronic it is painless and may be associated with overflow incontinence.

ASSESSMENT AND MANAGEMENT

In patients presenting with inability to pass urine a careful history and physical examination is very helpful in establishing the etiology and choosing appropriate course of management. Retention no doubt can occur at any age group and in both sex but predominantly it is seen in elderly male. In children most likely cause for retention are phimosis, meatal stenosis, urethral stone and posterior urethral valve. Therefore a thorough examination of genitalia is must. In all those patients who are unable to pass urine and bladder is not palpable and having features of uremia, a medical renal disease should be suspected and treated accordingly.

In cases of retention with palpable bladder and having phimosis, a prepucial slit or circumcision may be undertaken. In case of stone in the urethra, suprapubic catheterization can be done if the bladder is found to be full on percussion.

In other conditions, transurethral catheter may be tried and if that fails, suprapubic catheterization should be done and patient is kept for further investigations and management at a later date.

In young adults, a thorough examination, careful history to be taken for trauma, history of contact and pyuria. Urethra on palpation may give the evidence of stricture, which could be post-traumatic or after gonococcal urethritis. Retention is to be relieved by suprapubic catheterization and patient should be called for micturiting cystourethrogram and retrograde urethrogram to know the detail of stricture (Fig. 21.5). Patient can be subjected to dilatation or intraoptic urethrotomy or urethroplasty at later date, based on the findings in urethrogram.

In elderly male, a thorough examination of genitalia and abdomen is to be done to see the palpable kidney or bladder. Digital rectal examination should be done to evaluate the prostate enlargement. In case the bladder is palpable and prostate is significantly enlarged, effort should be made to pass the Foley

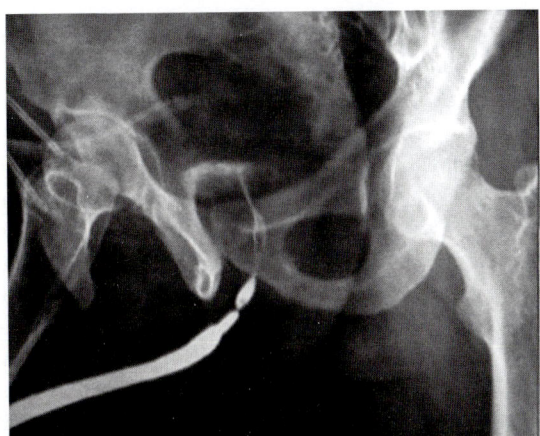

Fig. 21.5: Retrograde urethrogram in a patient with suprapubic cystostomy showing stricture at the membranous urethra

Percutaneous Cystostomy

Distended urinary bladder is confirmed by palpation and percussion. Wide-bore needle connected to a syringe is then inserted into the bladder 2 cm above the symphysis pubis to reconfirm the position of bladder by aspirating urine. Local anesthesia is administered, thereafter in the midline, 2 cm above the symphysis pubis a small 1 cm incision is made and through that the trochar and cannula is inserted and advanced vertically with care (Fig. 21.6A). After meeting some resistance, they will pass easily into the cavity of the bladder, as confirmed by the flow of urine when the trocar is withdrawn from the cannula. Introduce the catheter well into the bladder through the cannula (Fig. 21.6B). Once urine flows freely from the catheter, withdraw the cannula (Fig. 21.6C). Fix the catheter to the skin and connect it to a bag.

catheter in strict aseptic manner. If the catheter is not easily negotiating, then Gibbon's catheter may be tried as it is more stiff and can overcome the obstruction at the prostatic urethra. Alternatively Foley can be negotiated with help of catheter introducer. It should be done by expert hand without causing any urethral injury or false passages. During difficulties in catheterization, one should not use any force or inflate the balloon until urine has started flowing from the catheter. Catheter introducer should be used cautiously and gently.

In case the catheter cannot be negotiated with all possible means, percutaneous cystostomy (supracath/cystofix) under local anesthesia is to be done to relief the retention. Thereafter, the patient is admitted for further evaluation of benign prostatic hyperplasia (BPH) which is the most common cause of retention of urine in elderly male.

Many times in elderly male having prostatic enlargement, urinary retention may get precipitated in following situations
- Perineal surgery
- Painful anal condition
- Excess bout of alcohol
- Drugs like diuretic, anticholinergics, antidepressants and sympathomimetics
- CVA

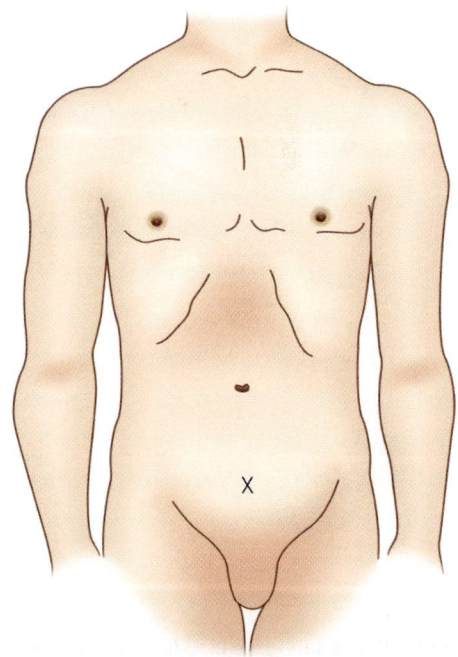

Fig. 21.6A: Site for insertion of trocar and cannula (2 cm above the symphysis pubis in the midline)

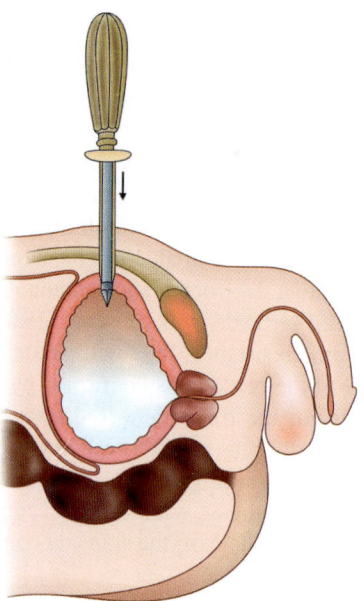

Fig. 21.6B: Trocar and cannula inserted vertically into the bladder

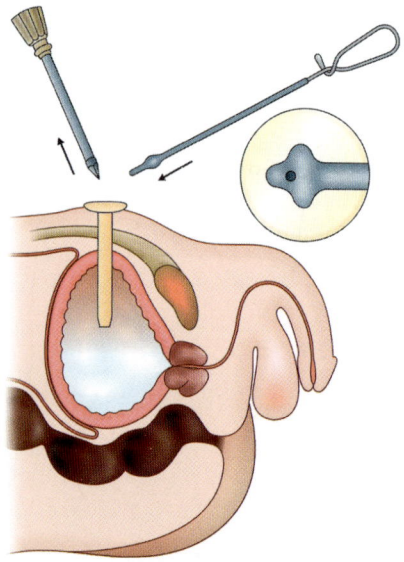

Fig. 21.6C: After entering the bladder trocar is removed. Flow of urine from the cannula confirms that the cannula is in bladder. Catheter is inserted through the cannula into the bladder

Suprapubic Cystostomy (Fig. 21.6D)

Lower midline incision is given under regional anesthesia, linea alba is incised and pyramidalis muscle is split (Figs 21.7A and 7B). Peritoneum is swept upwards to expose the urinary bladder which is identified by the presence of engorged veins (Fig. 21.7C). Two stay sutures are taken on the anterior surface of the bladder and stab is made in between preferably at a high point of bladder (Fig. 21.7D). A Malecot/Foley catheter is inserted through the opening thus made and secured in place by absorbable suture (Figs 21.7E and F). The catheter

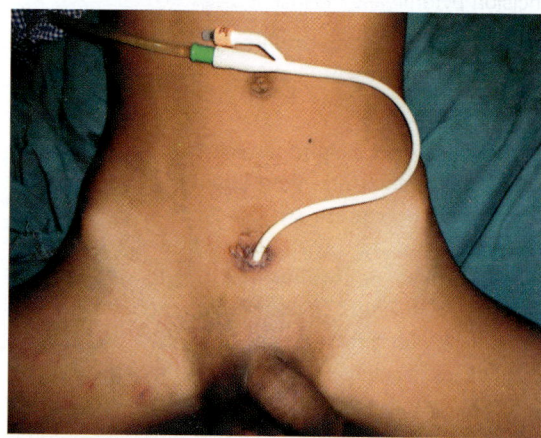

Fig. 21.6D: Suprapubic cystostomy in a patient with urethral stricture

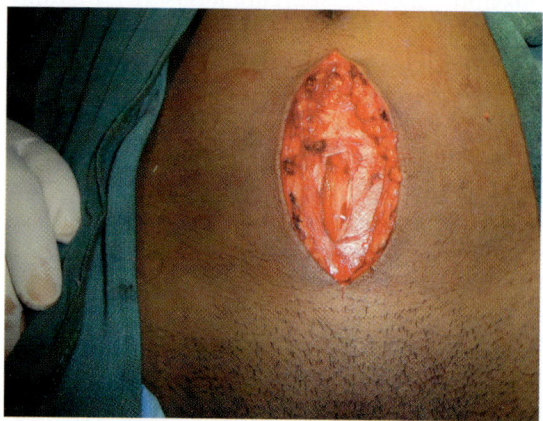

Fig. 21.7A: Lower midline incision

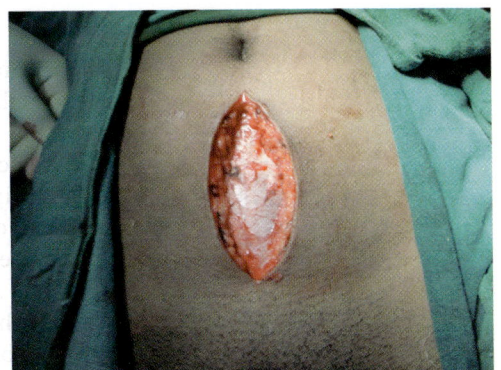

Fig. 21.7B: Incision at linea alba. In lower part of the incision pyramidalis muscle is split

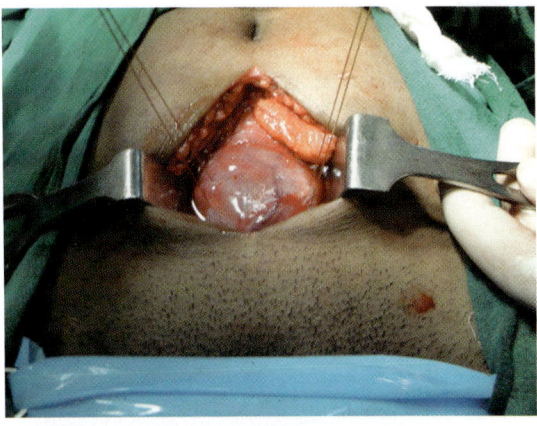

Fig. 21.7E: Stab is made between the stay sutures

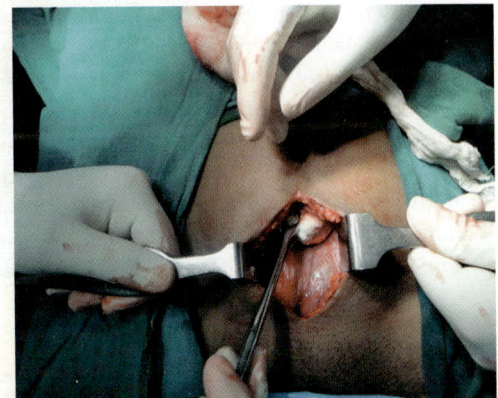

Fig. 21.7C: Bladder is exposed (identified by presence of prominent veins on its surface)

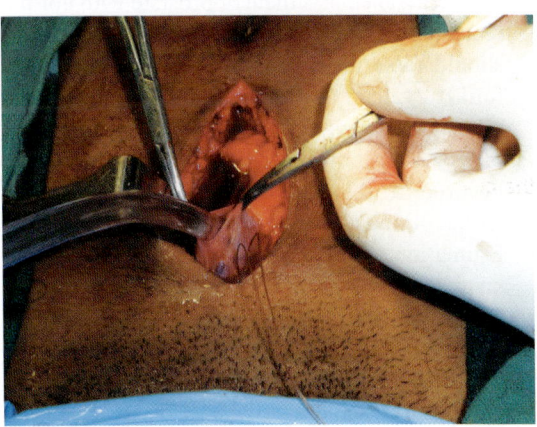

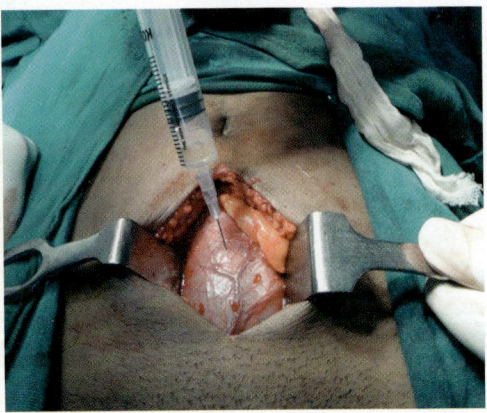

Fig. 21.7D: Stay suture taken over the bladder

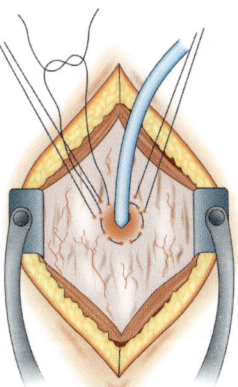

Fig. 21.7F: Malecot catheter inserted and tied by taking a purse string suture around it

is then brought out through the abdomen through a separate stab incision and fixed in the place with silk suture. Linea alba and skin are then subsequently closed.

Evaluation in Patients with Lower Urinary Tract Symptoms (LUTS)

- Quantification of symptom with IPSS (international prostate symptom score) Box 21.1.
- Adequate medical history about urinary tract symptoms, medications, previous surgical procedures and fitness for possible surgery
- Digital rectal examination (DRE) which in case of BPH reveals a smooth firm and typically symmetrical enlargement of prostate with normal rectal mucosa over it. Any nodularity or hardness should raise the suspicion of malignancy and further evaluation should be done by transrectal ultrasonography, PSA estimation and prostatic biopsy.
- Focused neurological examination
- Urine routine microscopy, culture and sensitivity
- Estimation of blood urea and serum creatinine to know the status of renal function
- Digital X-ray KUB to rule out any calculus causing obstructive symptoms
- *Serum PSA:* It is an organ specific antigen that is produced by the epithelial cell of acini and the duct of prostate gland. Normal value of PSA is (0.04–4.0 ng/ml) and the value may be variable with the age of the patient and other conditions of the prostate gland like BPH, prostatic malignancy, prostatitis and prostatic calculi. Any value more than 10 ng/ml should arouse suspicion of malignancy and should be taken care by detailed DRE/transrectal ultrasonography and biopsy. Rise in PSA at times can also be seen after DRE, prostatic biopsy, after sexual intercourse, after cystoscopy and TURP. Therefore, sufficient time gap should be given before estimating the baseline PSA value.
- All elderly male with features of BPH should have uroflowmetry as well as urethrocystoscopy. Uroflowmetry is a non-invasive procedure and

can assess bladder emptying efficiency by measuring the rate at which urine passes through the urethra. This urine flow is dependent on the volume of the urine voided. Uroflowmetry finding supports the clinical diagnosis of outflow obstruction secondary to BPH. Cysto urtethroscopic findings help in determining the length of prostatic urethra, degree of obstruction and its impact on bladder (Fig. 21.8). It also helps in evaluating the bladder for presence of trabeculation, diverticuli and calculi.

BPH

BPH is a major health problem in aging male. Very little is known regarding the biological process contributing the pathogenesis of benign hyperplasia of prostate. BPH and carcinoma prostate both the disease involve overgrowth of epithelial cells and may cause retention of urine. Unlike carcinoma prostate, BPH is rarely linked with genetic abnormalities and is an overgrowth of normal epithelium. Patients with symptomatic BPH are often treated now with alpha-blockers which take care of

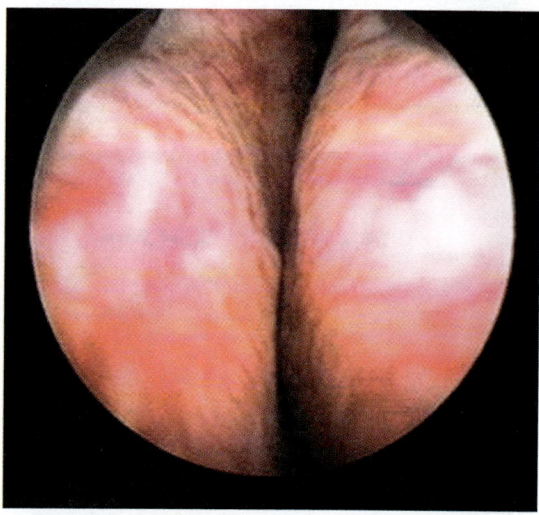

Fig. 21.8: Cystoscopic view showing bilaterally enlarged lobes of prostate

Box 21.1: International Prostate Symptom Score (IPSS)							
	Not at all	Less than 1 time in 5	Less than half the time	About half the time	More than half the time	Almost always	
1. Over the past month, how often have you had a sensation of not emptying your bladder completely after you finished urinating?	0	1	2	3	4	5	
2. Over the past month, how often have you had to urinate again less than two hours after you finished urinating?	0	1	2	3	4	5	
3. Over the past month, how often have you found you stopped and statted again several times when you urinated?	0	1	2	3	4	5	
4. Over the past month, how often have you found it difficult to postpone urination?	0	1	2	3	4	5	
5. Over the past month, how often have you had a weak urinary stream?	0	1	2	3	4	5	
6. Over the past month, how often have you had to push or strain to begin urination?	0	1	2	3	4	5	
	None	1 time	2 times	3 times	4 times	5 or more times	
7. Over the past month, how many times did you most typically get up to urinate from the time you went to bed at night until the time you got up in the morning?	0	1	2	3	4	5	
						Total I-PSS Score S=	
Quality of life due to urinary symptoms							
	Delighted	Pleased	Mostly satisfied	Mixed about equally satisfied and dissatisfied	Mostly Dissatisfied	Unhappy	Terrible
1. If you were to spend the rest of your life with you urinary condition just the way it is now, how would you feel about that?	0	1	2	3	4	5	
					Quality of life assessment index L =		

If available enter data for Q_{max} (CC/sec), R_{ml} (residual urine) and $V_{ml\ or\ gr}$ (prostate volume): S ___ L ___ Q ___ R ___ V ___
(Code for R and V : TA = Transabdominal, TR = Transrectal Ultrasound, MRI, CAT = CT scan, IVU, REC = Rectal, END = Endoscopy I&O = Catheterization, X = Other).

dynamic component of BPH that is the tension of the prostatic smooth muscle, which is mediated primarily via alpha-adenoreceptors (Fig. 21.9). Where as 5-alpha reductase inhibitor affects the static component of BPH by blocking the conversion of testosterone to dihydrotestosterone responsible for hyperplasia of prostatic tissue. Alpha-blocker relieves the symptoms and improves the urinary flow rate, whereas the 5-alpha reductase inhibitor prevents the further progression of BPH. Although both the drugs can be used separately but long-term effect of combination of both the drugs is found to be better in reducing the progression of BPH. Recently introduced combination of Dutastride and most selective alpha-blocker tamsulosin taken for twenty-four weeks provides considerable relief of symptoms. Dutastride reduce the total serum PSA concentration by approximately 50% in six month duration of treatment. Dutastride is a new, dual 5-alpha reductase inhibitor designed to treat BPH. The drug inhibits the 5-alpha reductase isoenzyme (type I and II) that mediates the synthesis of dihydro-testosterone, the primary androgen responsible for hyperplastic growth of BPH. Finestride, first 5-alpha

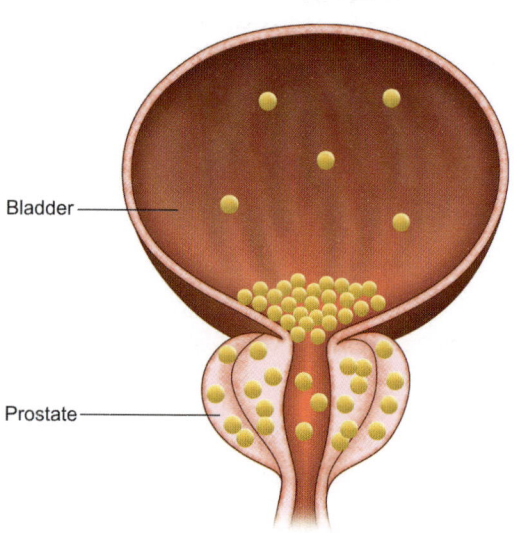

Fig. 21.9: Distribution of alpha 1-adenoreceptors in the bladder neck, prostate and bladder body

reductase inhibitor only inhibits type II isoenzyme. With the recent study it is observed that the inhibition of type I isoenzyme may be of significance in future in prevention/treatment of prostatic cancer.

Patients showing no symptomatic relief should be subjected to surgical treatment. Transurethral resection of prostate (TURP) is considered to be the gold standard treatment for relief of symptoms of LUTS. There are various other surgical approaches to deal the BPH.

I. **Transurethral Microwave Thermal Therapy:** It provides durable improvement in symptoms, quality of life, and flow rates for at least 5 years after treatment.

II. **Transurethral Needle Ablation of Prostate (TUNA):** It is effective and offers good long term clinical improvement in treatment of BPH.

III. **Transurethral Electro Vaporization Prostate (TUVP):** This procedure is one of the most promising alternatives to TURP. The efficacy, safety and durability are comparable to that of TURP.

IV. **Holmium Laser Enucleation of Prostate (HoLEP):** It is performed with minimal complication and blood loss. This procedure requires an overnight hospital stay and patient can be discharged without any indwelling catheter. The only drawback of this procedure is nonavailability of tissue for histopathological examination.

In case the prostatic Bx comes as adenocarcinoma and the disease is localized in a healthy male with life expectancy more than ten years, Radical prostatectomy can be offered.

Other modalities of treatment can be radiotherapy/brachytherapy or transurethral resection of prostate with bilateral orchiectomy alongwith anti-testosterone hormonal therapy.

ACUTE RENAL FAILURE

INTRODUCTION AND TYPES

Acute renal failure is characterized by sudden reduction in urine output. It could be anuria where there is complete absence of urine formation or oliguria where there is less than 300 ml of urine formation in 24 hours.

Urine production from kidney is dependent on good renal perfusion by adequately oxygenated blood. Therefore hypotension and hypoxia adversely affect urine formation.

Renal failure can either be pre-renal, renal, or post-renal. Pre-renal is mostly by impaired renal perfusion, which could be due to several factors like-hypovolemia, hemorrhage, and severe dehydration, cardiac condition like myocardial infarction, cardiac tamponade, and sepsis. All these conditions lead to systemic azotemia.

Renal type of failure several conditions which affects the nephron, glomeruli and tubules of the kidney causing reduction in urine formation are:

- Prolonged hypotension
- Certain nephrotoxic drugs like aminoglycoside, cephalosporin, amphotericin
- Radiological contrast media
- Myoglobinuria
- DIC
- Mismatch blood transfusion.

Post-renal cases involve obstruction to the urinary pathway like renal calculus disease, accidental ligation of ureter during surgery, retroperitoneal fibrosis effecting both the ureter and pelvic malignancy obstructing the ureter.

Acute renal failure is of utmost important for surgeon because of its common association with many complicated operative procedures like renal transplant, cardiopulmonary bypass, major operative procedures in septic shock, major vascular procedures like aroto-femoral bypass and aortic aneurysm. It is also seen in major blunt and life-threatening abdominal trauma and multiple organ failure. In blunt trauma with associated crush injury the raised label of myoglobin and hematin, in major surgery of obstructive jaundice release of bilirubin, all of these are nephrotoxic and they affect the renal tubule and leads to renal failure. Patient having pre-existing renal dysfunction with raised creatinin label are more susceptible to acute tubular necrosis, therefore need

to manage carefully by good hydration and avoidance of the use of any nephrotoxic drugs.

Another important condition in the surgical practice is acute abdominal compartment syndrome where the increase intra-abdominal pressure with massive edema of the intra-abdominal organ leads to decrease renal perfusion. If it is not managed in the earlier stage then it become irreversible and will lead to acute tubular necrosis.

PRESENTATION AND MANAGEMENT

At times it becomes difficult to differentiate between pre-renal and renal azotemia. Both these conditions are associated with decreased urine output less than 15–20 ml/hr with increase in BUN and creatinin. In cases of conditions of pre-renal origin it has been observed that the BUN rise is more compare to the creatinin rise. These patients on examination there is evidence of failing heart (causing decreased renal perfusion) with engorged neck vein, crepitation in lungs and cardiac gallop. In pre-renal condition the concentrating ability of nephrons are normal. Therefore, normal urine osmolarity with the fractional excretion of sodium less than 1% whereas in renal failure, acute tubular necrosis the concentrating ability of the nephrons is markedly decreased resulting urine equal to serum. The fractional excretion of sodium is more than 3%. Investigation of fractional excretion of sodium is a good criteria in differentiating azotemia of pre-renal and post-renal origin.

Patients having no previous history of cardiac disease, administration of normal saline or ringer lactate and in cases of hemorrhage blood should be given. The fluid is continued till the urine output is 30–40 ml/hr. Patients with hypovolemia with sepsis, ionotropic support with dopamine should be given which increase the renal perfusion and cardiac contractility. At many times with good fluid supplementation, furosemide could be tried to achieve the diuresis. Mannitol may also be used as plasma expander and osmotic diuretics but care must be taken to avoid overloading the circulation.

In cases where the fluid challenge fails, diuresis not achieved and hypotension is continued it leads to damage the renal epithelium and the condition passed on to acute renal anuria on account of tubular necrosis. Whenever the surgical patient goes into the renal failure the management mainly on supportive care as there is no definitive pharmacological treatment. The prevention of acute renal injury should always be taken care by every clinician.

During the oliguric phase which last about seven to ten days, urine is very scanty and dark in color. Patient develops anorexia with hiccups. Abdominal distension is common. If untreated or treated incorrectly at this stage the blood urea goes on increasing with rise in systolic in blood pressure. In all these cases the fluid should be restricted. Daily fluid intake should be limited to 500 ml plus the amount equal to that of the volume vomited, or lost by gastric aspiration, diarrhea or from fistulas. Clinician should see the moisture of the tongue or skin turgor as they are the excellent guide to the state of the hydration. Dietary sodium should be restricted to 2 gm/day. All these patients have got a tendency to develop systemic acidosis. Reversing acidosis by giving the sodium bicarbonate should always be avoided. The greatest danger to the patients at this stage is the rising serum potassium because of the risk of cardiac arrhythmia and need the immediate management. In conditions of life-threatening oliguria, frequent measurement of serum potassium and ECG changes should be done at frequent intervals. ECG shows prolong PR interval and tall T-wave in cases of hyperkalemia. In such condition administration of 10% of calcium gluconate over 15 minutes along with IV glucose with insulin (30 U of regular insulin in one liter of 10% glucose) will help in lowering the serum potassium level. Use of ion exchange resins (kayexelate) may be used in enema form to reduce the level of potassium.

In these condition patient's general nursing care be taken and if require in cases of sepsis, a non-nephrotoxic antibiotic should be used. In failure of all the above efforts renal support in the form of peritoneal or hemodialysis should be undertaken especially in the following conditions.

Indication of Hemodialysis

- Serum potassium> 5.5 meq/l
- BUN>80–90 mg/dl
- Persistence acidosis
- Uremic symptoms
- Fluid overload.

In the reversible lesions after 8–10 days the epithelium of the lower nephron starts regenerating and little urine is passed. When the diuresis commences then the amount of fluid equal to the output of urine of the previous 24 hr is added. Frequent serum electrolyte estimation should always be done and the loss of sodium and potassium during this diuretic phase should appropriately be replaced. When the renal excretion exceeds more than a liter per day, the blood urea level starts to fall. The goal of nutritional support is to preserve the lean body mass and maintain immunocompetence. All these patients are in hypercatabolic stage both due to surgery as well as acute renal failure. They are to be given hypercaloric diet. Patient's general condition must be taken care by giving a high calorie, low protein diet containing adequate daily amount of mineral salts.

POST-RENAL OBSTRUCTIVE ANURIA

A through clinical examination is to be done by clinician. One should palpate the bladder for fullness and catheterize to exclude retention. USG is helpful to demonstrate the dilated pelvis and calyces. Plain X-ray may show the obstructive calculus. In such cases management should be done by passage of catheter or irrigation of catheter if blocked, percutaneous nephrostomy or insertion of double J-stent. Definitive surgical management of obstructive etiology should be done after the stabilization of patients at later date.

TORSION OF TESTIS (SPERMATIC CORD)

Twist of the spermatic cord on account of violent contractions of cremasteric muscle jeopardizing the blood supply of testis is a true surgical emergency and needs to be tackle at the earliest, failing which a irreversible ischemic injury of testis may occur. Symptoms of torsion of testis depends upon the degree and site of torsion of the spermatic cord. The abnormal contraction of cremasteric muscle is generally seen after the precipitating factors like straining during defecation, lifting of heavy weight, and during vigorous act of coitus. Patients generally present as sudden agonizing pain in the scrotum, groin and lower abdomen and may be associated with vomiting. This condition can mimic strangulated hernia.

On examination if the scrotum on the side of pain is found to be empty and edematous with a tender lump at the external abdominal ring then the possibility of torsion of testis should be considered. In young adults with fully developed testis, complains of severe pain with inflamed scrotal skin and temperature can mimic epididymitis or epididymo-orchitis. Elevation of scrotum relieves the pain of epididymo-orchitis but the pain gets aggravated in cases of torsion of testis. Features of urinary tract infection are generally absent in torsion, whereas it may be present in epididymo-orchitis.

Inversion of testis, high investment of tunica vaginalis (testis hangs in the tunica as clapper in bell) and cases where testis is separated from epididymis are the common predisposing factors for causing torsion of testis.

Management

Whenever the diagnosis of torsion of testis is suspected, in the beginning a gentle manual derotation should be attempted. If it is in the right direction it will relieve the pain but if it is in the wrong direction it will aggravate the pain. If manual detorsion fails, then a prompt surgical exploration of testis is mandatory. During exploration the viability of testis must be examined, cord should be derotated to establish the blood flow of testis. Warm sponges should be tried in doubtful cases of viability of testis. When testis is to be preserved it should be kept in dartos pouch and fixed with suture. If testis is gangrenous then it is removed (Fig. 21.10). It is always advisable to fix the contralateral testis due to possible anatomical variation.

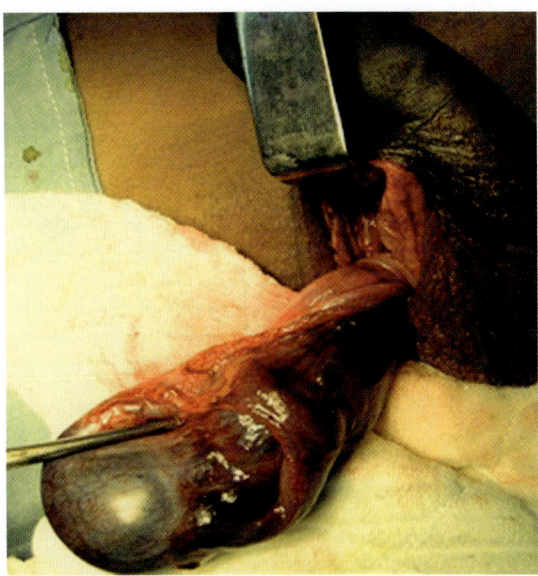

Fig. 21.10: Torsion testis showing gangrenous testis on exploration

On certain occasion twist is seen in appendix of epididymis. This condition is often mistaken for acute epididymo-orchitis and difficult to distinguish from torsion of testis. Immediate exploration for excision of torsioned appendix should be undertaken.

PENILE FRACTURE

A traumatic rupture of tunica albuginea of erected peni with immediate loss of penile rigidity and swelling is known as penile fracture. It is generally seen when the erected penis strikes wrongly against the pubis and perineum during coitus.

The penis is composed of three bodies of erectile tissue: the corpus cavernosum (left and right) and the corpus spongiosum. Both corpora cavernosa are covered by the tunica albuginea. All three corpora are surrounded by Buck's fascia (Fig. 21.11). Sudden direct trauma to the penis or an abnormal bending of the penis in an erect state can cause a tear of the tunica albuginea, with injury to the underlying

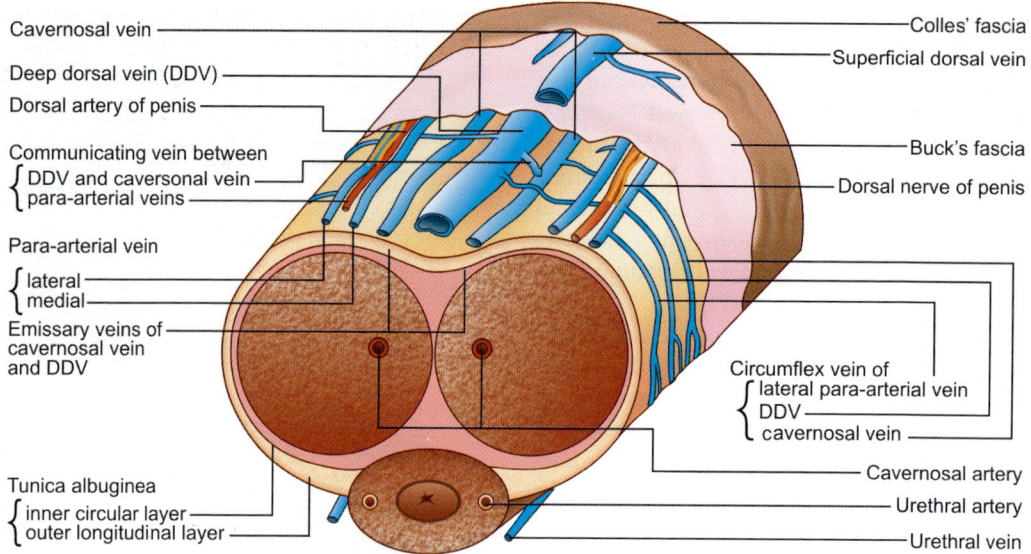

Cavernosal vein
Deep dorsal vein (DDV)
Dorsal artery of penis
Communicating vein between
{ DDV and caversonal vein
{ para-arterial veins
Para-arterial vein
{ lateral
{ medial
Emissary veins of cavernosal vein and DDV
Tunica albuginea
{ inner circular layer
{ outer longitudinal layer

Colles' fascia
Superficial dorsal vein
Buck's fascia
Dorsal nerve of penis
Circumflex vein of
{ lateral para-arterial vein
DDV
{ cavernosal vein
Cavernosal artery
Urethral artery
Urethral vein

Fig. 21.11: Cross-section of penis

corpus cavernosum. Patients generally describe a popping, cracking, or snapping sound with immediate detumescence.

On physical examination in fracture penis, the normal external penile appearance is completely obliterated because of significant penile deformity, swelling, and ecchymosis (egg plant deformity) (Fig. 21.12).The penis is abnormally curved, often in an S-shape. The penis is often deviated away from the site of the tear secondary to mass effect of the hematoma. If the urethra has also been damaged, blood is present at the meatus. If the Buck's fascia is intact, penile ecchymosis is confined to the penile shaft. If the Buck's fascia has been violated, the swelling and ecchymosis are contained within the Colles' fascia. In this instance, a "butterfly-pattern" ecchymosis may be observed over the perineum, scrotum, and lower abdominal wall.

MANAGEMENT

Principles of surgical treatment are as follows:
• Optimize the surgical exposure
• Evacuate the hematoma

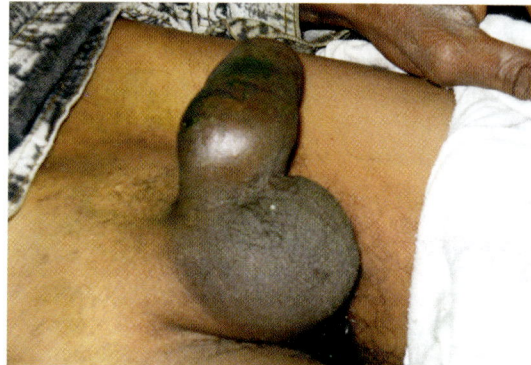

Fig. 21.12: Fracture penis showing egg plant deformity

• Identify the site of injury
• Correct the defect in the tunica albuginea
• Repair the urethral injury if present.

In general or regional anesthesia a circumferential incision is made at the corona. The incision is carried through the dartos fascia up to the Buck's fascia. The penis is degloved up to the base of the penis, taking care not to injure the dorsal neurovascular bundle. Both corpora cavernosa and the corpus spongiosum are thoroughly inspected.

Upon encountering a corporal hematoma, the Buck's fascia is opened and the hematoma is evacuated. After evacuating the hematoma, a defect in the tunica will be apparent (Fig. 21.13) which is repaired. Urethral transections if present are repaired primary over a catheter.

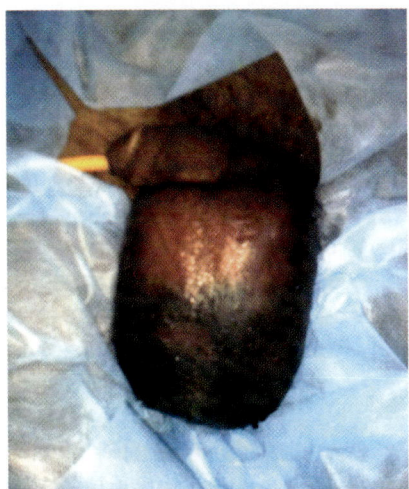

Fig. 21.14: Fournier's gangrene

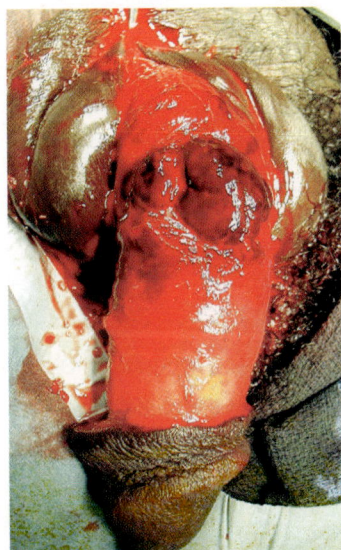

Fig. 21.13: Torn tunica albuginea in fracture penis

FOURNIER'S GANGRENE

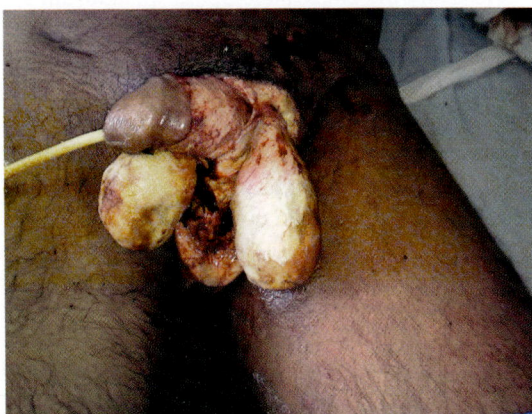

Fig. 21.15: Exposed testis after debridement

It is the fulminating inflammation of the subcutaneous tissue of scrotum resulting in the vascular disaster of infective origin. The infection leads to the obliterative arteritis of the scrotal skin resulting in the rapid onset of the gangrene (Fig. 21.14). It is synergistic infection and common organisms involved are hemolytic Streptococci, *Staphylococcus*, *E coli* and *Clostridium welchii*. Patient presents with scrotal inflammation and gangrene and at times exposure of both the testis (Fig. 21.15).

The condition usually follow after a minor bruise or injury to the scrotum. It is also reported after urethral dilatation and drainage of periurethral abscess. Diabetic patients are specially prone to Fournier's gangrene.

Treatment

Appropriate treatment is wide excision of involved skin with administration of broad spectrum antibiotics and regular dressings. The exposed testes can be covered in scrotum once the inflammation is fully settled or can be repositioned in thigh.

Fournier's gangrene if not dealt carefully, may result in death of the patient.

Fournier's gangrene is very much similar to necrotizing fascitis of the anterior abdominal wall. Mixed pattern of organism like that of Fournier's gangrene are involved in this case as well. This is also called as Meleney's synergistic spreading gangrene. Wide excision, thorough debridement and appropriate antibiotics are the treatment of choice. Patient who survive may require large areas of skin grafts (Fig. 21.16).

PRIAPISM

In this condition, penis persistently remains erect and is painful. This erection is found to be on account of idiopathic thrombosis occurring in the prostatic venous plexus.

Normally the glans and corpora spongiosum are not involved in priapism. The peak incidence is seen between 5 to 10 and 20 to 50 years of age.

Priapism could be either of low flow (veno-occlusive) Type I, where there is priapism is generally associated with painful erected penis. Common causes for low flow priapism are
- Sickle cell trait and disease
- Drugs like sildenafil
- Malignant penile infiltration
- Spinal cord injury
- Spinal anesthesia.

Another Type II high flow priapism is associated with increase arterial inflow, but without increase in venous outflow resistance. This type is seen generally seen in perineal or penile trauma cases. In high outflow priapism erect penis is not tender and glans is also soft and non-tender.

Management

Ischemic priapism are frequently associated with irreversible cavernosal tissue damage and

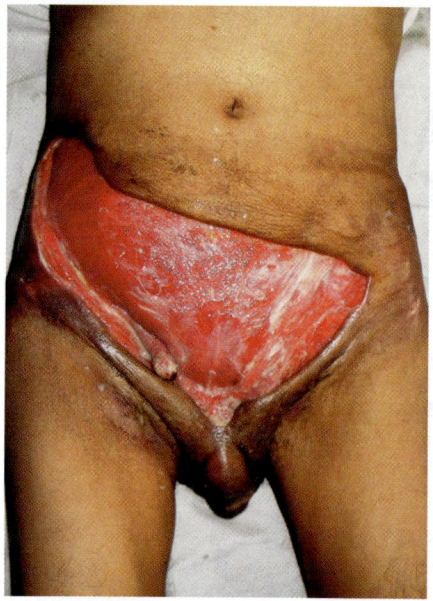

Fig. 21.16: Large raw area over the abdominal wall after Meleney's gangrene

subsequently erectile function loss, whereas in non-ischemic priapism, they preserve the erectile ability, therefore ischemic priapism warrants emergency management, where as non-ischemic priapism do not.

Low flow ischemic priapism require corporal irrigation with normal saline. The first line treatment should consist of evacuation of blood, and irrigation of corpora cavernous alongwith intracavernous injection of an α-adrenergic sympathomimetic agent. In case, these management fail than it becomes necessary to divert the occluded corporal blood flow by shunt procedures either corpora spongiosal or corpora saphenous.

High flow priapism is treated by arterial embolization or at times open surgical arterial ligation.

Gynecological Emergencies in Surgical Practice

INTRODUCTION

The term "acute abdomen" carries with it a sense of urgency, rarely found in other areas of medical practice. A correct diagnosis is critical. Most patients with such symptoms are first seen by the general surgeon and, in this setting, the etiology may include gastrointestinal, urologic, gynecologic or obstetric considerations. Hence, when confronted with an acute abdomen in a female patient, the surgeon must keep in mind that the problem may be related to the female pelvic viscera. In most such cases, the preoperative diagnosis is clear-cut and management is transferred to a gynecologist who is better qualified to deal with the problem. However, not infrequently, the differential diagnosis is difficult and the surgeon may encounter a gynecological condition unexpectedly at laparotomy.

ACUTE ABDOMEN IN OBSTETRICS AND GYNECOLOGY

The important differential diagnoses are abortion, ectopic pregnancy, an ovarian accident, acute salpingitis and pelvic peritonitis. The most pertinent question in the mind of any clinician: managing a woman in the reproductive age group should be – "is this woman pregnant? Does she has a pregnancy related complication?" In India despite legalization of abortion for more than three decades septic induced abortion and its associated complications in the form of perforation of uterus and bowel continue to occur. The management of this condition is multidisciplinary requiring the participation

gynecologist, surgeon, anesthesiologist, and nephrologist for optimal outcome.

We have attempted to classify acute abdomen related to gynecologic causes as those with a positive pregnancy test and those with a negative test (Tables 22.1 and 22.2). However, an overlap does occur and sometimes in a chronic ectopic, pregnancy test may be negative while a woman with a corpus luteum rupture may not be pregnant. Conditions like placental abruption, rupture uterus and intraperitoneal bleeding due to placenta percreta, although encountered in late pregnancy, are not infrequently seen in the late second trimester (20–28 weeks of gestation).

Ectopic Pregnancy

Pregnancy occurring outside the uterine cavity is ectopic and occurs in 2% of all spontaneous

Table 22.1: Acute pelvic pain and positive pregnancy test
Ectopic pregnancy
Abortion: threatened, incomplete, inevitable miscarriage
Pelvic peritonitis/pyoperitoneum following septic induced abortion
Ruptured corpus luteum of pregnancy
Pregnancy with ovarian cyst
Red degeneration of leiomyomatous uterus
Rupture uterus
Placental abruption
Placenta percreta with intraperitoneal bleeding
Coincidental pathology—UTI, appendicitis, cholecystitis, pancreatitis

Table 22.2: Acute pelvic pain and negative pregnancy test

1. Vascular complications
   - Torsion ovarian cyst
   - Torsion fallopian tube
   - Torsion pedunculated subserous leiomyoma
2. Hemoperitoneum
   - Uterine perforation following D&C
   - Rupture of functional ovarian cyst
3. Neoplasm
   - Rupture/Bleeding
   - Rapid growth
4. Endometriosis
5. Infection
   - Pelvic inflammatory disease
   - Tubo-ovarian abscess

conceptions. Majority of ectopic pregnancies are tubal, occurring commonly in the ampullary followed by isthmic part of the tube (Fig. 22.1). The most common cause of an ectopic pregnancy is prior salpingitis. Acute or chronic inflammation decreases the luminal diameter, thereby the fertilized ovum has difficulty in navigating the tubal length. If the delay in passage exceeds 7 days, then implantation occurs in the fallopian tube rather than the uterus. Other causes include altered tubal motility, associated with tobacco use, or due to the inhibitory effect of progestins associated with progestin only contraceptive pill. Use of intrauterine contraceptive device (IUCD), tubal adhesions from prior surgery and prior tubal ligation are also important risk factors for ectopic pregnancy

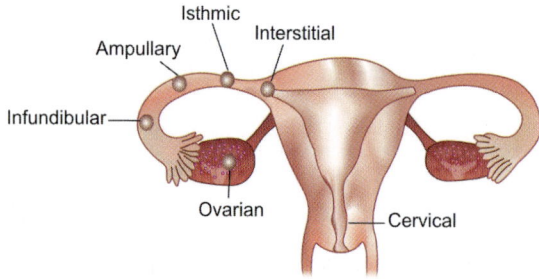

Fig. 22.1: Sites of ectopic pregnancy

A tubal pregnancy is highly unstable and the likely outcome is either a tubal abortion or tubal rupture (Fig. 22.2). In tubal abortion, the conceptus gets extruded through the fimbriated end of the tube, accompanied by a variable degree of bleeding and pain. When this bleeding is slow, blood accumulates to produce a pelvic hematocele, but a rapid hemorrhage can also occur. In tubal rupture, the conceptus burrows through the wall of the tube and finally breaks through the peritoneal surface causing a very rapid hemorrhage.

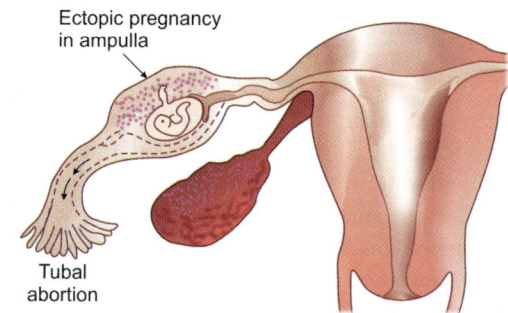

Fig. 22.2: Outcome of tubal pregnancy

In case of tubal rupture, the patient usually presents with severe abdominal pain often with fainting attack followed by collapse (Fig. 22.3). In tubal abortion, bleeding is more gradual and consequently the degree of collapse is less severe. Initially there is a dull ache from tubal distension followed by colicky pain.

When implantation occurs in the isthmus, the narrowest part of the tube, rupture nearly always occurs. These are the patients who bleed in the third and fourth week of pregnancy and who do not give history of missed period because this has not had time to occur.

Abortion

Abortion is the termination of pregnancy either spontaneously or intentionally prior to period of viability. More than 80% of abortions occur in first

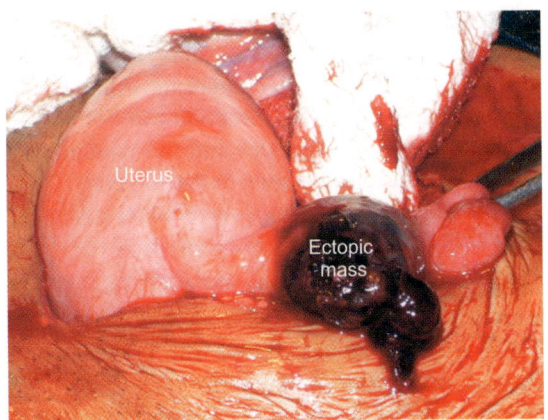

Fig. 22.3: Intraoperative photograph showing ampullary tubal rupture

12 weeks of pregnancy. Miscarriage is a term popular in the UK.

Threatened Abortion

The patient presents with amenorrhea followed by slight bleeding or a bloody vaginal discharge. Pain is usually not a feature although backache or mild abdominal pain may occur after a variable period of time. The patient's condition is generally good and on examination, the cervical os is closed and size of uterus corresponds to the period of gestation.

Inevitable/Incomplete Abortion

These patients usually present with history of amenorrhea followed by excessive bleeding per-vaginum and severe cramping abdominal pain. A history of passage of fleshy mass (products of conception) per-vaginum may be elicited.

General condition of the patient is proportionate to the amount of blood loss and on examination the internal os is open and products of conception may be found protruding through it.

Septic Abortion

Abortion associated with evidence of infection of the uterus and its content is called a septic abortion.

About 10% of abortions requiring admission to hospital are septic. In majority of cases, the infection follows illegal induced abortion, but infection can also occur after a spontaneous abortion. Such an abortion is a life-threatening emergency not only because of the sepsis, but also because major blood loss has often occurred, and uterine and bowel injury may be associated complications.

The microorganisms involved in a septic abortion are usually those normally present in the vagina (endogenous), and include both aerobic and anerobic bacteria.

Clinically cases are graded as:

Grade I: Infection localized to the uterus
Grade II: Infection spreads beyond the uterus to the parametrium, tubes, ovaries or pelvic peritoneum
Grade III: Generalized peritonitis, endotoxic shock, acute renal failure with multi-organ dysfunction.

The patient often appears toxic with a high grade fever. There may be a foul smelling discharge per-vaginum and continuous bleeding since the D&C (although history of D&C may be concealed because of illegal nature). Occasionally the patient may present with bowel prolapsing through the vagina. On examination the lower abdomen is diffusely tender and guarding and rigidity may be present. The cervix is usually open with a mucopurulent discharge exuding through it and the uterus and adnexae tender.

Ruptured Corpus Luteum of Pregnancy

A corpus luteal cyst tends to rupture either towards the end of menstrual cycle or during pregnancy. There is sudden onset of lower abdominal pain which is severe and continuous; often located at first to one iliac fossa but may spread to both sides if hemorrhage is progressive and severe. Nausea and vomiting may occur. Pregnancy test may be negative but clinical presentation is like a ruptured ectopic pregnancy with acute presentation. Pelvic findings may be normal.

Twisted Ovarian Cyst in Pregnancy

The incidence of adnexal torsion in pregnancy is 1 in 5000 cases. Torsion usually occurs around 10–12 weeks when the enlarging uterus rises out of the pelvis and pushes the ovaries anteriorly causing torsion. The most common tumor to undergo torsion during pregnancy is a mature cystic teratoma. The presentation is that of an acute abdomen with severe colicky pain usually located in one iliac fossa, although the site of pain may be variable because the gravid uterus might displace the ovarian cyst high up to the hypochondrium. Due to variable location of pain as well as reluctance on the part of the surgeon to operate on a pregnant patient, there is often a delay in diagnosis and surgical intervention, leading to greater morbidity.

Red Degeneration of Leiomyomatous Uterus

It usually occurs in the late first or early second trimester of pregnancy corresponding with the maximum growth of the uterus. The leiomyoma suffers from relative ischemia as the blood supply is preferentially diverted to the rest of the pregnant uterus, resulting in necrosis within the fibroid. Fibroids of more than 5 cm, with their precarious blood supply, are more liable to degenerate.

The condition is characterized by onset of abdominal pain of all grades of severity. Vomiting is frequently associated, and both temperature and pulse are likely to be raised. On examination, the most characteristic feature is the localization of tenderness at the site of the leiomyoma. Diagnosis is assisted by knowing that a fibroid existed previously.

Rupture Uterus

A previous cesarean section scar, particularly of the classical variety, injudicious use of oxytocics, past history of D&C and manual removal of placenta predispose to rupture uterus. Rarely rupture can occur by direct violence (road traffic accidents) or even spontaneously.

The patient classically presents with severe pain abdomen. If the patient is in labor, contractions usually cease. Fainting is common and usually there is some external bleeding. Rupture can occur even in the late second trimester and the patient may present as an acute abdomen to the surgeon.

Placental Abruption

In this condition there is hemorrhagic separation of a normally situated placenta from the uterine wall. There is a definite association with pre-eclampsia so the patient may have hypertension and albuminuria but this is not always so.

In a typical case, a patient, late in pregnancy, develops severe abdominal pain. The uterus is tense and tender and fetal heart sound may not be detected.

Placenta Percreta with Intraperitoneal Bleeding

Morbidly adherent placenta occurs when there is a defect in decidua basalis, resulting in an abnormally invasive placentation. Prior uterine surgery, myomectomy, curettage and cesarean section are risk factors. In case of placenta percreta, the placenta penetrates through the uterine serosa resulting in severe abdominal pain, hemoperitoneum and shock. Although usually encountered in late pregnancy, this condition can present in the late second trimester. In the last 20 years of the author's practice three cases of intraperitoneal bleeding due to placenta percreta were opened by the surgeon (Fig. 22.4). In one case the bleeding vessels on the surface of the uterus were sutured, patient closed and referred to gynecologist, only to be reopened the next day!

In recent years with an increase in cesarean section, a parallel precipitous rise in morbidly adherent placenta has been noted. Hence, this differential diagnosis must always be kept in mind in patients with acute abdomen with a previous uterine scar.

Torsion Ovarian Cyst

Torsion only occurs in ovarian tumors with a long pedicle. The risk is greatest when the tumor

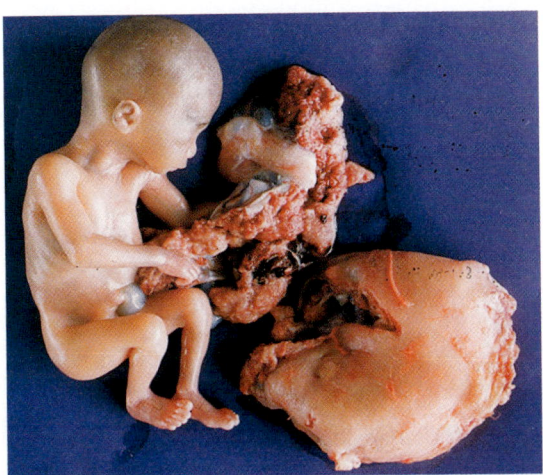

Fig. 22.4: Supracervical hysterectomy specimen showing fundal rupture with placental penetration beyond the serosa in a 35-year-old $G_3P_2L_2$ who presented with acute abdomen and shock at 20 weeks gestation

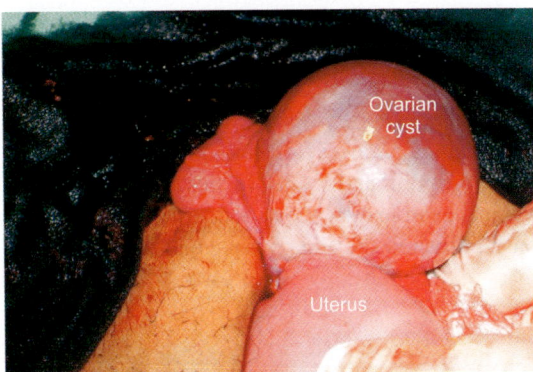

Fig. 22.5: Intraoperative photograph showing torsion ovarian cyst

measures 8–12 cm. The majority of ovarian tumors that undergo torsion are benign ovarian cysts, the most common being a mucinous cystadenoma. These tumors are usually unilateral, multiloculated and often have a long pedicle so their rotation can occur easily. Papillary cystadenomas usually do not have a pedicle and are not prone to torsion. Dermoid cysts, because of their long pedicle, favorable size and sebaceous content, which make them 'float', are also notorious for twisting. Torsion causes vascular obstruction leading to a rapid (Fig. 22.5) increase in size of the cyst, an acute hyperemic reaction followed by gangrene. Untreated, the ischemic cyst may become adherent to surrounding structures or rarely may detach to form a peritoneal loose body.

Bilateral torsion of ovarian cysts occurs with large theca lutein cysts seen in patients with a molar pregnancy and in these patients a simple untwisting and fixing at laparoscopy/laparotomy suffices. A good practice point here would be to examine both ovaries before a decision for cystectomy/oophorectomy is taken.

Often the onset is acute with severe pain abdomen and variable degree of constitutional upset.

Torsion Fallopian Tube

With a reported incidence of 1 in 1,500,000 women, this condition is an uncommon cause of acute abdominal pain. It has been noted that the right tube is more liable to twist. Torsion of a healthy tube seems related to unusual length and mobility. Moreover, any abnormality of the fallopian tube, e.g. pyosalpinx or hydrosalpinx can predispose to torsion. The twist is seldom more than thrice and changes vary from venous congestion to ischemia and gangrene (Fig. 22.6).

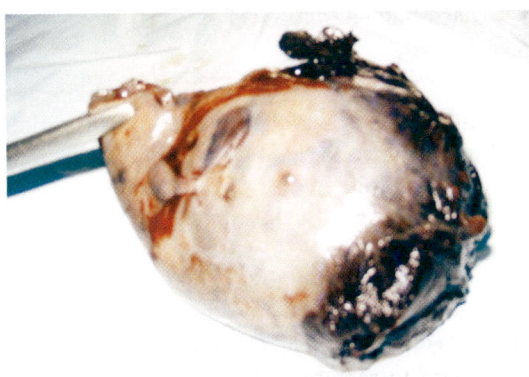

Fig. 22.6: Gangrenous salpingectomy specimen of twisted fallopian tube in a young girl

As in the much commoner torsion of an ovarian cyst, onset is acute and the pain colicky, sited in the lower abdomen, and usually localized to one or other iliac fossa. Rigidity and tenderness are variable. Examination often reveals a maximal tender spot just above the pubis and about 2 inches from the midline. Vaginal examination shows tenderness in the fornix on the affected site and on bimanual examination, a mass may be felt.

Torsion Pedunculated Subserous Leiomyoma

The condition may occur spontaneously, following injury or during pregnancy when a rising uterus predisposes to torsion. In untreated cases, gangrene and infection may supervene. Alternatively, the ischemic myoma may become fibrosed, calcified, adherent to adjacent viscera or detached to form a peritoneal loose body. The patient usually gives history of intermittent attacks of acute abdominal pain, which gradually becomes continuous.

Uterine Perforation Following D&C

This is a potentially serious but infrequent complication of D&C. The patient usually presents with history of D&C followed by severe pain abdomen and bleeding per vaginum. There may be varying degree of shock with features of hemoperitoneum. Bowel injury may also be an associated finding (Fig. 22.7).

Rupture Functional Ovarian Cyst

Functional cysts which rupture can be either follicular or corpus luteal cysts. While follicular cysts rupture around the middle of the menstrual cycle, corpus luteal cysts usually rupture premenstrually or during pregnancy.

Acute mid-menstrual lower abdominal pain with tenderness localized to one side of the pelvis has long been diagnosed as a syndrome (*Mittelschmerz*), which, if of short duration, is readily diagnosed but if prolonged or unduly severe may be confused with other acute intraperitoneal diseases. Unnecessary

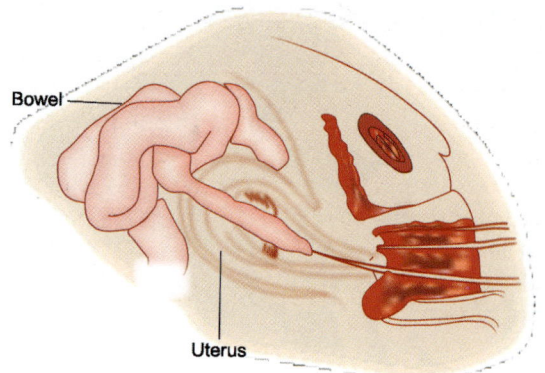

Fig. 22.7: Uterine perforation with bowel injury during suction evacuation

operations may be avoided if the symptoms and signs of this condition are well recognized by the general surgeon.

Following rupture of a tense retention cyst, hemorrhage may be sufficient to cause peritoneal irritation with acute local signs and symptoms.

Rupture/Rapid Growth of a Neoplastic Ovarian Mass

Rupture usually follows trauma, torsion or compression during labor. In certain cases, there is no known cause of rupture and it is assumed that a rapidly expanding neoplasm has outgrown its stromal support. Rupture of an ovarian neoplasm results in acute abdominal pain with varying degree of shock. The clinical picture is confusing with widespread peritoneal irritation. The diagnosis is further confused by the fact that the tumor is often not palpable because it becomes flaccid. Fluid may be detected in the flanks. However, diagnosis may be greatly assisted by knowing that the tumor, which now is no longer palpable, existed previously.

Endometriosis

It is an occasional cause of an abdominal emergency, though rarely presents in a way which allows preoperative diagnosis.

Ovarian Endometriosis

This is the commonest site of endometriosis and leads to the formation of "chocolate cysts". Such cysts take months or years to form and a careful history may reveal that the patient has suffered from dysmenorrhea of increasing severity, dyspareunia, actual or relative sterility and menorrhagia. Rupture of an endometriotic cyst causes a severe pain which characteristically occurs during the first or second day of menstruation.

Intestinal Endometriosis

Less often endometriosis affects the intestines and the emergency likely to arise is acute intestinal obstruction. Obstruction of the large intestine is uncommon because its lumen is wide. The small intestine is not involved as often as the colon and rectum with only the lower ileum being involved in reported cases. However, the relatively small caliber of the ileum makes an obstruction more probable than in the relatively wide rectum.

Pelvic Inflammatory Disease and Tubo-Ovarian Abscess

These result in significant morbidity, not only in the initial presentation, but also and more importantly concerning long-term sequelae. The route of infection is an upward spread from the vagina and through the uterus. The most common infecting organisms are *Chlamydia trachomatis* and *Neisseria gonorrhoea*. The difference between an abscess and tubo-ovarian abscess is that while in an abscess pus collects in a newly created space, the tubo-ovarian abscess is a collection of pus contained by adherence of adjacent organs. The patient usually presents sudden onset of acute lower abdominal pain associated with pyrexia and headache. There may be history of discharge per-vaginum. Past history of PID, especially where the partner was not treated simultaneously, is a strong predisposing factor. On examination, there is a mucopurulent cervical discharge and the uterus is tender and pain greatly aggravated by cervical movement. If a tubo-ovarian abscess has formed an adnexal swelling may be felt per vaginum.

DIAGNOSIS

History

Diagnosis starts with a focused and precise history. A thorough clinical examination and investigations especially a transvaginal sonography and in some cases radiography will clinch the diagnosis.

Establish the date of LMP and whether it was normal in nature and timing. As mentioned previously with a history of amenorrhea, one must keep ectopic pregnancy and complications of intrauterine pregnancy in mind. However, it is paramount to remember that urologic and gastrointestinal causes of pelvic pain may coexist with a normal intrauterine pregnancy. Moreover, an ectopic pregnancy may rupture even prior to a missed period.

Timing and nature of the pain, its site, any radiation, and any aggravating and relieving factors must be elicited. The pain in ectopic pregnancy is usually severe and associated with fainting attacks or giddiness. It is unilateral, colicky (due to tubal distension) and located in one of the iliac fossa prior to rupture. Once rupture or tubal abortion occurs, the pain is diffuse in the lower abdomen. Fainting attacks are peculiar to an ectopic pregnancy, although it can occur in any condition which produces massive intraperitoneal hemorrhage and collapse.

In case of an incomplete abortion, pain is cramp like and intermittent and usually described as either period or labor like due to uterine contractions trying to expel the remaining products. Unilateral pain, which is of sudden onset, acute and intermittent is usually suggestive of an adnexal torsion. This pain is colicky and may be exacerbated by positional change. Classically, the pain may have persisted intermittently for the past few days to weeks as the adnexa repeatedly twists and untwists itself.

Pain due to intraperitoneal bleeding and PID is usually bilateral and diffuse throughout the lower abdomen. Pain of PID may be chronic interspersed with acute exacerbations. With significant intraperitoneal bleeding the blood tracks under the diaphragm and causes referred shoulder tip pain.

Bright red, fresh and profuse bleeding is characteristic of an incomplete abortion while dark brown and scant bleeding is seen with an ectopic pregnancy or a missed abortion. One must enquire whether bleeding occurred before or after the pain. In case of ectopic pregnancy, bleeding usually occurs after the onset of pain while in an abortion bleeding and pain may occur together. Bleeding in late pregnancy accompanied by acute pain abdomen is seen with placental abruption and rupture uterus.

History of a recent D&C or interference by untrained personnel should be specifically asked for as it would give clues to the possibility of a septic abortion or uterine perforation. However in a patient presenting in a toxic condition with fever, foul smelling vaginal discharge and peritoneal signs, septic induced abortion must be suspected even when history is denied. Similar presentation occurs in acute PID or tubo-ovarian abscess.

Nausea and vomiting may be present in 70% of patients with adnexal torsion. Here acute pain with tachycardia, minimal pallor and a palpable lump usually clinches the diagnosis. Tenesmus may be seen with an ectopic pregnancy due to collection of blood in the pouch of Douglas. Failure to pass flatus, constipation and vomiting suggest bowel involvement.

Current use of IUCD or progesterone only pills and previous surgery are important predisposing factors for a tubal pregnancy. Past history of PID also predisposes to further attacks of PID as well as ectopic pregnancy and both these should be kept in mind.

Dysmenorrhea, dyspareunia, infertility and menorrhagia are important clues to the possible diagnosis of endometriosis.

History of previous cesarean section or D&C in a patient with severe pain abdomen in second or third trimester of pregnancy should alert the surgeon to the possibility of rupture uterus or placenta percreta with intraperitoneal hemorrhage.

EXAMINATION

Examination should start alongside history taking by observing the patient, whether she lies still, suggestive of peritonitis or is restless and unable to be comfortable in any position which is usually seen with pain associated with an abortion or adnexal torsion. Tachycardia with a low blood pressure suggests hypovolemia. Extreme pallor can be seen in acute hemorrhagic conditions like ruptured ectopic pregnancy, incomplete abortion, a ruptured ovarian cyst with intraperitoneal bleeding. Fever in excess of 38°C in a woman with acute pelvic pain is due to salpingitis, septic abortion, appendicitis, UTI or some other extragenital infection. Lesser degrees of fever may, however, occur with adnexal torsion. If subnormal temperature is present, it may be an ominous feature of endotoxic shock.

Lower abdominal tenderness and guarding indicate significant pelvic pathology. Unilateral signs usually indicate an unruptured ectopic pregnancy, adnexal torsion or extragenital pathology such as appendicitis. Bilateral signs indicate PID, but do not exclude any of the above diagnosis. When hemoperitoneum occurs, the tenderness and guarding are usually diffuse. Upper quadrant tenderness will be found in PID with accompanying Fitz Hugh Curtis syndrome.

A tender lump arising from the pelvis more towards the iliac fossae, suggests an ovarian mass while a normal pregnant uterus is in the midline, soft, non-tender with ballottement.

In late pregnancy, the findings of a tense, tender uterus with absent fetal heart sounds are suggestive of an abruption. In case of rupture uterus, contractions which were occurring earlier usually cease. The uterine contour is lost and fetal parts may be felt superficially.

Vaginal Examination

Speculum Examination

Purulent vaginal discharge is suggestive of septic abortion, PID or tubo-ovarian abscess. One should note whether bleeding is through the os and whether the os is open or closed. Slightly bleeding per-vaginum with a closed os is suggestive of threatened abortion while heavier bleeding through an open os implies inevitable abortion. Products of conception are seen protruding through the os in case of incomplete abortion. Occasionally bowel may be seen prolapsing through the cervix following perforation of uterus during suction evacuation or in a septic abortion.

Vaginal Examination

Pain on movement of cervix-the so-called "cervical excitation" pain is typical of an ectopic pregnancy or PID. However, it may also be observed when there is pus or blood in the pelvis causing peritonism.

On bimanual examination, the uterus is usually slightly enlarged, and softened with both an ectopic pregnancy and an intrauterine pregnancy.

The presence of an adnexal mass separate from uterus indicates an ectopic pregnancy, ovarian tumor, pyosalpinx, a tubo-ovarian mass or a subserous fibroid. Occasionally a tubo-ovarian abscess may be palpated in the cul-de-sac. Fullness of the pouch of Douglas may also be noted with an ectopic pregnancy.

In case of rupture uterus, a characteristic sign noted per-vaginum is the loss of the presenting part from its former position within the pelvis.

Diagnostic Aids

A *urine pregnancy test* is the first line investigation in any sexually active woman with acute pelvic pain. It becomes positive at the time of first missed period and a positive test result indicates an absolute need to determine whether the pregnancy is intrauterine or extrauterine. A negative test result, however, does not exclude an ectopic pregnancy especially a chronic ectopic.

Transvaginal sonography (TVS) is invaluable in diagnosing an intrauterine pregnancy and other pelvic pathology. Presence of an intrauterine gestational sac virtually rules out an ectopic pregnancy although rarely a heterotopic pregnancy may be present. Ultrasound criteria for diagnosis of ectopic pregnancy are visualization of a living extrauterine pregnancy, yolk sac, or embryo. A complex adnexal mass, an empty uterus and fluid in the pelvis in a patient with a positive pregnancy test is also suggestive of an ectopic pregnancy.

In intrauterine pregnancy with bleeding per-vaginum certain milestones can be measured on TVS to ascertain normal embryological development. If measurements of the gestational sac are irregular or fetal pole or cardiac activity are not visualized more than one week beyond their expected appearance termination of pregnancy may be offered.

TVS helps visualize any retained products of conception in septic and incomplete abortion. Occasionally a foreign body may be seen which could have been used for the criminal abortion. In addition tubo-ovarian masses or fluid around the uterus/POD suggest a pyoperitoneum.

In red degeneration of a leiomyoma ultrasound helps localize the tenderness to the site of myoma which clinches the diagnosis. Ovarian cysts and neoplasms can be easily diagnosed and characterized by ultrasound as being simple, benign or complex with features of malignancy. Color Doppler may greatly assist the diagnosis of adnexal torsion. A tubo-ovarian mass with complex internal echoes with presence of fluid in the POD is suggestive of PID.

In a suspected case of abruption, ultrasound findings are placenta located in the upper segment with evidence of a retroplacental clot (RPC). However, abruption may be present even when RPCs are not visualized. The classic features of placenta accreta on ultrasound are loss of retroplacental hypo-echoic zone, thinning and disruption of uterine serosal bladder interface and presence of fall out areas and lakes in the placenta. In patients with previous cesarean or D&C, these findings must be specifically looked for.

Although ultrasound has minimized the need for *culdocentesis*, this simple procedure can help triage patients requiring surgical intervention. During vaginal examination, a spinal needle is inserted through the posterior vaginal fornix into the cul-de-sac. If non-clotting blood is aspirated, the likelihood of an ectopic pregnancy is high.

Diagnostic laparoscopy should only be undertaken in a hemodynamically stable patient when other investigations fail to provide a definitive diagnosis. During laparoscopy, a careful and methodical approach should be followed. The anterior and posterior surface of uterus, both fallopian tubes and ovaries should be visualized. If there is evidence of infection, fluid can be aspirated and swabs taken from the fallopian tubes for bacteriological examination. The ovaries should be lifted up to allow the whole surface to be examined. Finally the parietal peritoneum, the appendix, the gallbladder and the perihepatic area should be inspected and findings documented accurately for future reference.

When laparoscopy is performed in women with acute pelvic pain, approximately 35% have acute or chronic PID, 20% ectopic pregnancy, 15% ovarian cyst, 5% adhesions not associated with PID and 2% appendicitis. In the remaining cases no cause will be identified.

TREATMENT

During patient evaluation, if a gynecological cause is found, the case should be referred to a gynecologist for appropriate care. Even when encountered unexpectedly at laparotomy, the gynecologist's expertise should be sought. It is important to be as conservative as possible in a young sexually active woman to preserve fertility. In the event that an ovarian neoplasm is encountered a staging laparotomy is necessary and again conservative management is the rule.

In an unruptured ectopic pregnancy a salpingostomy (laparoscopic/laparotomy) rather than a salpingectomy is the procedure to be adopted (Figs 22.8A to C).

In a ruptured ectopic with a massive hemoperitoneum laparoscopy is contraindicated. At laparotomy time should not be wasted in removing blood from the abdominal cavity; the uterus should be palpated, lifted and the ruptured tube identified. With two clamps on the mesosalpinx the bleeding is controlled and salpingectomy done (Fig. 22.9). The peritoneal cavity is then toileted and a pelvic drain inserted.

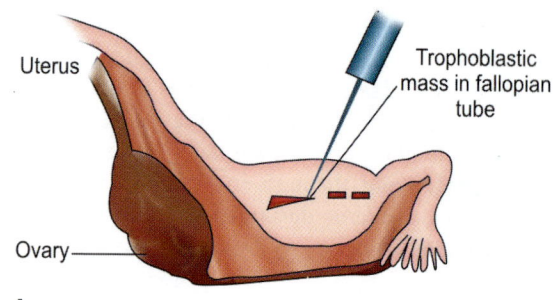

Uterus

Trophoblastic mass in fallopian tube

Ovary

A

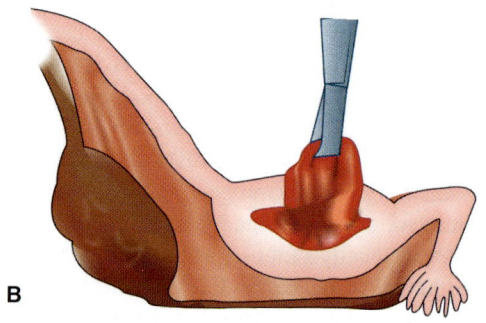

B

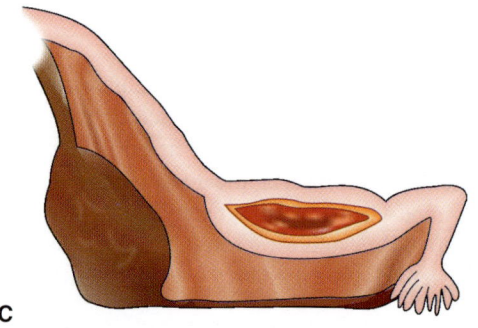

C

Figs 22.8A to C: Laparoscopic salpingostomy for ectopic pregnancy (A) Incision made with monopolar diathermy needle on trophoblastic mass (B) The mass is removed with forceps (C) The lumen is allowed to heal by secondary intention

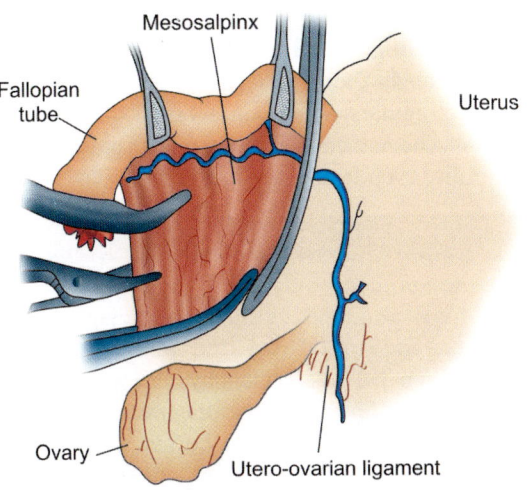

Mesosalpinx

Fallopian tube

Uterus

Ovary

Utero-ovarian ligament

Fig. 22.9: Technique of salpingectomy

In a ruptured corpus luteum a similar procedure as above is followed but here the tubes are normal. Small bleeding points on the ovary are identified and fine interrupted sutures applied. Rarely, it might be necessary to partly resect the ovary to arrest the hemorrhage. The oozing ovarian bed may be controlled with a few interrupted sutures in the mesoovarium.

In a *septic abortion* management involves intensive care. In grade I sepsis conservative management with broad spectrum antibiotics and fluid management usually suffice. When a decision to open is made based on examination and investigations, the uterus is carefully examined, perforation identified and uterine cavity evacuated abdominally. If the uterus is vascularized (pink), firm in consistency, not infected or gangrenous, it must be preserved. The wound is debrided and a few interrupted sutures are used to close the defect. Not infrequently a subtotal hysterectomy with conservation of ovaries may be required in a badly infected, gangrenous uterus. Both small and large bowel till the rectum must be explored and necessary procedures like resection/anastomosis and a ileostomy/colostomy may be required.

In a uterine perforation during a D&C or MTP, the dictum is to open and look for bowel injury if suction evacuation was performed. If perforation has occurred with a dilator, D&C may be completed under laparoscopic guidance and the uterus observed for bleeding which usually stops with evacuation of uterus and oxytocics.

In case of *twisted ovarian cyst* in a young woman for whom preservation of ovarian function is important, conservative treatment with unwinding of the adnexa and ovarian cystectomy/oophoropexy is preferred after untwisting and observing for reperfusion. This mode of management is only possible if the diagnosis is made promptly and laparotomy done, before irreversible changes occur. Oophoropexy involves surgically tacking the ovary to the pelvic side wall with absorbable sutures. This procedure has a success rate of approximately 88%. In the setting of severe vascular compromise or active bleeding, unilateral salpingo-oophorectomy should be performed. The same principle is followed for a twisted fallopian tube but conserving the ovary.

In women with ovarian endometriosis, the characteristic chocolate cyst containing viscous brown material will be seen at laparotomy. In younger women enucleation of the cyst with conservation of normal ovarian tissue is desirable. In older patients, hysterectomy with bilateral salpingo-oophorectomy should be performed. In case of patients with bowel endometriosis, the lesion appears similar to carcinoid and Crohn's disease at laparotomy. Use of frozen sections should be considered as this would enable endometriosis to be recognized and a limited resection to be performed.

Although *red degeneration of a leiomyoma* presents as acute abdomen the cornerstone of management is conservatism. Treatment consists of rest, analgesics and hydration. In extremely rare cases, where the pain is continuous and intractable, the need for myomectomy may arise especially in a twisted subserous myoma.

In suspected neoplasms, staging followed by cystectomy (Fig. 22.10)/salpingo-oophorectomy (Fig. 22.11) with intraoperative frozen section

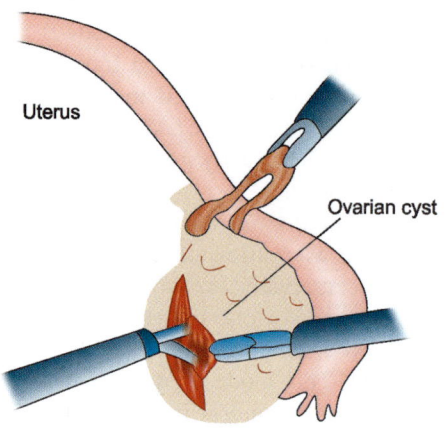

Fig. 22.10: Laparoscopic ovarian cystectomy: Ovarian incision given followed by enucleation of cyst

analysis is done. It is prudent to wait for a final histopathology before any radical surgery is contemplated. Young women usually present with germ cell tumors where conservative surgery with adjuvant chemotherapy is curative with preservation of fertility even in advanced stages.

<table>
<tr><td>Conclusion</td></tr>
</table>

For the surgeon confronted with acute lower abdominal pain, making the correct diagnosis is important and a mistake could be fatal. A high index of suspicion and involvement by both surgeon and gynaecologist may improve diagnosis and allow for appropriate treatment to be instituted at the earliest, thereby minimizing morbidity and conserving the fertility of the woman whenever possible.

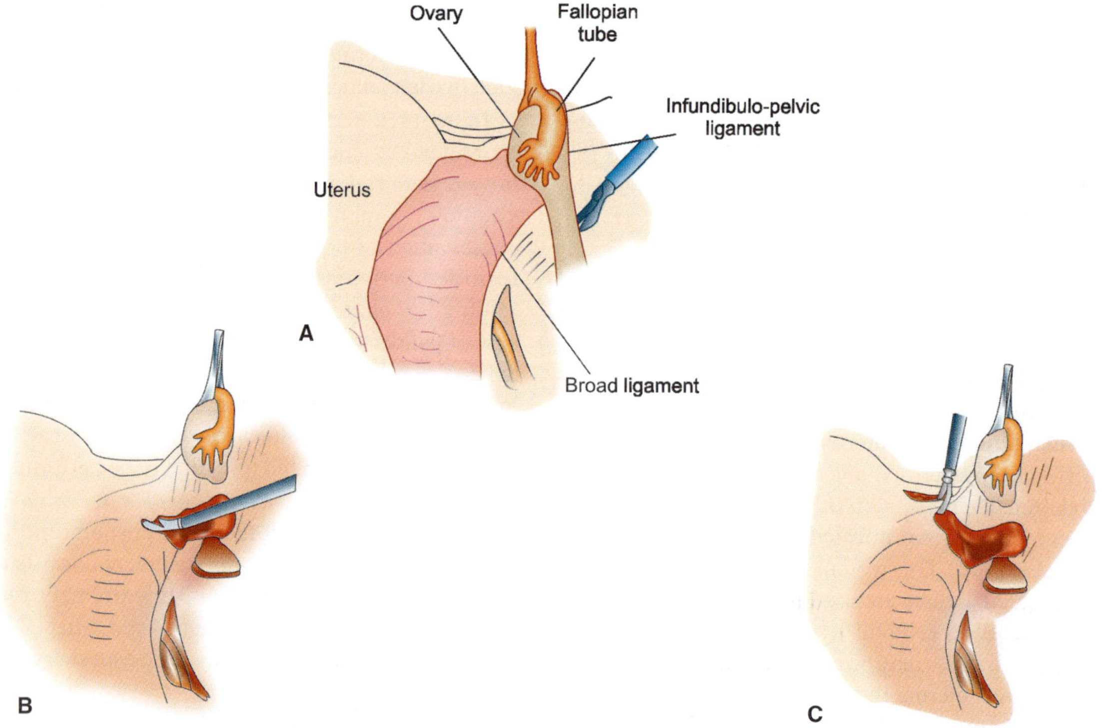

Figs 22.11A to C: Technique of laparoscopic salpingo-oophorectomy: (A) Infundibulo pelvic ligament coagulation (B) Opening of the broad ligament (C) Fallopian tube and utero-ovarian ligament coagulation

23 Acute Abdomen in Children

"Acute abdomen" is the medical term used for pain in the abdomen that usually comes on suddenly and is so severe that one may have to go to the hospital. As opposed to common abdominal pain, which can be caused by minor issues such as constipation, *acute* abdominal pain can signal a variety of more serious conditions, some of which require immediate medical care and/or surgery.

Acute abdomen in children can occur due to wide variety of causes. Evaluation of abdominal pain in children poses a major challenge for the clinician. The diagnosis in infants and small children can be really difficult due to lack of clarity in history and physical signs that are nonspecific and difficult to elicit. It is important to reach the diagnosis at the earliest so that need of surgery can be decided in order to avoid morbidity and mortality due to delay.

Pathophysiology

Acute abdominal pain arises from three neural pathways:

a. Parietal pain
b. Visceral pain and
c. Referred pain.

Parietal pain occurs due to noxious stimulation of the parietal peritoneum. This may occur due to ischemia, inflammation and stretching of parietal peritoneum. It is usually sharp, discrete, localized and increased by coughing or movement. The retroperitoneal lesions do not generate parietal pain.

Visceral pain occurs due to stimulation of a viscus by tension, stimulation or stretching. This pain is dull, poorly localized and felt in the midline.

Referred pain is felt in remote areas supplied by the same dermatome as the diseased organ. It is due to sharing of central pathways for afferent neurons from different sites.

Causes of Acute Abdomen

Most common causes of abdominal pain include medical problems while surgical causes are present in small percentage of cases. In infants and young children, complications of various congenital abnormalities are more common causes of abdominal pain, whereas acquired disorders are more common in older children and adolescents.

In first few years of life

1. Congenital abnormalities
2. Incarcerated inguinal hernia
3. Intussusception
4. Intestinal volvulus
5. Gastrointestinal perforation
6. Necrotizing enterocolitis in preterm neonates.

In older children

1. Trauma
2. Pancreatitis
3. Meckel's diverticulum
4. Primary peritonitis
5. Intestinal worm infestation.

In adolescents

1. Acute appendicitis
2. Cholecystitis (acalculus)
3. Testicular torsion
4. Rupture of ovarian cyst.

Non-surgical causes of abdominal pain include hyperthyroidism, Addison's disease, diabetic ketoacidosis, hypercalcemia, etc.

Non-specific abdominal pain: It is the most common cause of abdominal pain in late childhood and early adolescence. It is a colicky pain with some localization that becomes worse after meals. Bowel sounds may be increased and a palpable mass of feces may be present in right or left iliac fossa. The causes commonly are constipation, irritable bowel and chronic spasm.

Diagnosis

The three main considerations for clinician should be:
a. age and sex of the patient
b. duration of symptom
c. the presence of other symptoms/signs related to specific organ systems.

History

An accurate history and detailed examination will provide more information than a multitude of investigations. The chronological order of appearance and progress of each symptom must be obtained.

Age

Newborns to 2 years of age: Major surgical causes are midgut volvulus associated with malrotation and intussusception. Neonates, more so than older children, with unrecognized intestinal obstruction deteriorate rapidly, show an increase of associated morbidity and mortality and appropriate surgical treatment becomes more hazardous. Early diagnosis depends largely on the prompt detection of obstructive manifestations by the clinician and the subsequent accurate interpretation of radiographic findings and other investigations, leading to definitive treatment, which should always be preceded by appropriate resuscitation of the child.

Children (2–12 years of age): Acute appendicitis is the most important cause of acute abdomen in this age group.

Adolescents: Appendicitis still remains major diagnosis in this age group. In an adolescent female, mittelschmerz, pelvic inflammatory disease and ectopic pregnancy should be considered.

Pain: The nature of the pain and its onset should be elicited carefully. Children who cannot verbalize usually present late and associated symptoms may not be noticed. Many times, infants react to pain as a change in behavior, persistent crying, irritability, sleeplessness and poor feeding.

Colicky pain signifies obstruction of a gastrointestinal tract, urinary tract or hepatobiliary tract. Patients with severe pain lasting over 4–6 hours are more likely to have a surgical cause. Sudden pain that is aggravated by jerks or bumps while riding is suggestive of peritoneal irritation.

Associated symptoms: Pain usually precedes vomiting in surgical conditions. Any child with bilious vomiting should be considered to have acute intestinal obstruction unless proved otherwise. Urinary symptoms like dysuria, frequency and urgency suggest urinary tract infection.

Gynecologic history: In pubertal girls, complete gynecological history is important. History regarding menstrual history, sexual activity and contraception should be ascertained.

Drugs: Some drugs like erythromycin, salicylates and lead can cause abdominal pain and thus a history of past drug intake becomes important.

Physical Examination

Physical examination should be completed and should begin as the child walks into the room. Change in gait is suggestive of pain in the hip joint and psoas abscess. One should gain confidence of the child before examination. General physical examination should be completed first while procedures like pharyngeal examination and rectal examination should be done last. Hydration status and vital signs of the patient should be assessed. One should look for tongue furring, jaundice and characteristic spots of Henoch–Schönlein purpura.

Abdominal examination: The breathing pattern of the patient should be noted. On abdominal examination, note should be made of distension, any previous scars and visible bowel loops and peristalsis. The child is requested to point to site of maximum tenderness. The abdominal palpation is begun from the normal area. It is useful to distract the child by talking during examination to differentiate between voluntary guarding and rigidity. Abdominal examination is not complete without examination of hernial sites.

Rectal and pelvic examination: These should be performed only when these are likely to provide some information that is not elicited on abdominal examination. Rectal examination may provide information on tenderness, presence of mass, fecal matter, melena and sphincter tone. Intussusceptum may be felt on rectal examination. In an adolescent girl, purulent cervical discharge, tenderness and adenexal mass suggest pelvic inflammatory disease.

Investigations

Investigations help to confirm the diagnosis that is made on basis of detailed history and examination but cannot replace them. These should be done according to the history and clinical findings.

Laboratory Investigations

1. Complete blood count: Leukocytosis and toxic granulations suggest presence of infection in the body.
2. Urinalysis: It helps to diagnose urinary tract infection and stone.
3. Pregnancy test is advocated in post-menarchal girls.

Radiological investigations

Different radiological investigations can be used to ascertain the cause of acute abdomen.

Plain film radiograph of abdomen and chest is important in a case of acute abdomen. Distribution of gas in the bowel, free gas under dome of diaphragm (Fig. 23.1), air-fluid levels (Fig. 23.2), mass

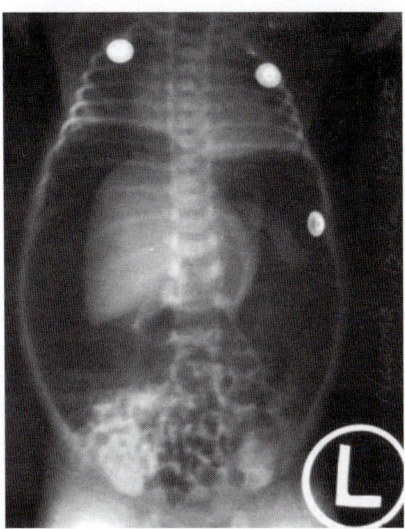

Fig. 23.1: Pneumoperitoneum indicating hollow viscus perforation

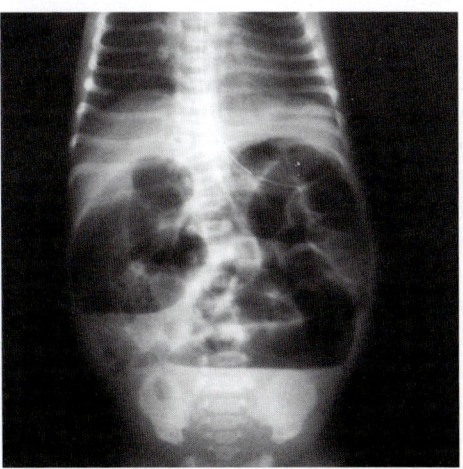

Fig. 23.2: Multiple air-fluid levels indicating intestinal obstruction

lesions, calcification and outline of psoas muscle are noted. A chest X-ray should be done to rule out pneumonia.

Ultrasonography has become the mainstay of diagnosis in emergency settings. It is readily available, is less expensive, does not cause radiation exposure and can be done at bedside in severely sick patient. But it is highly operator dependent and findings may be obscured by gaseous distension. Questions to be addressed are status of the organs, lymphadenopathy, free fluid, mass lesions, bowel wall thickness and intestinal peristalsis.

Computed tomography is more accurate but involves radiation and may require contrast. It should be done in selected settings. Mostly an intravenous contrast enhanced CT examination without oral contrast is carried out in case of acute abdomen.

Laparoscopy: Diagnostic laparoscopy plays a significant role in the evaluation of acute abdominal pain. In addition to confirming or ruling out a diagnosis, it has the advantage of performing definitive therapeutic intervention at the same time.

Management

The general measures that are taken in a patient with acute abdominal pain are:

1. Intravenous fluids are necessary when the pain is severe and associated with vomiting. Any child who is likely to be suffering from surgical cause is kept nil orally.
2. Nasogastric intubation is done where intestinal obstruction is suspected. Sometimes it may be indicated in acute pancreatitis.
3. Antibiotics may be administered as and when indicated. Routine use is not justified.
4. Pain relief: The practice of providing analgesia for children with acute abdominal pain is divergent between primary emergency physician and pediatric surgeons. Some surgeons are less likely to provide analgesia for children with acute abdominal pain. The perceived disapproval of providing analgesia to children with acute abdominal pain by pediatric surgeon is considered a barrier influencing primary emergency medicine practice. Intravenous morphine provides significant pain relief to children with acute abdominal pain without adversely affecting the examination and it does not affect the ability to identify patients with surgical conditions.

5. Definitive treatment depends on the final diagnosis and may require surgical intervention.

Different Conditions Causing Acute Abdomen

Infantile Colic

It is a common cause of abdominal pain in first month of life. Infants suffering from colic scream and draw up their legs up against their abdomen. Relief may occur after some time.

Malrotation and Volvulus

This condition is one of the most important emergencies in children especially neonates that requires a very high index of suspicion for early diagnosis in order to prevent bowel ischemia.

Rapid elongation of midgut is associated with herniation outside with subsequent return and fixation by the 12th week of gestational life. Failure of fixation results in mobile or subhepatic cecum. The bowel may undergo volvulus due to short mesentery. It is most commonly seen in the neonate but may occur at any age.

The generally healthy child presents with sudden onset of bilious vomiting. As the level of obstruction in midgut volvulus is high, abdominal distension does not occur in all cases. Untreated child rapidly goes into shock and peritonitis.

In absence of peritonitis, contrast studies may be done to confirm diagnosis. In case of a suspected volvulus, no time should be spent on diagnostic investigations and child taken up for urgent laparotomy after aggressive resuscitation. The rotated bowel is untwisted and base of mesentery is widened. There is no need to fix the cecum in right iliac fossa.

In case of frankly gangrenous bowel, resection and anastomosis is done.

Appendicitis

Acute appendicitis is the most common and important cause of acute abdomen in children. There is history of pain arising in the umbilical region which that shifts to right iliac fossa to be finally localized at McBurney's point. This indicates irritation of parietal peritoneum. The pain is associated with vomiting and fever, in that order. Vomiting preceding pain is more suggestive of gastroenteritis. Anorexia may be present. Perforation may occur in delayed diagnosis.

On examination, there is pain in the right iliac fossa and percussion may reveal rebound tenderness. In case of perforation of appendix, there will be diffuse tenderness suggestive of peritonitis. In late presentation, there may be formation of an appendicular mass. It may be required to re-examination may be required at intervals in doubtful cases. Complete blood counts and urinalysis are helpful at times but normal counts in presence of classical history and signs do not rule out appendicitis. The clinician has to weigh the significance of the signs and symptoms to differentiate between acute appendicitis and nonspecific abdominal pain.

Ultrasonography is useful diagnosis. It may demonstrate distended appendix, localized ileus and peri-appendiceal fluid. An appendicular abscess or mass can be diagnosed. Preoperative focused appendiceal CT with colonic contrast has not been found to increase the accuracy in diagnosis of appendicitis when compared with patients diagnosed by history and clinical examination and laboratory investigations. But it may be useful in presence of atypical history and examination. Treatment of acute appendicitis is emergency appendicectomy. This can be performed by open surgery or by laparoscopic method. A standard protocol for management of acute appendicitis helps to reduce hospital stay and complications. An appendicular mass is managed conservatively followed by interval appendicectomy 3–6 months later.

Intussusception

Intussusception is invagination of bowel (intussusceptum) in to lumen of adjacent bowel loop (intussuscipiens). This leads to intestinal obstruction and subsequent interference with mesenteric blood supply and necrosis if not treated (Fig. 23.3).

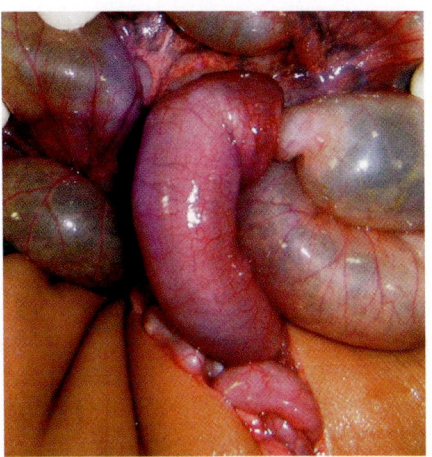

Fig. 23.3: Ileo-ileal intussusception

Various types include ileo-colic (most common), ileo-ileal and colo-colic. Peak age for intussusception is 6 to 12 months and it is uncommon in neonatal age. Most cases are idiopathic but history of preceding viral illness, gastroenteritis or respiratory illness may be available. Intussusception in older children is more likely to be associated with a lead point like Meckel's diverticulum, invaginated appendix or polyp.

The hitherto healthy child presents with sudden onset colicky abdominal pain that may be associated with facial pallor and bilious vomiting. In between attacks, the child is calm and healthy. Later, the child may pass blood mixed mucus (red currant jelly stools).

Abdominal examination may reveal a palpable mass in the abdomen in about 85% cases. In late stages, mass may be palpable on rectal examination or it may prolapse out of the anus. Bowel ischemia and necrosis leads to peritonitis and abdominal examination will reveal guarding and rigidity with rebound tenderness. Delayed presentation is associated with features of septicemia and shock.

Plain X-ray abdomen may show coiled spring sign due to air trapped between intussusceptum and intussuscipiens. Later, features of intestinal obstruction may be apparent. Ultrasonography is now considered a very good modality and when properly performed, it obviates the need of contrast studies. It can also be used to assess the completeness of reduction of intussusception by air or contrast. Contrast enema is still considered confirmatory investigation in many centers.

After correction of fluid and electrolyte imbalance, treatment aims at reduction of the intussusception. This may be done by non-operative means like air or barium reduction under radiological control. It should not be attempted when signs of peritonism are present. In case of failure or lack of facility, surgical exploration and reduction is done. Gangrene requires resection of the affected bowel.

Complicated Inguinal Hernia

Complicated inguinal hernia is the commonest cause of mechanical intestinal obstruction in children. Obstruction and strangulation of the bowel presents with abdominal pain and bilious vomiting. Delay in diagnosis can occur due to failure to look at the hernial sites and difficulty in making a diagnosis. Early diagnosis and emergency surgical reduction of hernia followed by herniotomy is necessary.

Meckel's Diverticulum

Meckel's diverticulum is the remnant of the vitello-intestinal duct on the antimesenteric border of the small intestine (Fig. 23.4). It is usually present within 2 feet of the ileocecal junction. It may present as acute abdomen at any age due to complications like acute inflammation; perforation and peritonitis; lead point for intussusception and acute intestinal obstruction due to volvulus around a band between Meckel's diverticulum and umbilicus. It is difficult to diagnosis this entity preoperatively and confirmation is usually made on exploratory laparotomy for intestinal obstruction. Complicated Meckel's diverticulum should be removed at surgery.

Acute Pancreatitis

Acute pancreatitis is inflammation of pancreas associated with variable local and systemic inflammatory response. Its incidence in childhood is

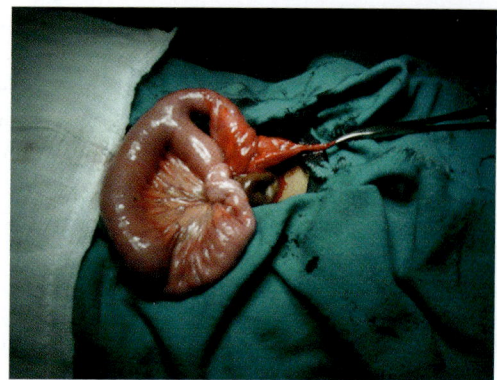

Fig. 23.4: Meckel's diverticulum

unknown. Diagnosis is difficult in small children because of non-specific clinical features.

Idiopathic pancreatitis is the commonest group seen although trauma is the most common recognized cause of pancreatitis in childhood. Other causes include infections, biliary tract disease, drugs, metabolic and hereditary diseases. Acute auto-digestion of pancreas leads to local and systemic inflammatory response.

Usual presenting feature is sudden onset severe abdominal pain in the epigastrium and upper lateral quadrants. The pain may radiate to back. Nausea and vomiting usually follow. Hypovolemia and shock can occur along with multiorgan failure in late cases.

Diagnosis is confirmed by hyperglycemia, hypocalcemia, elevated LDH and other liver function test. Serum amylase and lipase are markedly raised. Serum trypsinogen and alpha-1-antitrypsin have good sensitivity. Abdominal X-ray can be used to rule out other causes of acute abdomen. Ultrasound is useful but CT scan is the best investigation to assess and identify edema, necrosis, abscess and pseudocyst formation. Treatment is generally supportive with nasogastric drainage and intravenous fluids initially. Use of antibiotics is advocated in high risk groups. Enteral feeding should be started early and parenteral nutrition reserved for those who do not tolerate the former. Mortality is about 10–15%. Surgical intervention is needed for management of complications like pancreatic necrosis, abscess and pseudocyst.

Peptic Ulcer Disease

Peptic ulcer disease in childhood presents most commonly as abdominal pain and is responsible for about 15–20% cases of abdominal pain. It may be primary or secondary peptic ulcer disease. It is the secondary peptic ulcers, usually due to underlying disease or drugs that are more acute in onset. Peptic ulcers can present as complications including perforation.

Urinary Tract Infection

Urinary tract infection (UTI) is a common infection in children and causes acute morbidity. Its incidence is higher in girls than the boys. Majority of cases are caused by gram-negative bacteria. Some of the cases present as acute abdominal pain that can be associated with fever, vomiting, lethargy and symptoms of systemic sepsis. Urinary symptoms include burning, urgency, frequency and flank pain. Urine may be turbid or foul smelling. Untreated UTI can be associated with vesicoureteric reflux and results in renal scarring.

Urinalysis and urine culture examination are necessary for diagnosis. Antibiotic therapy is given according to culture sensitivity reports. Therapy may be oral in uncomplicated UTI while complicated UTI necessitates use of parenteral administration.

Patients should be evaluated by ultrasonography, micturating cystogram and Dimercaptosuccinic acid scan (DMSA) for assessment of renal damage after treatment of initial infection.

Miscellaneous Surgical Causes

Abdominal tuberculosis is a common cause of intestinal obstruction in India and may present as acute abdomen in case of acute intestinal obstruction or perforation of bowel.

Round worms are a common cause of acute abdomen in children. These can cause acute intestinal obstruction due to impaction of worms in the lumen. Untreated, there may be peritonitis due to pressure necrosis and perforation.

Primary pyogenic psoas abscess is an important cause of abdominal pain in India. It is associated with fever, inability to use the affected limb and fixed flexion deformity at the hip. Diagnosis is made by ultrasound examination. Treatment includes surgical drainage and appropriate antibiotics.

Hirschsprung's disease may present with enterocolitis and acute intestinal obstruction in neonatal age. If not treated, it may lead to perforation and peritonitis.

Acute cholecystitis and cholelithiasis can cause acute abdominal pain in some children.

Psychosomatic Disorders

The cause of acute and recurrent abdominal pain may not be identified in many children even after repeated examination and investigation. A careful psychosocial history and assessment by a psychologist is helpful in such cases. Caution should be exercised before labeling a child to be suffering from psychosomatic disorder. The acceptance by parents of a biopsychosocial model of illness is important for the resolution of recurrent abdominal pain in children.

Surgical Referral

Surgical consultation in patients with acute abdominal pain is indicated in following situations.

1. Severe increasing pain with progression
2. Deterioration in general condition
3. Bile stained or feculent vomiting
4. Involuntary abdominal guarding and rigidity
5. Rebound abdominal tenderness
6. Masking of liver dullness suggesting free gas
7. Signs of acute blood loss into abdomen
8. Significant abdominal trauma
9. Suspected surgical cause
10. Abdominal pain without obvious etiology.

When to operate immediately and when to observe and when not to operate at all represents the major challenge for the pediatric surgeon. The acute abdomen is a clinical diagnosis and other diagnostic modalities have only a supportive role. The decision to operate is based on the results and on repeated clinical examination.

24 | Septic Shock

Shock is a physiological condition in which there is inadequate tissue perfusion. Septic shock is defined as sepsis with hypotension not responding to adequate fluid resuscitation combined with perfusion abnormalities. Hypotension is defined as systolic blood pressure <90 mm Hg or reduction of more than 40 mm Hg from the base line reading.

Septic shock is a spectrum of clinical response to infection that begins with sepsis, progressing to severe sepsis leading to cellular hypoxia and disruption of necessary biochemical process with resultant organ dysfunction. In early stages with control of infection these alteration can be reversed but if remain untreated they may become irreversible leading to cell death and to MODS (multiple organ dysfunction syndrome).

Etiopathophysiology

The following groups of the patients are at great risk of developing the sepsis.
- Individuals over 65 years, due to age-related changes in the systemic inflammation and coagulopathic process.
- Neonates (particularly among the premature with low birth weight)
- Immunocompromised individuals (patients with cancer, diabetes, alcoholism and malnourishment)
- Invasive diagnostic and therapeutic procedure especially for lung, abdomen, and urinary tract.
- Patients in the intensive care unit

During the process of microbial invasion the human body responds with a complex immunological defense mechanism. In the event of poor immunological response, infection gets established. Many times the immune mechanism is poorly regulated and body may generate endogenously inflammatory compound leading to the uncontrolled cascade of inflammation and that is known as systemic inflammatory response syndrome.

SYSTEMIC INFLAMMATORY RESPONSE SYNDROME

Systemic inflammatory response syndrome (SIRS) is a wide spread systemic inflammatory response to a variety of primary insult to the body which could be due to infection, trauma (surgery), pancreatitis or even burns. SIRS can be diagnosed when two or more of the following criteria are present.
- Temperature >38°C or < 36°C
- Heart rate> 90 beats /min
- Respiratory rate > 20 breath /min
- WBC> 12,000/mm^3 or <4000 mm^3 or more than 10% of immature (band) cell in peripheral blood smear.

In SIRS there is increase in cytokine production, abnormal nitric oxide synthesis and coagulopathy. The cytokines are protein molecules produced by activated inflammatory cells and function as messengers to incite the production of intermediate metabolites, pro-inflammatory cytokines like tumor necrosis factor-alpha (TNF-alpha), interleukins like IL-1, IL-6, IL-8, IL-12, interferon and platelet activating factors. Cytokines also activates neutrophils that engulf the pathogens. Many times in the individual who are susceptible to sepsis, the anti-inflammatory cytokines fail to regulate the early response to the infection, and excessive amount of TNF-alpha, IL–1, IL–6 and interferon are released throughout the system leading to tissue and capillary injury, manifesting features of SIRS like fever, tachycardia, leukocytosis, etc.

Severe sepsis which occurs on account of infection is always associated with organ dysfunction, hypoperfusion and hypotension. If this hypotension persists in spite of adequate fluid resuscitation and require inotropic or vasopressor support it indicates the development of septic shock which is characterized by lactic acidosis, oliguria, altered mental state along with all other criterias of SIRS.

Infection starts with invasion and proliferation of microorganisms which is rapidly followed by host monocyte/macrophages recognition of specific microbial product by a family of pattern recognition receptors that include the toll-like receptors (TLRs). Lipopolysaccharides (LPS or endotoxin) is a component of cell wall of Gram-negative bacteria and is recognized by TLRs-4. TLRs-2 recognizes peptidoglycan and lipotechoic acid from Gram-positive bacteria and zymosan from yeast.

In response to different pathogen products, cells of the immunesystem also produce microbicidal agents and soluble mediators in an effort to eliminate the invading pathogen.

Sepsis thus is a process comprising of two major components, infectious and inflammatory. It has been observed that the patients with exaggerated inflammatory response to uncontrolled infection, progress from mild SIRS to sepsis then severe sepsis and finally lethal problem like septic shock. Patients with severe sepsis and shock suffer from hypotension due to arteriolar dilation. Typically in septic shock, patients have increased cardiac output due to hyperdynamic pattern of circulation. Although there is increase in cardiac output and there is a deficiency in effective perfusion of tissues of vital organ like heart, liver, or brain. Myocardial dysfunction is second major factor contributing to hypotension in septic shock. It is the endotoxin and exotoxin which release endogenous mediators of inflammation. When these toxins enter the circulation they cause impaired function of cardiac myocytes.

CLINICAL ASSESSMENT AND LABORATORY INVESTIGATION

- Physical examination and rapid assessment of patient's present condition. There are numerous clinical manifestations of sepsis, but most common are fever or hypothermia, unexplained tachycardia, hyperventilation or unexplained tachypnea, leukocytosis or leukopenia, thrombocytopenia or coagulopathy, altered blood pressure and altered mental status. Other symptoms of poor perfusion are oliguria and signs of delayed capillary filling, hypotension, cold skin, decreased level of consciousness.

- Differentiate from other types of shock like hypovolemic or cardiogenic shock.

- Laboratory studies based on clinical examination should include arterial blood gas, routine blood count and differential counts, lactate level estimation, serum amylase and lipase, liver function test, cardiac enzymes, fibrinogen and fibrin degradation products. Cortisone level should also be done to detect the adrenal insufficiency. X-ray chest and ECG are essential for the assessment of cardiopulmonary system. Plain and contrast radiological imaging to be done if required for the cases of visceral perforation and intra-abdominal abscess. USG, CT, and MRI to be done as and when required.

- Biochemical markers: Although they are not routinely monitored in the clinical setting but the elevated levels of these cytokines often correlates with the severity of the disease. Serum levels of C-reactive protein are normally low but may rise to ten to hundred folds in patients with SIRS. In cases of systemic infection higher serum concentration of procalcitonin (PCT) is also observed. The higher levels of these proteins have been predictive of sepsis and organ dysfunction. A recent study suggests that elevated serum PCT is considered to be a better marker of sepsis than C-reactive protein.

- Identify the causative organisms by culture and the site of infection by appropriate imaging studies. The lungs, abdomen, and urinary tracts are the common sites of infection, diagnosis of which can be made clinically but it is important for the clinician to confirm the diagnosis based on microbial studies by culture and sensitivity.

- Identification of organ dysfunction—For diagnosis of MODS in septic shock, one should always evaluate carefully the respiratory tract, cardiovascular, renal, gastrointestinal, hepatic, and central nervous system.

MANAGEMENT

It includes resuscitation, search for infective focus, suitable antibiotic coverage and control of infection.

Resuscitation

Shock of any kind is a medical emergency and hence all efforts are to be made to resuscitate the patient immediately. Like any other patient in critical condition the protocol of ABC (airway, breathing and circulation) should be followed. Airway should be assessed and supported. At times the patient with septic shock has reduced level of consciousness or encephalopathy that may require intubation and mechanical ventilation for airway protection. Circulatory assessment is done by recording the blood pressure and pulse rate. In septic shock most of the patients are in circulatory failure and are supported by vasopressor and ionotropes. Prompt care is necessary to avoid MODS. The hypotension seen in septic shock is multifactorial in origin. Sepsis leads to myocardial depression and decreased vasomotor tone. There is also a significant loss of plasma volume in the interstitial space resulting in intravascular hypovolemia. Therefore hypovolemia should be restored rapidly by intravenous fluids preferably by using crystalloid or colloid solution. It is observed that a given volume of colloid results in greater expansion of plasma volume than the equal volume of crystalloid. But use of crystalloid is economical and is generally adopted. Fluid resuscitation should be continued till CVP of 8–14 mm Hg is achieved. Successful resuscitation is demonstrated by preservation of

normal renal function and resolution of metabolic (lactic) acidosis.

Timely administration of antibiotics (within 4–6 hour of presentation) is very essential. Delay in administration of antibiotics in such patients lead to higher mortality in comparison to those who received appropriate therapy promptly. While choosing the antibiotic the clinician should consider the appropriate dose and dosing frequency, sensitivity of the microorganism, and timing of the drug administration.

Use of Vasopressor

In spite of adequate fluid resuscitation, if the patient still remains to be hypotensive, it necessitates the use of vasopressor and inotropic support. These drugs help in improving the cardiac function in patients with septic shock. The common vasopressor used in septic shock are dopamine, dobutamine, epinephrine and vasopressin. epinephrine and dobutamine increases the cardiac contractility. Dopamine and epinephrine causes tachycardia in comparison to norepinephrine. In the recent study, the use of norepinephrine is found to be more effective than dopamine in cases of refractory septic shock. The usual dose range of norepinephrine is 1–30 microgram/min intravenously. Vasopressin therapy also found to be useful in reversing the hypotension in case of septic shock. The intravenous dose of Vasopressin is limited to 0.01–0.04 U/min as high doses may lead to splanchnic and coronary ischemia and can also lead to decreased cardiac output. Dobutamine is equally effective in increasing the myocardial contractility by stimulating the β_1 adrenergic receptors. The usual dose range for dobutamine is 5–15 microgram/kg/min.

In a standard therapy after volume resuscitation keeping the CVP at 8–12 mm Hg later followed by vasopressor therapy to maintain the mean arterial pressure at 65 mm Hg. Recently an early goal-directed therapy includes the measurement of central venous oxyhemoglobin saturation (CVO_2 sat). If it is less than 70% then blood is given to achieve the hematocrit of 30%. If the CVO_2 saturation still remains less than 70% then dobutamine is added with a dose of 20 microgram/kg/min to achieve the CVO_2 saturation of 70%. This particular approach of therapy for septic shock appears to be promising but additional trials are forthcoming.

Role of Corticosteroids

The septic shock has been demonstrated to cause relative adrenal insufficiency. There has been number of trials for corticosteroid therapy in severe sepsis and septic shock but have failed to improve the survival rate in septic shock. The usual dose is hydrocortisone 100 mg thrice a day intravenously for five to seven days.

Role of Human Activated Protein-C

Human activated protein-C after a multi-centric trail found to be greatest benefit in most acutely ill patients with APACHE II score of more than equal to 25. The use of recombinant human activated protein-C (Drotrecogin-alpha) treatment found to be associated with rapid recovery of cardiac and pulmonary function and lower incidence of MODS. It is very expensive and not suitable for less acutely ill patients (APACHE II score of less than equal to 25). It has anticoagulant, anti-inflammatory and fibrinolytic property. The anticoagulant effects of activated protein-C include inactivation of coagulation factors Va, VIIa and inhibition of thrombin formation. Its anti-inflammatory effect includes a reduction of IL 1 and IL 6, TNF, and other pro-inflammatory cytokines. The fibrinolytic effect includes activation of endogenous tissue plasminogen activator.

Sepsis often depletes plasma protein-C levels, greater the depletion poorer the prognosis. It has been found that intravenous infusion of activated human protein-C has got potential therapeutic benefit in severe sepsis.

Surgical Therapy

All cases of sepsis having abscess external or intra-abdominal should be drained and debrided thoroughly. Generally these abscesses are formed when a local inflammatory response to the infection triggers a coagulation cascade that generates fibrin which then develops into capsule and fibrous tissue surrounding the infection. The contents of the capsule can be drained percutaneously or surgically to resolve the infection. Laparotomy at times becomes necessary for those abscesses which cannot be treated percutaneously.

COMPLICATIONS

Septic shock is itself a severe complication of many diseased process and major operative procedure with infection. It carries a high mortality rate because of multiple organ failure.

Pulmonary

Lungs are very much susceptible to injury in cases of septic shock. Acute lung failure with sepsis in surgical practice is known as acute respiratory distress syndrome (ARDS). It is usually associated with multiple organ failure. ARDS is a pulmonary manifestation of a wide spread abnormality of cellular metabolic function, precipitated most commonly by sepsis or trauma. In ARDS due to insult to the pulmonary vascular endothelium and alveolar epithelium there is an inflammatory reaction leading to the increase permeability of alveolar capillary membrane and pulmonary edema which ultimately leads to ventilation perfusion mismatch and refractory hypoxemia. Mechanical ventilation is an essential component in treating ARDS. Mortality is very high in ARDS due to sepsis than the other causes like multiple trauma, fat embolism, and gastric aspiration.

Renal

Hypoperfusion due to hypovolemia may lead to oliguric acute renal failure. Intermittent hemodialysis is the standard treatment in dealing such complication. It has been observed that daily hemodialysis lead to better control of uremia, fewer hypotensive episodes and more rapid resolution of acute renal failure.

Hematological

Bacterial products in sepsis activate the coagulation cascade. The cytokines like TNF-alpha and interleukins released during the host response also activate the coagulation and enhances the formation of thrombin and fibrin clots. All these factors together are responsible for disseminated intravascular coagulation and organ dysfunction.

Endocrine System

Hypoglycemia and insulin resistance has been commonly seen in patients with septic shock which further increases the risk of complications like severe infection, multiple organ failure and death.

Gastrointestinal System

Ileus and malabsorption are the common complications of septic shock. Enteral feeding is always found to be superior to total parenteral nutrition. Early jejunal feeding is helpful in maintaining the normal bacterial flora and GI tract barrier function thereby minimizing the bacterial and endotoxin translocation.

Patients with septicemic shock treated with antibiotics are generally at increase risk for development of pseudomembranous enterocolitis. Because of low perfusion in septicemic shock, patient may develop intestinal ischemia and pancreatitis. Cholestatic jaundice is also seen in severe septicemic shock. Cholestasis and hypoperfusion in septic shock are responsible for development of acalculous cholecystitis which should be treated urgently.

Central Nervous System

Sepsis commonly results to brain dystrophy and associated encephalopathy which can be either transient encephalopathy or irreversible brain damage.

Multi Organ Failure (MOF)

Severe sepsis and septicemia shock are the most common cause of MOF. It has been observed that single organ system failure is associated with 40% mortality, two organ system failure with 60% mortality, whereas three or more organ system failure lasting for more than three days is found to have 98% mortality. In cases of patients older than 65 years, then the mortality can rise by 20% in each category. Multiple organ failure is the final complication of critical illness and leading cause of death in cases of septicemic shock.

Recognition and management of septic shock with features of SIRS and MODS is very important as early treatment can prevent the morbidity and mortality. Rapid adequate volume resuscitation as well as aggressive support of dysfunctioning organ system is critical. Along with these majors the proper antibiotic coverage, control of infectious source, adequate nutrition and aggressive pulmonary management are important factors for not allowing the patients of septicemic shock to progress into multiple organ failure and death.

25 Painful Anorectal Conditions

SURGICAL ANATOMY

The anal canal (Fig. 25.1) is 1.5" (4 cm) long and is directed downward and backward from the rectum to the anal orifice. The mid of anal canal which represents the junction between endoderm and ectoderm is known as dentate line. The upper half is lined by columnar epithelium with splanchnic innervations and is insensitive to pain, whereas the lower half of the anal canal below the dentate line is lined by squamous epithelium and is supplied by somatic nerves and are very sensitive to pain. The painful anal sensation arises from the perianal skin, the anoderm, anal sphincters and the surrounding muscles. The common painful anorectal conditions are

I. Anorectal abscesses
II. Acute anal fissure
III. Strangulated hemorrhoid (acute thrombosis)
IV. Thrombosed external hemorrhoid (perianal hematoma)
V. Rectal procedentia.

The painful anal condition can be diagnosed by précise history taking and thorough examination. Not only the character of pain (throbbing, piercing, aching or sore) but also the timing and relation to defecation is important.

Inspection of anus and surrounding skin will immediately reveal the hematoma, painful thrombosed piles or painful, erythematous and tender fluctuating swelling indicating the anorectal abscess or prolapse of rectum. Everting the anal skin may expose the fissure in ano. One should also try if possible to do the proctoscopy and sigmoidoscopy to rule out any other anorectal lesion.

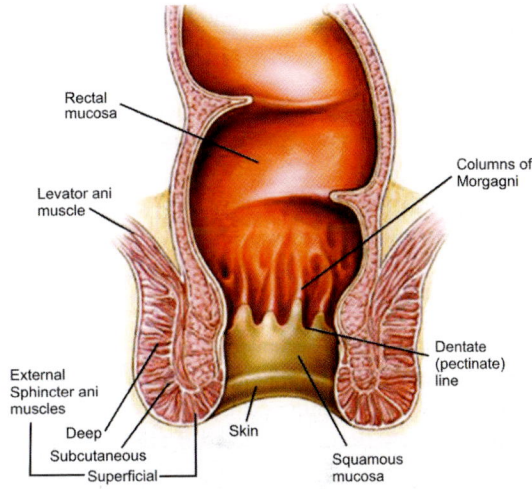

Fig. 25.1: Anatomy of anal canal

ANORECTAL ABSCESS

The anorectal abscess is more common in men than women. These abscesses (90% of the cases) commences as infection of anal gland. Large percentage of anorectal abscess coincides with fistula in ano. Other causes could be injury to the rectal wall, blood born infection or extension of a cutaneous boil. One should also keep in mind the possibility of underlying rectal neoplasm, Chron's disease and generalized disorders like diabetes and AIDS.

Common types of abscesses are (Fig. 25.2)
• Perianal abscess (most common)
• Ischiorectal abscess

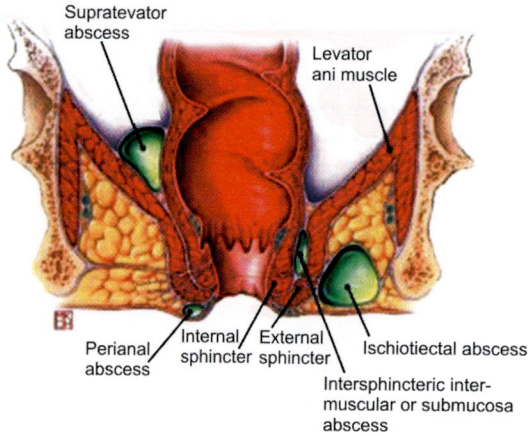

Fig. 25.2: Common types of anorectal abscess

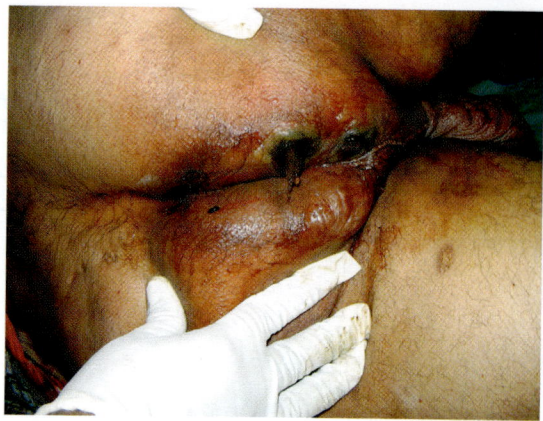

Fig. 25.3: Horseshoe ischiorectal abscess

- Submucous abscess
- Supralevator abscess.

Perianal Abscess

It is the most common abscess which occurs as a result of suppuration of anal gland. It may also occur as a result of thrombosed external piles. Such hematoma may become infected if not drained and lead to perianal abscess. Patient presents with acute painful perianal condition with throbbing pain and constitutional symptoms. On examination there may be redness, induration and swelling around anus. Tender painful cystic swelling will be present.

Ischiorectal Abscess

It is commonly due to lateral extension of the perianal abscess. It can also result from hematogenous or lymphatic spread of infection. The poor vascularization of ischiorectal fat makes this area vulnerable for abscess formation. Ischiorectal fossa communicates to the opposite site through post sphincteric space and hence abscess can spread to the opposite site in a horseshoe fashion (Fig. 25.3). On examination there is a tender erythematous induration, which at time may be fluctuant and palpable on the corresponding site of anal canal.

Submucous Abscess

It is generally formed after injection sclerotherapy for hemorrhoid and it resolves quickly. It is usually seen above the dentate line.

Supralevator Abscess

The supralevator abscess lies between the upper part of levator ani and pelvic peritoneum and is secondary to acute inflammatory condition like acute appendicitis, salpingitis, diverticulitis.

MANAGEMENT

No place for conservative management for any of these abscesses and should be treated as acute emergency. Abscesses should be drained under general or regional anesthesia in lithotomy position.

Surgery

Perianal Abscess

After skin is prepared with antiseptic solution, a cruciate incision is made over the most tender and fluctuating point as close to the anal verge as possible (Fig. 25.4). All the loculi in the abscess cavity are broken with an artery forceps to allow free drainage of pus. Skin edges must be excised to avoid the

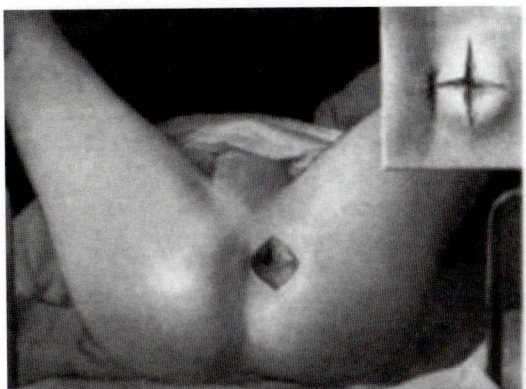

Fig. 25.4: Cruciate incision for drainage of perianal abscess

sealing of abscess opening. Minor bleeding can be controlled by pressure or electrocoagulation. Packing should not be done as it hinders free drainage of abscess. Incision is made close to anal verge because in case fistula develops, the external opening will remain close to the verge and can be treated simply by fistulotomy.

Ischiorectal Abscess

Unilateral abscess can be drained either by single incision or multiple counter incisions over the area of maximum tenderness or fluctuation close to the anal verge.

Submucosal Abscess

These should be drained internally by incising the mucosa over the abscess.

Supralevator

Overall management will depend upon the underlying pathology. If collections result from abdominopelvic disease, it may be drained transerectally or transabdominally. Collection that results from extension of intersphincteric abscess should be drained transrectally as trans-perineal drainage through ischiorectal fossa can result in supra-sphincteric fistula formation.

Post-Anal Abscess and Horseshoe Extension

It should be drained by deep posterior midline incision. All the muscle attached to coccyx, the superficial external sphincter and the lower edge of internal sphincter are divided. If there is a horseshoe extension to the ischiorectal fossa, multiple secondary incision are made in the skin overlying the ischiorectal space.

Postoperative Care

Patients are advised to take sitz bath three to four times a day. Analgesics are prescribed and antibiotic should be given according to pus-culture and sensitivity.

ANAL FISSURE

Acute anal fissure is a common cause of severe anal pain. There is acute pain during defecation associated with bleeding per anus. It is defined as a longitudinal tear/crack in the mucosa and skin of the anal canal. As this is present below the dentate line, it is very painful because of the somatic nerve supply (Fig. 25.5). It is commonly situated in the midline posteriorly although in 10% of the cases it may be present situated anteriorly also. The precise cause of anal fissure is yet to be determined. They occur

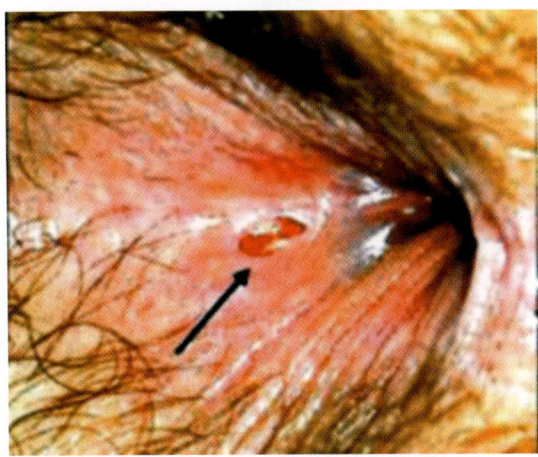

Fig. 25.5: Anal fissure

due to tear of anoderm at the time of defecation by passage of a bulky or constipated stool. The pain causes an intense protective spasm of the internal sphincter and increases resting anal canal pressure. Fissures may undergo spontaneous healing but resultant scar do break down again and can lead to chronic fissure. These chronic fissures have a fibrous base; edematous edges and hypertrophied skin tag which is also known as sentinel pile (Fig. 25.6). In long-standing cases the muscles of the internal sphincter become contracted by formation of fibrous tissue. These fissures can predispose to infection and abscess formation of the anal canal.

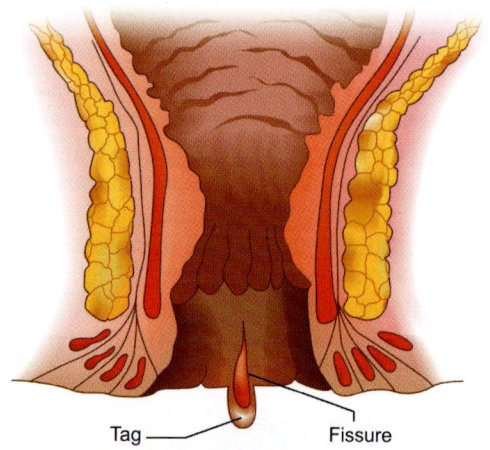

Fig. 25.6: Anal fissure and sentinel pile

Tag — Fissure

Clinical Symptoms

History is usually characteristic with severe pain in relation with defecation. Bleeding is often common during defecation but is seldom profuse. During examination, a sentinel tag may be noticed and fissure can be seen by parting the buttocks. In acute condition one should avoid digital rectal examination and proctoscopy as it is very painful. In chronic anal fissure, digital rectal examination and proctoscopy can be well tolerated. Digital rectal examination can reveal tenderness at the site of fissure if allowed. Induration of chronic fissure can be felt in digital examination.

Treatment

Treatment includes sitz bath, adequate analgesia, stool softening agents, high-fiber-diet and bulk-forming agents such as Isabgol. Application of local anesthetic cream (xylocaine ointment) prior to defecation may help in reducing pain during defecation.

Medical or Chemical Sphincterotomy

It has now become an important part in the management. 2% nitroglycerine ointment is applied in the anal canal twice a day. This relieves the sphincteric spasm by relaxing the anal sphincter due to release of nitric oxide, thereby allowing the fissure to heal. Diltiazem ointment and oral nifidipine are other agents which are used for chemical sphincterotomy. Majority of the acute fissures heal in four to six weeks of application of these ointments with dietary precautions. Any fissure which does not heal in six weeks time are termed as chronic fissure and are to be subjected to operative sphincterotomy.

Lateral Anal Sphincterotomy

In this procedure internal sphincter is divided away from the fissure either in the right or left side. This procedure can be performed by an open or closed method.

Open lateral sphincterotomy: Patients is placed in lithotomy position after spinal or general anesthesia, a small incision is made in 3 O' clock position (Fig. 25.7A). Using an artery forceps lower border of the internal sphincter is hooked (Fig. 25.7B) and divided with scalpel (Fig.25.7C). Skin closed with absorbable suture.

Closed Lateral sphincterotomy: Patient is placed in lithotomy position, left index finger is inserted in the anus and the left thumb pulp in the groove between internal and external sphincter. No 15 scalpel blade is inserted into this groove (Fig. 25.8A) and the cutting edge of blade is turned medially and sphincter is incised towards the left index finger (Fig. 25.8B). Small skin wound is left open to allow drainage and to prevent hematoma formation.

Anal dilatation (Lord's procedure) is no more recommended due to high chances of incontinence and recurrence.

Skin incision made external to and verge

External sphincter

A

Internal sphincter

External sphincter

B

Internal sphincter

C

Figs 25.7A to C: Open method of lateral anal sphincterotomy

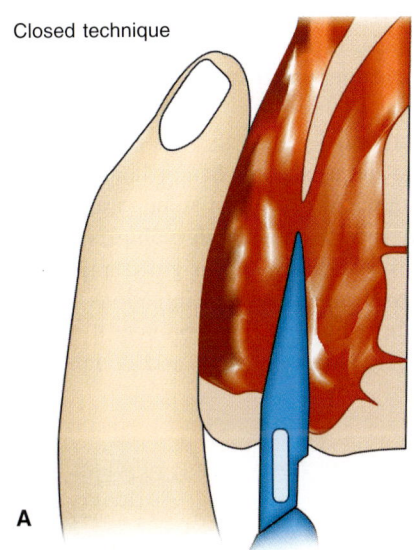

Closed technique

A

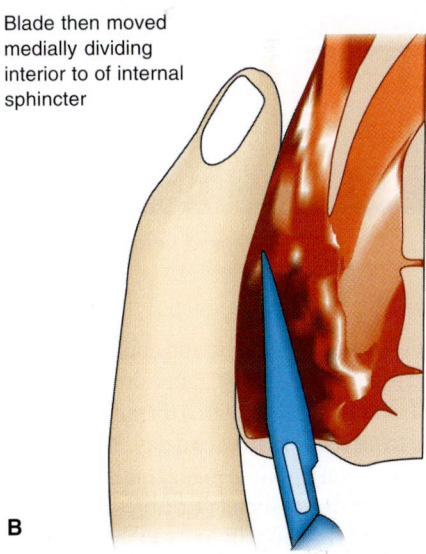

Blade then moved medially dividing interior to of internal sphincter

B

Figs 25.8A and B: Closed method of lateral anal sphincterotomy

ACUTE THROMBOSIS OF PROLAPSED HEMORRHOID

Definition

Thrombosis is one of the complications of the hemorrhoids. It occurs when one or more internal hemorrhoids get prolapsed and strangulated by the sphincter.

Patients usually presents with a painful, edematous, firm and irreducible hemorrhoidal mass at the anal margin (Fig. 25.9). In some cases the edema gradually subsides and the thrombus is absorbed in two weeks of time. It can get complicated by formation of ulceration and infections which may lead to formations of the submucosal abscess. At times it may turn gangrenous and sloughs off.

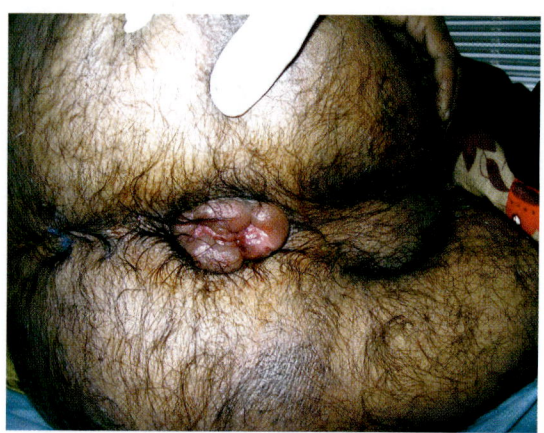

Fig. 25.9: Prolapsed hemorrhoids

Treatment

Patient is placed on bed rest and analgesics are given for pain relief. Large moist gauze dressing is applied on, and is held at place with a T-bandage. Patient is advised to take sitz bath twice a day. The mass slowly shrinks with conservative management. Thrombosis with passage of time leads to fibrosis and cure the symptoms. If patient is not relieved with conservative management patient is subjected to hemorrhoidectomy.

RECTAL PROLAPSE

Rectal prolapse is the protrusion of entire thickness of rectal wall through the anal sphincter. As the rectum descends, it intussuscepts upon itself. Rectal prolapse can be partial or complete. Partial prolapse involves the protrusion of only mucosa and submucosa and generally occurs in old age and children. Complete prolapse is less common and the protrusion consists of all layers of rectal wall. Presence of concentric rings is characteristic of rectal prolapse which is not found in prolapsed internal hemorrhoids and mucosal prolapse (Fig. 25.10). Rectal prolapse should always be distinguished with intussusception. In rectosigmoid intussusception there is a deep groove between the emerging mass and margin of anus into which finger can be entered, which is not the case in partial or complete rectal prolapse.

Treatment

Patients with rectal prolapse may present in the emergency because of incarceration or bleeding due

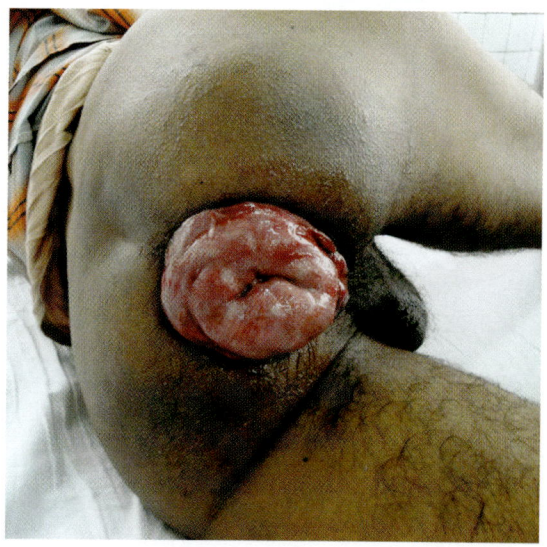

Fig. 25.10: Complete rectal prolapse

to erosion of the protruded bowel. In cases of irreducible or incarcerated rectal prolapse, the prolapsed segment is covered with moist pads soaked with hypertonic saline to reduce the edema. After sometime, when the edema has reduced attempt should be made to manually reduce the prolapsed segment into anal canal preferably under general anesthesia. All such patients should be admitted for complete evaluation and appropriate operative management which can be either done from abdominal or perineal route.

Abdominal Approach

Principle of all abdominal operation for rectal prolapse is to replace and to hold the rectum in its proper position.

Wells Procedure

In the Wells procedure the rectum is dissected from the sacrum in the usual way and the rectum is fixed to the sacrum by inserting a mesh in between. The mesh is sutured to the periosteum of the sacrum in the midline and then wrapped on either side of rectum leaving the anterior wall free.

Ripstein's Procedure

In Ripstein's operation the rectosigmoid junction is hitched up to the sacrum with a teflon sling just in front of sacral promontory.

Perineal Approach

There are two commonly performed operations in perineal approach.

Delorme's Procedure

In this procedure mucosa of the prolapsed rectum is removed and underlying muscle is plicated with a series of sutures. When the sutures are tied, rectal muscle gets concertinaed towards the anal canal. Thereafter anal canal mucosa is sutured circumferentially.

Thiersch Operation

In this technique after reduction of prolapse, encirclement of anal orifice is achieved with steel wire or non-absorbable suture. It is a simple procedure and has a definite place where patient cannot undergo other operations.

INTRODUCTION

Post-surgical pain is a widespread recognized clinical entity. The clinical-practical guidelines for the management of acute postoperative pain have been developed by the agency for health care quality and research of US Department of Health and Human Services. These clinical-practical guidelines included acknowledgment of historical inadequacies in perioperative pain management, importance of good pain control, need for accountability for adequate provisions of perioperative analgesia by health care institution. In addition, several other professional societies (e.g. American society of anesthesiologists) have also developed clinical-practical guidelines for acute pain management. Anesthesiologists are leaders in the development of acute postoperative pain services and application of evidence-based practice to acute pain management. Pain is a consistent and predominant complaint of most individuals following most surgical interventions. "Failure to relieve pain is morally and ethically unacceptable." Adequate pain relief could be considered a basic human right.

Definition of Pain

Acute pain has been defined as normal, predicted, physiological response to associated chemical, thermal or mechanical noxious stimulus. Generally acute pain resolves within 1 month. Acute pain-induced change in central nervous system is known as neuronal plasticity. This results in sensitization of nervous system resulting in allodynia (a painful response to typically non-painful stimulus) and

hyperalgesia (an exaggerated pain response to a normally painful stimulus). Various surgical procedures that can lead to chronic painful conditions include hernioplasty, thoracotomies, nephrectomies, modified radical mastectomy, etc.

Incidence

Pain is a common human experience, a symptom frequently encountered in clinical practice that is usually associated with actual or impending tissue damage. The true enormity of the problem can only be surmised, as epidemiological data are lacking. Clinical surveys dating back to 1950s suggest that there is an ongoing pandemic of poorly managed acute postoperative pain, with up to 75% patients describing their pain as moderate to severe in these circumstances.

Factors Affecting Variability of Clinical Pain Complaint, Behavior and Response to Management

1. *Biological factors*

   The flow of nociceptive impulses is dynamic and modifiable by:

   • Sensitization of peripheral and central nociceptors in response to prolonged or excessive noxious stimuli, so amplifying the response characteristics of the system to subsequent noxious stimulus.

   • Modulation or "dampening" of nociceptors at various points along their passage to consciousness.

- Eliciting local and general motor and autonomic reflexes.

2. *Psychological factors*
   - Affective: The intrinsic emotional response to a noxious stimulus is influenced by preexisting affective dysfunction and personality traits.
   - Cognitive: Understanding the nature, cause, purpose and consequence of the pain, together with learned influences (copying style, previous pain experiences and culture).

3. *Social/environmental factors*
   The gain derived from an individual with family, work, community and health carers, together with immediate context.

4. *Pharmacological factors*
   Pharmacokinetics and pharmacodynamic variability.

Consequences of Inadequate Acute Pain Relief

1. *Cardiovascular:* Tachycardia, hypertension and increase in cardiac workload.
2. *Pulmonary:* Respiratory muscle spasm (splinting), decrease in vital capacity, atelectasis, hypoxia, and increased risk of pulmonary infection.
3. *Gastrointestinal:* Postoperative ileus.
4. *Renal:* Increased risk of oliguria and urinary retention.
5. *Coagulation:* Increased incidence of thrombo-emboli.
6. *Immunologic:* Impaired immune function.
7. *Muscular:* Muscle weakness and fatigue, increased risk of thromboembolism due to limited mobility.
8. *Psychosocial:* Anxiety, fear and frustration results in poor patient satisfaction.
9. *Chronic pain:* Acute pain in cases of hernioplasty, thoracotomies, nephrectomies, modified radical mastectomy, etc. can lead to development of chronic neuropathic pain in a variable proportion of patients having been operated for these surgeries. About 15–35% of hernioplasty patients, 20–40% of mastectomy patients and 35–55% of

patients undergoing thoracotomy have been reported to have chronic neuropathic pain (with typical allodynia and hyperalgesia, Fig. 26.1) at 6 and 12 months of follow-up.

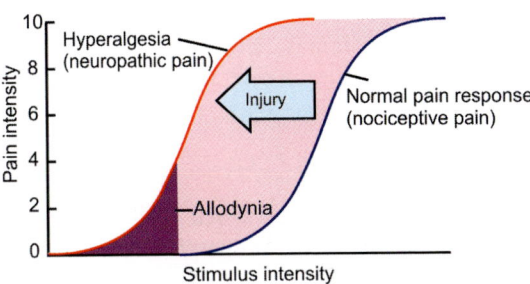

Fig. 26.1: Nociceptive pain and postoperative neuropathic pain

Pain Pathways

The nociceptive pathway is an afferent three neuron dual ascending system, with descending modulation from cortex, thalamus and brainstem. Nociceptors are free nerve endings located in skin, muscle, bone and connective tissue with cell bodies located on the dorsal root ganglia. The first order neurons of pain pathway have their origin in the periphery as A and polymodal 'C' fibers. A fibers transmit "first pain" which is described as sharp or stinging in character and is well localized. Polymodal 'C' fibers transmit "second pain", which is more diffuse in character and is associated with the affective and motivational aspects of pain.

First order neurons synapse with second order neurons in dorsal horn primarily within lamina I, II and V where they release excitatory amino acids and neuropeptides. Some fibers can ascend or descend in Lissauer tract prior to terminating on neurons that project to higher centres. Second order neurons consist of nociceptive specific and wide dynamic range (WDR) neurons. Nociceptive neurons located primarily in lamina I, respond only to noxious stimuli. WDR neurons are predominantly located in lamina IV, V and VI respond to both noxious and non-noxious input and are involved with affective motivational components of the pain. Axons of both nociceptive specific and WDR neuron ascend the spinal cord via dorsal column, medial lamniscus and anterior lateral spinothalamic tract to synapse on third order neurons in the contralateral thalamus, which then projects to somatosensory cortex where nociceptive input is perceived as pain (Fig. 26.2).

Pain Processing

Pain pathway is not "hard wired" and nociceptive input is not passively transmitted from periphery to brain. Tissue injury tends to fuel neuroplastic changes within the nervous system which results in both peripheral and central sensitization. Clinically this can manifest as hyperalgesia and allodynia.

Four elements of pain processing consist of:
1. *Transduction:* An event whereby noxious thermal, chemical or mechanical stimuli are converted into an action potential.
2. *Transmission:* This is conduction of that transduced action potential from the site of stimuli to higher cortex.
3. *Modulation:* Involves alterations of afferent neural transmission along the pain pathways. The dorsal horn of the spinal cord is the most common site for modulation of pain pathways. Modulation can be achieved by either inhibition or augmentation of the pain signals.
4. *Perception:* Process which involves the perception of the pain signal.

Physiology of Nociception

Tissue damage following surgical procedures leads to activation of small nociceptive nerve endings and

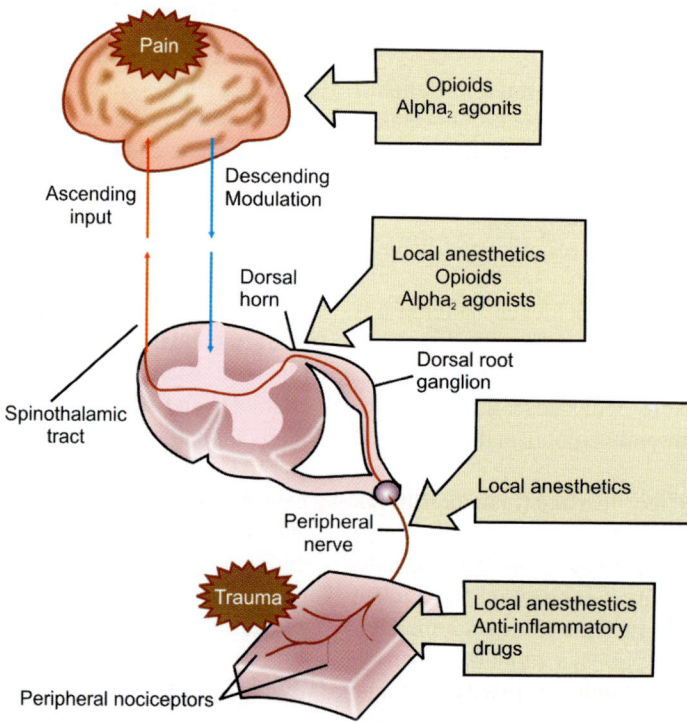

Fig. 26.2: Pain pathways and multimodal analgesic approach

local inflammatory cells (e.g. macrophages, mast cells, lymphocytes and platelets) in the periphery. Antidromic release of substance P and glutamate from small nociceptive afferents results in vasodilatation, extravasation of plasma proteins and stimulation of inflammatory cells to release numerous algogenic substances. This chemical milieu will both directly produce pain transduction via nociceptor stimulation and facilitate transduction by increasing the excitability of nociceptors. The chemical mediators of nociceptions are being given in Table 26.1.

Therefore, a **multimodal approach to pain therapy** (Fig. 26.2) should target all four elements of the pain processing pathway. All these four elements of pain processing are carried upon through chemical mediators.

Assessment of Acute Postoperative Pain

We know pain is a uniquely personal symptom with no reliable objective signs. So one has to accept individual's "self-report" of the severity of pain they are expressing. So to assess pain severity there are various "self-reporting" pain severity, pain scoring systems in adult patients. They correlate well and are generally reliable. Postoperative acute pain severity should be scored and recorded both at rest and on movement at regular intervals. Pain severity score has been declared as fifth vital sign along with BP, PR, RR and temperature. When these five vital signs are recorded along with sedation scoring constitutes a minimum data set which should be observed in a surgical ward on a bedside chart.

Simple Pain Scoring System

1. *Visual analogue scale (VAS):* Employs a 10-cm drawnline with the left anchor pain descriptors labeled "no pain" and right-sided equivalent labeled "worst possible pain". It require patients to move their current pain severity on the continuum. VAS score is the measured distance from no pain point to the pain estimate.

2. *Verbal numerical rating scale (VNRS):* Ask patients to estimate their pain severity as a number

Table 26.1: Algogenic substances		
Substance	*Source*	*Effect*
Bradykinin	Macrophages and plasma kininogen	Activates nociceptors
Serotonin	Platelets	Activates nociceptors
Histamine	Platelets and mast cells	Produces vasodilatation, edema and pruritus
		Potentiates the response of nociceptors to bradykinin
Prostaglandin	Tissue injury and cyclooxygenase pathway	Sensitizes nociceptors
Leukotriene	Tissue injury and lipooxygenase pathway	Sensitizes nociceptors
Excess H^+ ion	Tissue injury and ischemia	Increases pain and hyperalgesia associated with inflammation
Cytokines, e.g. interleukins and tissue necrosis factor	Macrophages	Excite and sensitize nociceptors
Adenisone	Tissue injury	Pain and hyperalgesia
Neurotransmitters, e.g. glutamate and substance P	Antidromic release by peripheral nerve terminals following tissue injury	Substance P activates macrophages and mast cells
		Glutamate activates nociceptors
Nerve growth factor	Macrophages	Stimulates mast cells to release histamine and serotonin
		Sensitizes nociceptors

'0' being no pain and '10' being the worst possible pain (Fig. 26.3).

Simple Method of Scoring Acute Pain

- Believe your patient for the severity of the pain he or she is experiencing.
- Score the pain by asking the patient to estimate the pain at rest and during deep breathing or on performing a standard movement as either
  - 0 = none
  - 1 = mild
  - 2 = moderate
  - 3 = severe.

Facies Pain Rating Scale

- This scale is used in pediatric patients who cannot express the severity of pain. So the severity of pain is assessed by their facial expression.

Minimum Assessment Intervals

- Every 5 min following
  - IV bolus local anesthetic or opioids or both
  - After top ups
- Every two hours for 24–48 hours postoperatively
- Every four hours thereafter.

Description of Acute Surgical Pain

- Onset of pain
- Temporal patterns of pain
- Site of pain
- Radiation of pain
- Character of pain
- Severity of pain
- Frequency of pain
- Exacerbating factor
- Relieving factors
- Response to analgesics
- Response to other interventions
- Associated physical symptoms
- Associated psychological symptoms
- Interference with daily activities.

Pre-emptive or Preventive Analgesia

The aim of pre-emptive analgesia is to prevent NMDA receptor activation in dorsal horn, which causes wind up, facilitation, central sensitization, expansion of receptive field and long-term potential all of which can lead to a chronic pain state.

In order for pre-emptive analgesia to be successful three critical principles must be adhered to:

1. The depth of analgesia must be adequate enough to block all nociceptive input during surgery.
2. The analgesic technique must be extensive enough to include the entire surgical field.
3. The duration of analgesia must include both intraoperative and postoperative period.

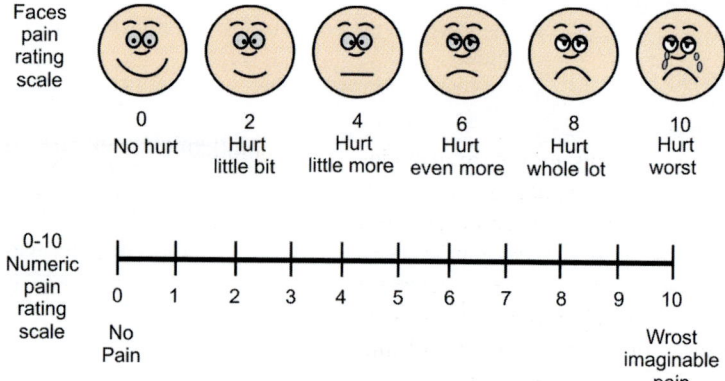

Fig. 26.3: Pain severity scale

There are lot of studies on pre-emptive analgesia with variable outcomes. So the credibility of this modality of analgesia is still to be proved.

Treatment Options for Acute Pain

Many options are available for the treatment of postoperative pain, including systemic (i.e. opioid and non-opioid) analgesia and regional (i.e. neuraxial and peripheral) analgesia. Techniques must be multimodal and according to the feasibility in a given clinical scenario.

PHARMACOLOGICAL STRATEGIES TO MANAGE ACUTE PAIN

Systemic Analgesic Techniques

Opioids

Advantages and characteristics: Opioid analgesics are one of the cornerstone options for the treatment of postoperative pain. These agents generally exert their analgesic effects through μ-receptors in the CNS, although there is evidence that opioids may also act at peripheral opioid receptor. A theoretical advantage of opioid analgesics is that there is no analgesic ceiling. Actually, analgesic efficacy of opioid is typically limited by the development of tolerance or opioid-related side effects.

Opioids may be administered by the subcutaneous, transdermal, transcutaneous, transmucosal or intramuscular route but the most common routes of postoperative systemic opioid analgesic administration are oral and intravenous. Opioids may also be administered at specific anatomic sites such as the intrathecal or epidural space.

Serum drug concentrations may exhibit wider variability with certain routes of administration (e.g. intramuscular) than with others (e.g. intravenous). In general, opioids are administered parenterally (intravenous or intramuscularly) for the treatment of moderate to severe postoperative pain, in part because these routes provide a more rapid and reliable onset of analgesic action than the oral route doses. The transition from parenteral to oral administration of opioids usually occurs after the patient initiates oral intake and postoperative pain has been stabilized with parenteral opioids. A newer version involving patient activated electrically facilitates delivery of transdermal fentanyl, has been introduced for use in hospitalized adult patients (Table 26.2).

Intravenous Patient Controlled Analgesia

Various factors including wide interpatient and intrapatient variability in analgesic needs, variability in serum drug levels and administrative delays, may result in inadequate postoperative analgesia. Therefore, to overcome some of these issues intravenous patient controlled analgesia (IVPCA) optimizes delivery of analgesic opioids and minimizes the effect of pharmacokinetics and pharmacodynamics variability in individual patients. A PCA device is programmed for several variables, including the demand (bolus) dose, lockout interval, and background infusion (Fig. 26.4). An optimal demand on bolus is integral to the efficacy of intravenous PCA or a suboptimal demand dose may result in inadequate analgesia whereas an excessive demand dose may result in a higher incidence of undesirable side effects such as respiratory depression.

The optimal dose for morphine is 1 mg and 40 μg for fentanyl in opioid naïve patient. The lockout interval may also affect the analgesic efficacy of intravenous PCA. If lockout interval is too short it may contribute to an increase in

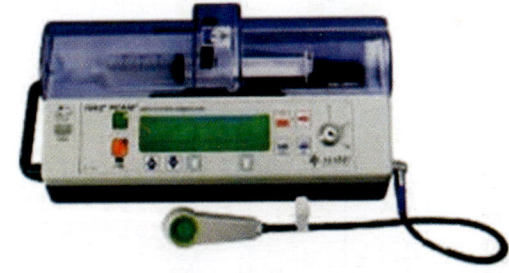

Fig. 26.4: Intravenous patient controlled pump used for continuous infusion of analgesics

Table 26.2: Opioid analgesic pharmacokinetics

Drug	Onset of effect	Peak effect	Duration of effect	Elimination t½	Protein binding (%)	Metabolism pathway	Active metabolism	Major excretion pathway
Alfentanil	Immediate	1.5–2 min	<10 min	1.5–1.85 hr	92%	Liver	–	Urine
Fentanyl injection	IV: immediate, IM: 7–8 min	–	IV: 0.5–1 hr, IM: 1–2 hr	3.65 hr	Alters with increasing ionization	Liver	–	Urine
Fentanyl transdermal	–	24–72 hr	72 hr	~17 hr	Decreases with increasing ionization	Liver: CYP3A4	–	Urine
Fentanyl transmucosal	–	–	–	7 hr	80–85%	Liver: CYP3A4	–	Urine
Hydromorphone	IM/subcutaneous: 15 min, Oral: 30 min	0.5–1 hr	IR: 4–5 hr, ER: 24 hr, IM/subcutaneous: 4–5 hr	IR: 2.3 hr, ER: 18.6 hr, IM/subcutaneous: 2.6 hr	8–20%	Liver: glucuronidation	–	Urine
Levorphanol	IM: 15–30 min	Oral: 1 hr	–	IV: 11–16 hr	40%	–	–	–
Meperidine	–	–	2–4 hr	3–6 (parent), <20 hr (nor-meperidine)	60–80%	Liver	Norme-peridine	–
Methadone	Parenteral: 10–20 min, Oral: 30–60 min	–	4 hr	8–59 hr	85–90%	Liver primarily: CYP3A4 and to lesser extent CYP2D6	–	Urine and fecal
Morphine sulfate	IM/subcutaneous: 10–30 min	Epidural: 10–15 min, Oral: 1 hr	Subcutaneous/IM: 4–5 hr	1.5–2 hr	20–35%	Liver: glucuronidation	Morphine and glucuronide	Urine
Oxycodone	Within 60 min	–	IR: 3–4 hr, CR: 12 hr	IR: 3.2 hr, CR: 4.5 hr	45%	Liver: somewhat involves CYP2D6	Noroxycodone and urine oxymorphone	Urine
Oxymorphone	Parenteral: 5–10 min	–	Parenteral: 3–6 hr	1.3 hr	–	Liver	–	Urine
Propoxyphene	–	2–2.5 hr	–	6–12 hr (parent), 30–36 hr (norpropoxyphene)70%	80%	Liver	Norpropoxyphene	Urine
Remifentanil	Rapid	–	–	10–20 min	91–93%, 79% in neonates	Hydrolysis by esterases	–	Urine
Sufentanil	IV: immediate Epidural: 10 min	–	Epidural: 1.7 hr	2.7 hr	20%	Liver and small intestine	–	–
Tramadol	–	–	2 hr (tramadol), 3 hr (M1, active metabolite)	6.3 hr (tramadol), 7.4 hr (M1, active metabolite)	20%	Liver: CYP2D6 and CYP3A4	O-desmethyl-tramadol (M1) via CYP2D6	Urine

medication-related side effects and if it is too long, it may result in inadequate analgesia and decrease the effectiveness of intravenous PCA. In essence, the lockout interval is a safety feature of IVPCA and although the optimal lockout interval is unknown, most intervals range from 5 to 10 minutes. Many studies show that use of background infusion only increases the analgesic dosage used and the incidence of side effects such as respiratory depression. Therefore, routine use of continuous or background infusion as part of intravenous PCA in adult opioid naïve patients is not recommended. There may be a role of background infusion in opioid tolerance or pediatric patient (Table 26.3).

The incidence of opioid-related adverse events from IVPCA does not seem to differ significantly from that of other methods of administration. Factors that may be associated with occurrence of respiratory depression with intravenous PCA include use of a background infusion, advanced age, concomitant administration of sedative or hypnotic agents and coexisting pulmonary disease such as sleep apnea.

Tramadol

Tramadol is a synthetic opioid that exhibits μ agonist activity and inhibits reuptake of serotonin and norepinephrine. Although tramadol exerts its analgesic effects primarily through central mechanism, it may have peripheral local anesthetic properties and comparable in analgesic efficacy to aspirin (650 mg) and codeine (60 mg) or ibuprofen (400 mg). Advantages of tramadol in postoperative analgesia include a relative lack of respiratory depression, major organ toxicity and depression of gastric intestinal mobility and a low potential for abuse. Common side effects include dizziness, drowsiness, sweating, nausea, vomiting, dry mouth and headache. Tramadol should be used with precaution in patients with seizures or increased intracranial pressure and contraindicated in those taking monoamine oxidase inhibitors [if its side effects are prominent, a combination of tramadol (37.5 mg) and paracetamol (325 mg), Ultracet can be given twice or thrice daily].

Table 26.3: Intravenous patient controlled analgesia regimens			
Drug concentration	Size of bolus	Lockout interval (min)	Continuous infusion
Agonists			
Morphine (1 mg/ml)			
Adult	0.5–2.5 mg	5–10	–
Pediatric	0.01–0.03 mg/kg (max, 0.15 mg/kg/hr)	5–10	0.01–0.03 mg/kg/hr
Fentanyl (0.01 mg/ml			
Adult	10–20 µg	4–10	–
Pediatric	0.5–1 µg/kg (max, 4 µg/kg/hr)	5–10	0.5–1 µg/kg/hr
Hydromorphone (0.2 mg/ml)			
Adult	0.05–0.25 mg	5–10	–
Pediatric	0.003–0.005 mg/kg (max, 0.02 mg/kg/hr)	5–10	0.003–0.005 mg/kg/hr
Alfentanil (0.1 mg/ml)	0.1–0.2 mg	5–8	–
Methadone (1 mg/ml)	0.5–2.5 mg	8–20	–
Meperidine (10 mg/ml)	5–25 mg	5–10	–
Oxymorphone (0.25 mg/ml)	0.2–0.4 mg	8–10	–
Sufentanil (0.002 mg/ml)	2–5 µg	4–10	–
Agonist-Antagonists			
Buprenorphine (0.03 mg/ml)	0.03–0.1 mg	8–20	–
Nalbuphine (1 mg/ml)	1.5 mg	5–15	–
Pentazocine (10 mg/ml)	5–30 mg	5–15	–

Nonopioid Analgesic Adjuncts

NSAIDs

The analgesics of this class are the most commonly used drugs because of their anti-inflammatory, analgesic and antipyretic effects (Table 26.4). The analgesic effect of NSAIDs is mediated through the inhibition of cyclo-oxygenase (COX) enzyme, types 1 and 2, which convert arachidonic acid to prostaglandins. COX 1 is the enzyme that produces prostaglandins, which are important for general 'house keeping' functions such as gastric protection and hemostasis. COX 2 is the inducible enzyme that produces prostaglandins that mediate pain, inflammation, fever and carcinogenesis. Prostaglandin E2 is the key mediator of both peripheral and central sensitization: Peripherally prostaglandins do not directly mediate pain, rather, they contribute to hyperalgesia by sensitizing nociceptors to other mediators of pain sensation such as histamine and bradykinin. Centrally prostaglandin enzymes facilitate pain transmission at the level of dorsal horn by:
- Increasing the release of substance P and glutamate from the five order neurons.
- Increasing the sensitivity of second order neurons.
- Inhibiting the release of neurotransmitters from descending pain modulating pathways.

NSAIDs have proved effective in the treatment of postoperative pain. In addition, they are opioid sparing, can significantly decrease the incidence of opioid-related side effects such as postoperative nausea, vomiting and sedation. Unlike opioids, NSAIDs exhibit a "ceiling effect" with respect to maximum analgesic effects. Parenteral NSAIDs such as ketorolac are commonly used as part of multimodal approach for acute postoperative pain management. The common significant side effects of NSAIDs seen in clinical practice are platelet dysfunction, gastrointestinal ulceration, an increased risk of nephrotoxicity, hypovolemia, congestive heart failure and chronic renal insufficiency. To avoid these side effects it is better to avoid non-selective NSAIDs in perioperative period.

The COX2 selective inhibitors were developed in an attempt to minimizing their side effects. Four COX2 inhibitors are available for clinical use—celecoxib, rofecoxib valdecoxib and parecoxib. The COX2 specific inhibitors offer the potential advantages of reduced incidence of gastrointestinal ulceration and they do not inhibit platelet function. Because prostaglandins play a crucial role in renal function through their affect on blood flow, natriuresis and glomerular filtration, traditional NSAIDs and COX2 inhibitors can cause fluid retention and hypertension. Short-term use of parecoxib and valdecoxib in patients following coronary artery bypass surgery is associated with an increased risk of thromboembolism. Both COX-1 and COX-2 play a significant role in bone fusion following fractures and the traditional NSAIDs have been involved to inhibit the healing process particularly following lumbar spine fusion surgery. The COX-2 inhibitor should not be prescribed in known case of coronary artery disease, known hypersensitivity to drugs, and patients with Samter's triad (asthma, aspirin insensitivity and nasal polyposis). Finally, avoid celecoxib and valdecoxib in patients with allergic type reactions to sulfonamides.

Paraminophenol derivative acetaminophen has both analgesic and antipyretic properties but is devoid of any anti-inflammatory effect. The mechanism of action of the drug is considered to be the inhibition of a putative control cyclooxygenase, COX-3 that results in decreased production of prostaglandin in CNS. There may be modulation of descending inhibitory serotonergic pathways and the drug may act on the opioidergic system and NMDA receptors. It is devoid of all side effects of NSAIDs. Acetaminophen is opioid sparing and can be used in conjunction with an NSAID as part of a multimodal analgesic regimen (Table 26.4). Paracetamol intravenous formulation is available which can be used as 500–1000 mg Q6H. It is also available in the form of suppositories which is useful for pediatric patients.

Table 26.4: Nonopioid analgesic (adult dosing guidelines)				
Drug	*Route*	*Half-life (hr)*	*Dose (mg)*	*Comments*
Phenylacetic acids				
Diclofenac potassium	Po	2	50 mg q8 hr	MDD = 150 mg
Pyrrolacetic acids				
Ketorolac	IV	6	30 mg initially followed by 15–30 mg q6–8 hr not to exceed 5 days	MDD = 120 mg, Hypovolemia should be corrected prior to administration. Decrease the dose in the elderly (>65 years of age) and in renal failure
Propionic acids				
Ibuprofen	Po	2	400 mg q4–6 hr	MDD os 2,400 mg
Naproxen	Po	12–15	250 mg q6–8 hr	LD = 500 mg, MDD ~ 1500 mg
Ketoprofen	Po	2.1	25–50 mg q6–8 hr	MDD = 300 mg
Oxaprozin	Po	42–50	600 mg q12–24 hr	MDD = 12200 mg
Enolic acids (Oxicams)				
Meloxicam	Po	15–20	7.5–15 mg q24 hr	
Poroxicam	Po	50	20–40 mg q24 hr	
Indolacetic acids				
Inomethacin	Po	2	25 mg q8–12 hr	MDD = 200 mg
Sulindac	Po	7.8	150 mg q12 hr	MDD = 400 mg, Active metabolite has a half-life of 16 hr
Etodolac	Po	7.3	300–400 mg q8–12 hr	MDD = 1000 mg
COX-2 inhibitors				
Celecoxib	Po	11	100–200 mg q12 hr	LD = 400 mg, MDD = 400 mg, Avoid this drug in patients allergic to sulfonamide

NMDA Receptors Antagonists

Ketamine and dextromethorphan may be useful analgesic adjuncts. Excitatory neurotransmitter stimulation of NMDA receptors is supposed to be involved in the development and maintenance of several phenomena (1) persistent postoperative pain, (2) hypersensitivity, wind up and allodynia, (3) opioid induced tolerance. Therefore, low dose ketamine (0.25 to 0.5 mg) intravenous bolus followed by an infusion of 2 to 4 µg/kg/min can provide significant analgesia and opioid sparing. The mechanism of action of ketamine is NMDA receptor blockade but in addition, the drug interacts with opioidergic, cholinergic and monoaminergic receptors and block sodium channels. Also, NMDA receptor antagonists may act synergistically when combined with an opioid. The ideal intravenous PCA morphine ketamine ratio is 1:1 with an 8-minute lockout.

Dextromethorphan, the isomer of the codeine analogue levorphanol, is a noncompetitive NMDA receptor antagonist that acts through NMDA antagonism. It can be administered through oral, intravenous and intramuscular routes. Intramuscular route is best because large dosages through intravenous route cause hypotension and bradycardia. The preoperative administration of 150 mg of oral dextrometheophan can reduce PCA morphine requirements of patients undergoing abdominal hysterectomy and preincisional administration of 120 mg of intramuscular dextromethorphan provides pre-emptive analgesia in patients undergoing elective upper abdominal surgeries.

α2 Adrenergic Agonist

α2 adrenergic agonist, clonidine (half-life 9 to 12 hours) and dexmedetomidine (half-life 2 hours) may be administered perioperatively to provide analgesia, sedation and anxiolysis. The presynaptic activation of α_2 receptors that results in the decreased release of norepinephrine is employed in mediating analgesia. Clonidine is a partial selective agonist for the α2 adrenoreceptor, dexmedetomidine is super selective for the receptor.

Their respective α_2/α_1 binding ratios are 220:1 for clonidine versus 1620:1 for dexmedetomidine. Analgesia is mediated supraspinally (locus coeruleus), spinally (substantia gelatinosa), and peripherally. Dexmedetomidine is superior analgesic because of its greater affinity for 2A subtype of the receptors. Clonidine has been used through intravenous, intramuscular, oral, intraarticular, epidural, intrathecal routes. 2–3 µg/kg of clonidine has shown decreased consumption of morphine in several studies. Sedation, hypotension, bradycardia are the main side effects of clonidine.

Dexmedetomidine is d-enantiomer of medetomidine. It is a highly selective α_2 agonist that does not interact with GABA mimetic system and so does not depress respiratory drive. Other advantages are analgesia, titrable sedation (cooperative sedation) and anxiously, its cardioprotective effect is through decreasing sympathetic tone centrally. There are low incidences of hypotension and bradycardia which can be treated with atropine, epinephrine or volume infusion. Dexmedetomidine is a useful adjunct to both opioid and non-opioid analgesia as part of a multimodal analgesic approach. The recommended dose of dexmedetomidine is a loading dose of 1 µg/kg IV over 10 min followed by an infusion of 0.2–0.7 µg/kg/hr. A dexmedetomidine infusion (0.2–0.7 µg/kg/hr) combined with peripheral nerve blockade may provide superb analgesia, anxiolysis and sedation during prolonged procedure.

$\alpha_2\delta$ ligands

$\alpha_2\delta$ subunit calcium channel ligands (e.g. gabapentin and pregabalin) are effective analgesics not only for neuropathic pain syndrome but also for the postoperative pain. When these drugs are combined with NSAIDs, it has been shown to be synergistic in attenuating the hyperalgesia associated with peripheral inflammation. **Gabapentin** prevents the development of central excitability and is antihyperalgesic. The meta-analysis of analgesic effects of gabapentin suggests that it should be part of multimodal analgesic regimen for perioperative pain management. The recommended adult dose of gabapentin for postoperative pain is 900 mg orally 1 to 2 hours before surgery. Pregabalin is another GABA analogue, that may be useful for perioperative pain. The perioperative administration of celecoxib and pregabalin, in combination provides analgesia that is superior to that of either drug used alone, following spinal fusion surgery. Side effects associated with these drugs include somnolence, dizziness, confusion and ataxia.

Glucocorticoids

The glucocorticoids are well known for their analgesic, anti-inflammatory and antiemetic effects. Inhibition of cytosolic phospholipase A2 upstream from the lipooxygenase and COX enzymes in the prostaglandin cascade most certainly accounts for both their anti-inflammatory and analgesic effects by inhibiting leukotriene and prostaglandins production. Recent studies, suggest that combination of dexamethasone (8 mg intravenous) and gabapentin (800 mg orally) administered 1 hour prior to varicocele surgery improves postoperative analgesia and decreases the incidence of nausea and vomiting. However, because of the small doses used perioperatively corticosteroids are considered to be relatively safe.

Regional Analgesic Techniques

A variety of neuraxial (primarily epidural) and peripheral regional analgesic techniques may be used for effective treatment of postoperative pain. In general, the analgesia provided by epidural and peripheral techniques is superior to that with systemic opioids and use of these techniques may even decrease morbidity and mortality.

Single-dose Neuraxial Opioids

Administration of single dose of opioids may be efficacious as a sole or adjuvant analgesic agent when administered intrathecally or epidurally. One of the most important factors in determining the clinical pharmacology for a particular opioid is its degree of lipophilicity (versus hydrophilicity). Hydrophilic opioids act for longer duration of analgesia once they have reached CSF, but associated with high incidence of side effects because of cephalic or supraspinal spread of these compounds. Whereas lipophilic opioids (fentanyl and sufentanyl) tend to provide a rapid onset of analgesia and their rapid clearance from CSF may limit cephalic spread and less incidence of side effects such as delayed respiratory depression.

A single bolus of epidural fentanyl may be administered to provide rapid postoperative analgesia. However, diluting the epidural dose of fentanyl (50–100 µg) in at least 1 ml of preservative-free normal saline is suggested to decrease the onset, and prolong the duration of analgesia, possibly as a result of an increase in initial spread and diffusion of the lypophilic opioids. Use of a single dose of hydrophilic (morphine) is specially helpful in providing postoperative epidural analgesia.

An extended release formulation of (single dose) epidural morphine encapsulated within liposomes that results in up to 48 hours of analgesic has recently been introduced. Concurrent administration of liposomal extended release morphine and local anesthetics may increase peak concentration of morphine.

Continuous Epidural Analgesia

Analgesia delivered through an indwelling epidural catheter is a safe and effective method for management of acute postoperative pain. Intraoperative use of the epidural catheter as part of a combined epidural-general anesthetic technique results in less pain and faster patient recovery immediately after surgery than general anesthesia followed by systemic opioids.

Analgesic Drugs

i. *Local anesthetics:* Epidural infusion of local anesthetic alone may be used for postoperative analgesia but in general it is not as effective in controlling pain as local anesthetic-opioid combinations are. Epidural infusion of local anesthetic alone may be warranted for postoperative analgesia in an attempt to avoid opioid-related side effects; however, the sole use of local anesthetic is less common than the use of a local anesthetic-opioid combination because of significant failure rate (from regression of sensory blockade and inadequate analgesia) and relatively high incidence of motor blockade and hypotension.

ii. *Opioids for epidural infusion*: Opioids may be used alone for postoperative epidural infusion and do not generally cause motor block or hypotension from sympathetic blockade. The analgesic site of action for continuous hydrophilic opioid infusion is primarily spinal. Use of a continuous infusion rather than intermittent boluses of morphine may result in superior analgesia with fewer side effects.

iii. *Local anesthetic opioid combination*: When compared with a local anesthetic or opioid alone, a local anesthetic-opioid combination provides superior postoperative analgesia (including improved dynamic pain relief), limits regression of sensory blockade and possibly decreases the dose of local anesthetic administered. Continuous epidural infusion of local anesthetic-opioid combination also provides analgesia superior to that of intravenous PCA with opioid.

The choice of local anesthetic for continuous epidural infusion varies. In general, bupivacaine ropivacaine or levobupivacaine is chosen because of the differential or preferential clinical sensory blockade with minimal impairment of motor function. Concentration for postoperative analgesia

(≤0.125% bupivacaine or levobupivacaine or ≤2% ropivacaine) are lower than those used for intra-operative anesthesia. The choice of opioid also varies. Most clinicians prefer a lipophilic opioid (fentanyl, 2 to 5 μg/ml or sufentanyl, 0.5 to 1 μg/ml) to allow rapid titration of analgesia. The use of hydrophilic opioid (morphine, 0.05 to 0.1 mg/ml or hydromorphine, 0.01 to 0.05 mg/ml) as part of a local anesthetic-opioid epidural analgesic regimen (Table 26.5).

Adjuvant Drugs

Few of the adjuvants may be added to epidural infusions to enhance analgesia while minimizing side effects. Two of the studied adjuvants are clonidine and epinephrine. Clonidine mediates its analgesic effect primarily through the spinal dorsal horn α_2 receptors on primary afferents and interneurons as well as descending noradrenergic pathway. Epidural dose typically range from 5 to 20 μg/hr. Clinical application of clonidine is limited by its side effects: hypotension, bradycardia and sedation. Hypotension and bradycardia are both dose-dependent.

Epinephrine may improve epidural analgesia, can increase sensory blockade and is generally adminis-tered at a concentration of 2–5 μg/ml. Epidural administration of NMDA antagonists, such as ketamine, can theoretically be useful in attenuating central sensitization and potentiating the analgesic effect of epidural opioids, but additional safety and analgesic data are needed.

Side Effects of Neuraxial Drugs Many medication-related (opioid-local anesthetic) side effects can occur with the use of postoperative epidural analgesia but before automatically ascribing the cause to the epidural analgesic regimen, it is important to first consider other causes, such as low intravascular volume, bleeding and low cardiac output leading to hypotension and cardiovascular accident, pulmonary edema and evolving sepsis leading to respiratory depression.

Following can be attributed as side effects of neuraxial local anesthetic opioid combination regimen:

* Hypotension
* Motor blockade
* Nausea and vomiting
* Pruritus
* Respiratory depression
* Urinary retention

Table 26.5: Patient-controlled epidural analgesia regimens			
Analgesic solution	Continuous rate (ml/hr)	Demand dose (ml)	Lockout interval (min)
General regimens			
0.05% bupivacaine + 4 μg/ml fentanyl	4	2	10
0.0625% bupivacaine + 5 μg/ml fentanyl	4–6	3–4	10–15
0.1% bupivacaine + 5 μg/ml fentanyl	6	2	10–15
0.2% ropivacaine + 5 μg/ml fentanyl	5	2	20
Thoracic surgery			
0.0625%–0.125% bupivacaine + 5 μg/ml fentanyl	3–4	2–3	10–15
Abdominal surgery			
0.0625% bupivacaine + 5 μg/ml fentanyl	4–6	3–4	10–15
0.125% bupivacaine + 0.5 μg/ml sufantanil	3–5	2–3	12
0.1%-0.2% ropivacaine + 2 μg/ml fentanyl	3–5	2–5	10–20
Lower extremity surgery			
0.0625%–0.125% bupivacaine + 5 μg/ml fentanyl	4–6	3–4	10-15
0.125% levobupivacaine + 4 μg/ml fentanyl	4	2	10

- Slowing of gastrointestinal function
- Metabolic toxicity
- Allergy, physical tolerance
- Euphoria
- Hallucination
- Miosis
- Muscle rigidity.

Patient Controlled Epidural Analgesia (PCEA)

Like intravenous PCA, PCEA follows individualization (see IV PCA) of postoperative analgesia requirements and may have several advantages over continuous epidural infusion (CEI), including lower drug use and greater patient satisfaction. PCEA may also provide analgesia superior to that afforded by IV PCA. PCEA is a safe and effective technique for postoperative analgesia in routine surgical wards (Fig. 26.5).

Peripheral Regional Analgesia

The use of peripheral analgesic techniques as a simple injection or continuous infusion can provide analgesia superior to that with systemic opioids. A variety of wound injection and peripheral regional techniques (e.g. brachial plexus, lumbar plexus, femoral, sciatic-popliteal and scalp nerve blocks) can be used to enhance postoperative analgesia. Advantages of peripheral regional analgesia include

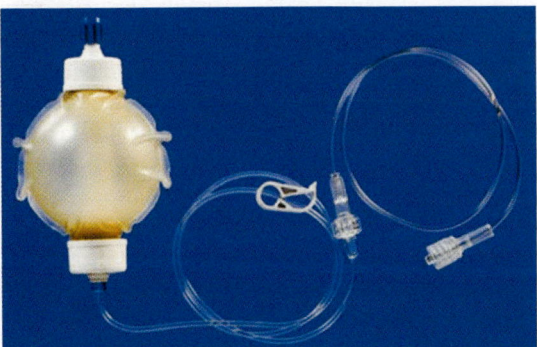

Fig. 26.5: Elastomeric pump used for continuous infusions of analgesic (intravenous or epidural infusion)

superior analgesia, decreased opioid-related side effects, decreased risk for spinal hematoma. The duration of postoperative analgesia resulting from local anesthetic in peripheral nerve block varies but may last up to 24 hours after single injection. Continuous infusions of local anesthetic can be administered through peripheral nerve catheters.

Non-neuraxial Analgesia

Several non-epidural regional analgesia techniques can be used for the management of postoperative thoracic pain, including paravertebral and intercostal blocks, interpleural (intrapleural); analgesia and cryoanalgesia. The most promising technique appears to be a thoracic paravertebral block which has been used for thoracic, breast and upper abdominal surgery and for the treatment of rib fracture pain. The possible sites of analgesia for a thoracic paravertebral block include direct somatic nerve, sympathetic nerve and epidural block. A thoracic paravertebral block can be administered as a simple injection or as continuous infusion through a catheter, may provide analgesia equal or superior to that of thoracic epidural analgesia.

The analgesic efficacy of interpleural analgesia is controversial, due to its mechanism of action. Intercostal blocks may provide short-term postoperative analgesia and may be repeated postoperatively. The incidence of pneumothorax increases with each intercostals nerve blocked. Cryoanalgesia used for postoperative analgesia after thoracotomy, does not appear to provide any analgesic advantage over epidural analgesia.

Intra-articular Analgesia

Local peripheral administration of opioids (e.g. intra-articular after knee surgery) may provide analgesia for up to 24 hours after surgery and decrease the incidence of chronic pain. Peripheral opioid receptors are found on the peripheral terminals of primary afferent nerves and are upregulated during inflammation of peripheral tissues. Use of higher dose of intra-articular morphine (5 versus 1 ml) result in superior analgesia; however, there may be no advantage in the degree of analgesia provided between intra-articular injection of local anesthetic may provide a limited duration of postoperative analgesia but the clinical benefit from the intra-articular injection of local anesthetic is unclear.

NON-PHARMACOLOGICAL STRATEGIES TO MANAGE ACUTE PAIN

Non-pharmacological techniques such as trans-cutaneous electrical nerve stimulation (TENS), acupuncture and psychological approaches can be used in an attempt to alleviate postoperative pain. The mechanism of TENS producing analgesia is not clear but may be related to modulation of nociceptive impulses in spinal cord, release of endogenous encephalins or a combination of these. Although, the analgesic efficacy of these techniques is controversial, TENS and acupuncture may provide postoperative analgesia, decrease postoperative opioid requirements, reduce opioid-related side effect and attenuate activation of the sympathoadrenal system.

The differential behavior response to surgical incision may be related to global (personality, gender, age and culture) and specific (i.e. fear, depression, anger and coping) psychological factors. Cognitive behavior therapy and biofeedback therapy may be efficacious in reducing pain and alleviating psychological factors associated with pain. Identifying and addressing psychological factors can reduce pain, improve the efficacy of pharmacologic analgesics and diminish patient's distress in part through enhancement of placebo effect. Although the placebo effect has traditionally been thought to have a psychological origin, the placebo response may exert part of its effects through activation of endogenous opioids and be useful in reducing intensity of pain.

Postoperative Analgesia in Special Populations

Ambulatory Surgical Patients

The optimizing treatment of postoperative and post-discharge pain is especially important in patients undergoing outpatient surgery because inadequate control of postoperative pain is one of the leading causes of prolonged stays or readmission after outpatient surgery. The traditional reliance on opioid analgesic may not be appropriate for ambulatory surgical patient, because of opioid-related side effects, delayed hospital discharge and post-discharge recovery. A multimodal or 'balanced' analgesic approach using a combination of opioid and non-opioid technique (i.e. NSAIDs or acetaminophen, local anesthetic and other non-pharmacologic therapies) may be more appropriate in this surgical population. Most outpatients rely on a combination of short-acting analgesics (e.g. opioid and acetaminophen) for postoperative pain. However, there are several strategies to optimize post discharge pain, including routine use of NSAIDs, small doses of sustained release opioids and routinely acetaminophen is added.

Elderly Patients

Changes in the physiology, pharmacodynamics, pharmacokinetics and processing of nociceptive information that occur with aging may influence the effectiveness of postoperative pain control in elderly. This group may have communicative, affective, cognitive, social and ideologic barriers to effective postoperative pain control. There is a clinically significant reduction in the intensity of pain perception or symptoms with increasing age. However, elderly may have an increased response to higher intensity, noxious stimuli, decrease pain tolerance and decreased descending modulation, which may contribute to the relatively high incidence of chronic pain in elderly patients. In general, analgesic requirements increase with increasing age. Use of intravenous PCA in elderly is appropriate to compensate for the wide inter-patient variability, although postoperative titration of intravenous morphine can also allow successful and safe administration to elderly patient. Use of postoperative epidural analgesia for elderly patients, especially those with decreased physiologic reserve, may attenuate the postoperative pathophysiology and is reported to improve postoperative outcomes, such as facilitating return of gastrointestinal function after abdominal surgery, lowering pain scores and decreasing pulmonary complications.

Elderly patients have higher incidence of affective or cognitive impairment (e.g. depression, dementia) that may interfere with effective pain management. One of the most devastating complications in elderly surgical patients is postoperative delirium which is associated with increased mortality rates and longer hospital stays. Higher pain scores predict a decline in mental status and an increased risk for delirium. The postoperative use of epidural analgesia may diminish postoperative delirium in part through superior analgesia and a decrease in pulmonary complications.

Pediatric Patients

Optimum control of postoperative pain is important in pediatric patients because poor pain control may result in increased morbidity and mortality. Because of developmental, cognitive and emotional differences, assessment of pain in pediatric patients can be difficult. Special scales are available to assist young children in self-reporting of pain. However, interpretation of behavior and physiologic parameters can be used to assess pain intensity in preverbal children or those who cannot self report their pain. A plan for postoperative pain management should be discussed with family and patient before surgery because pediatric patient may have many anxieties about pain and analgesic used after surgery. In general, oral route of analgesic is used for mild to moderate pain. Intravenous or regional analgesia is appropriate for moderate to severe postoperative pain. Use of intramuscular injections is strongly discouraged in this population. Children as young as 4 years have the cognitive and physical capability to properly use an intravenous PCA device. If opioids are used, children should be closely monitored because of their sensitivity for respiratory depression. Short-acting fentanyl is the choice of analgesic for the group of children who cannot handle intravenous PCA. Use of non-opioid analgesic agents such as NSAIDs is allowed in the

children of ≥ 2 years. Acetaminophen can be used in the children below 2 years. Some data suggest that rectal administration of acetaminophen postoperatively in a higher dose (40 mg/kg followed by three doses of 20 mg/kg at 6 hour intervals) than that previously recommended may result in appropriate serum analgesic levels.

Peripheral and neuraxial regional analgesic techniques are commonly used and effective for acute pain management in pediatric patients. One of the most common techniques is epidural analgesic, which can be delivered by a simple dose or using a continuous infusion catheter technique. The epidural analgesia can be executed at any level along the epidural space (thoracic, lumbar and caudal) but the caudal site is most commonly used in pediatric patients. Regional analgesia techniques may be useful in providing analgesia for wound invasion (e.g. herniotomy or orchidopexy), thoracotomy and orthopedic procedures, even intrathecal analgesia can be used in pediatric patient. Local anesthetic may also be administered topically to provide analgesia. Use of epidural analgesia is associated with improvement in some outcomes such as earlier tracheal extubation, return of gastrointestinal function and length of hospital stay.

Obesity, Obstructive Sleep Apnea (OSA) and Sleep

Although obese patients do not necessarily have OSA, yet obesity is the most important physical characteristic associated with OSA. Approximately 60 to 90% of OSA patients are obese. OSA is defined as more than five episodes per hour of cessation of airflow or more than 10 seconds despite continued ventilatory effort. Patients with OSA are generally at high risk for chronic cognitive impairment, pulmonary hypertension, cardiomyopathy, systemic hypertension and possibly myocardial infarction. Patients with OSA are at higher risk for respiratory arrest. Use of sedative doses of benzodiazepines and opioids may result in frequent hypoxemia and aponea which may be specially dangerous in OSA patients. Regional techniques (neuraxial blocks and peripheral analgesia) rather than systemic opioids be used in an attempt to reduce the likelihood of adverse outcomes. Importantly there is paucity of randomized clinical trial data to provide definitive high quality evidence-based recommendation for provision of postoperative analgesia to OSA patients.

CANCER PAIN MANAGEMENT

Introduction

An estimated 8 million (in 2009) people around the world are dying of cancer. Report from WHO is alarming that global cancer rate could increase by 50% to 15 million in 2009. Cancer pain can be nociceptive (1/3rd) or neuropathic (1/3rd) or a mixed (1/3rd) in origin. Pain can occur in any part during the course of cancer illness. Approximately 50–75% of patients in advance stage of cancer do experience cancer pain. Pain due to bone metastasis is of neuropathic origin, may be worst case scenario in a pain clinic, due to their refractoriness to opioids. A detailed systematic assessment of caner pain is crucial for identifying the etiology and developing a treatment plan, e.g. breast cancer can result in pain due to multiple etiologies during the course of illness right from the site of primary tumor to the metastatic spread to the bones, lung and liver. Approximately 25% of breast cancer spread to the bones first than spine, ribs, pelvis and long bones. The oral analgesic drugs are the mainstay of treatment of cancer pain. Between 75 and 85% of cancer patients can be controlled with oral medication. Adequate pain relief can be achieved by the combination of opioids, NSAIDs with or without adjuncts. In rest of the 15–25% patients whose pain cannot be optimized with oral medications can be offered percutaneous interventions.

Advances in the cancer treatment continue to lengthen survival among cancer patient. As patients lives are prolonged, the need for effective pain control to improve the quality of life has gained increased importance. There are four essential different causes of pain in cancer patients: acute cancer-related pain, chronic cancer-related pain, chronic non-malignant pain in opioid-tolerant patients, and end of life pain. Approximately 60–80% of all patients have tumor-related pain. Between 20 and 30% have treatment-related pain and 10–15% have pain un-related to cancer.

Cancer pain could be somatic, visceral, neuropathic, central and sympathetic pain. In most cases, pain initially can be adequately relieved by administration of either pharmacologic or invasive therapy and by adopting a multidisciplinary approach to supportive care. First line of drugs used for pain control are oral medications including NSAIDs, opioid analgesics and adjuvants agents. The analgesic ladder was originally developed by the cancer relief program of the World Health Organization and has become widely accepted method of drug selection (Fig. 26.6). NSAIDs are usually used in mild to moderate cancer pain. NSAIDs should be used cautiously in patients with peptic ulcer disease or bleeding tendencies.

Recently cyclooxygenase 2 (COX2) inhibitor, e.g. celecoxib, are also available especially for the patients in whom regular NSAIDs are contraindicated due to gastritis, ulcerations, or platelet dysfunction. Acetaminophen's analgesic action is by inhibition of nitric oxide synthetase; it works at both central and spinal sites.

Opioid analgesics are the mainstay therapy for cancer pain. Agonists-antagonist agents are not effective in treatment of cancer pain because of their ceiling effect of analgesia, potential to precipitate withdrawal and associated psychotropic side effects with increasing dosages. The pure opioid agonists should be used exclusively.

Adjuvant Therapy

Adjuvant agents may have inherent analgesic action, potentiate the effects of opioid analgesic or improve mood, sleep, nausea, anxiety, and somnolence. The tricyclic antidepressants are known to have analgesic action, treat depression, improve sleep and benefit patients with neuropathic pain, especially those with dysesthesias. Tertiary amines (e.g. amitriptyline, doxepin) are often first line of therapy owing to a great analogies effect. Anticonvulsant drugs (e.g.

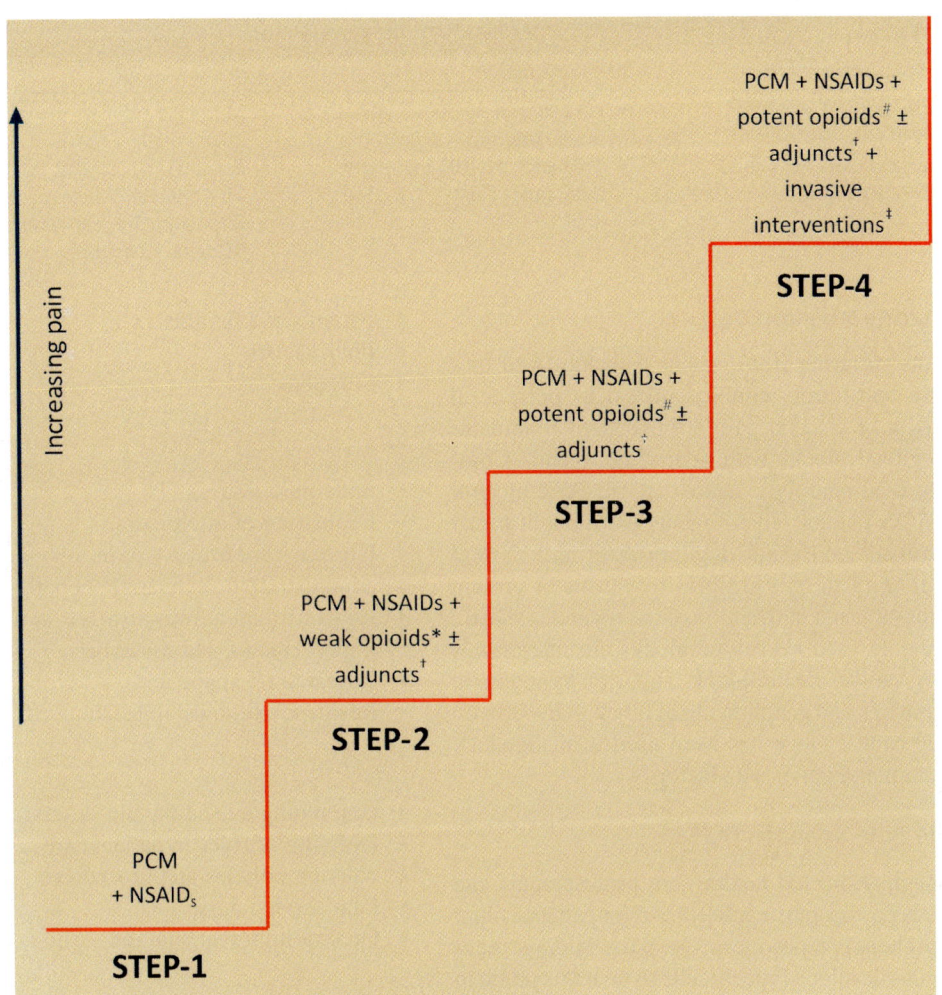

Increasing pain

PCM + NSAIDs +
potent opioids# ±
adjuncts† +
invasive
interventions‡

STEP-4

PCM + NSAIDs +
potent opioids# ±
adjuncts‡

STEP-3

PCM + NSAIDs +
weak opioids* ±
adjuncts†

STEP-2

PCM
+ NSAIDs

STEP-1

Fig. 26.6: WHO pain ladder

PCM Paracetamol; NSAIDs Non-steroidal anti-inflammatory drugs
*Tramdol, Codeine, Dihydrocodeine
#Morphine, Fentanyl, Methadone, Buprenorphine
†Amitryptyline, Duloxetine, Gabapentin, Pregabalin, Baclofen, Clonidine, Bisphosphonates
‡Celiac plexus block superior hypogastric block, ganglion impar block, hyperbaric phenol saddle block

pregabalin, gabapentin, carbamazepine, clonezepam, phenytoin) and antispasmodic drugs (baclofen) are helpful for lancinating pain. Other medications that can be useful sometimes are benzodiazepines, haloperidol and phenothiazides (Table 26.6).

Drugs for Neuropathic Pain

- Amitriptyline 25–75 mg orally, once a day
- Gabapentin 300–600 mg orally, 3 times a day
- Pregabalin 150–300 mg orally, twice a day or 600 mg sustained release preparation twice a day

Table 26.6: Usual starting doses of commonly used analgesics in cancer patients		
Step 1 analgesia	*Step 2 analgesia*	*Step 3 analgesia*
• Paracetamol, 1 g only four times a day • Ibuprofen, 400 mg orally, four times a day	• Co-codamol 30/500, 2 tablets orally, four times a day • Tramadol, 50–100 mg orally three times a day	• Morphine sulphate modified-released, 20 mg orally 12 hourly • Fentanyl transdermal patch, 12–25 µg/hr 72 hourly • Buprenorphine transdermal patch, 35 µg/hr 72 hourly

Percutaneous Interventions

Patients suffering from cancer pain localized to a certain body area which manifest as peripheral neuralgia or visceral pain are excellent candidates for regional blocks with neurolytic agents. Commonly used neurolytic agents are 50–95% alcohol or 6–12% phenol. These agents are thought to act by causing wallerian degeneration and axonal disruption of the nerve fibers by means of protein denaturation and destruction of the myelines sheath. Commonly used neurolytic blocks are intercostals blocks, celiac plexus block, superior hypogastric plexus block and ganglion impar block. A hyperbaric phenol caudal block has been used in malignancy of rectum and pelvis satisfactorily.

Acute Pain Services (APSs)

Although dedicated health care professionals can improve postoperative pain control for patients, more comprehensive preoperative pain management programs developed specifically to treat this problem can address need for all patients with an institution. The organizational aspect of such services are considerable and necessary for effective and safe care and may include issues such as education, administration, nursing and documentation.

Organizational Aspect of Acute Pain Services

Educational Activity

• Anesthesiologists
• Health insurance carriers
• Hospital administrators
• Nurses
• Patients and families
• Pharmacists
• Surgeons.

Administrative Activity

• Economic issues
• Evaluation of equipment
• Human resources—pain service personnel, administrative secretarial support
• Institutional administrative activity, quality improvements and assurance
• Research (if applicable)
• Residency fellowship teaching (if applicable).

Nursing

• Continuing education and in service training
• Defining of roles in patient care
• Nursing policies and procedures
• Pain service nurse
• Quality improvement and assurance.

Documentation

• Bedside pain management assessment flow sheet
• Daily consultation notes
• Educational packages
• Policies and procedures
• Preprinted orders.

Whether acute pain services actually improve outcomes is unclear. Two systemic reviews have examined the impact of acute pain services on patient outcomes, both the systemic reviews suggest that the introduction of acute pain services is associated with a decrease in pain scores and the effect of APS on analgesic-related side effects (e.g. nausea, vomiting), satisfaction and overall cost is uncertain.

27 Occupational Risk in Surgery and its Prevention

During the course of offering the surgical care and performance of operative procedures, exposure to patient's blood and body fluids has always been major surgical concerns for the surgeons and health care workers. It has been well documented that HIV, hepatitis B and C can be transmitted in the operating theater. Therefore, surgeons and health professionals should be fully aware of this occupational hazard.

AIDS patients have increased frequency for acute abdominal pain syndrome and on occasions they are subjected to emergency surgical procedures. Acute appendicitis in AIDS patient is normally due to occlusion of appendiceal lumen with fecalith, but sometimes it can occur because of Kaposi's sarcoma lesion or cytomegalo virus (CMV) infection. Presentation of appendicitis is generally classical but WBC count is normal in majority of the patients. Recently the perforation of the GI tract has also increased due to CMV infection. Kaposi's sarcoma, GI lymphoma and severe ileocolitis are additional causes of AIDS-related perforation of GI tract. Intestinal obstruction in HIV-infected patients is found to be due to pyloric obstruction secondary to lymphoma, small bowel obstruction due to myco-bacterial diseases and intestinal intussusception due to Kaposi's sarcoma. Hepatobiliary diseases like acute cholecystitis, cholangitis and jaundice are other common conditions seen in AIDS patients. On many occasions anorectal diseases may be present like condyloma acuminatum, abscess anorectal, etc. which may require surgical treatment.

Surgeons and other health care professionals are at high risk from the infected patients they treat by virtue of their exposure to penetrating injuries. The routine testing for HIV has evoked considerable legal and emotional responses to the discovery of a positive test in an individual on grounds that such findings may devastate the individual. A policy of routine testing would also be extremely costly.

HIV Transmission

Methods of HIV transmission have been well described and include sexual contact, sharing of needles among the intravenous drug users, exposure to infected blood and blood products, mother to child and infected blood transfusion. The exposures that take place to the health care professionals and surgeons are the percutaneous injury by needle prick or cut by a sharp instrument, contact of mucous membrane or non-intact skin with blood or other body fluids which are potentially infectious. In additional to blood and visible bloody body fluids, semen, vaginal secretions CSF, synovial, pleural, peritoneal, pericardial and amniotic fluids are considered infectious. Faeces, nasal secretions, saliva, sputum, sweat, tears, urine and vomitus are not considered potentially infectious unless they have visible blood. The risk varies with the type and severity of the exposure.

Risk of Transmission after needle injury

Hepatitis B virus	6–30%
Hepatitis C virus	1.8%
HIV	0.3%

The human immunodeficiency virus (HIV) after entering the bloodstream either through the mucous membrane or from blood to blood contact, infects CD4$^+$ T cells and begins to replicate rapidly. CD4$^+$ T cells are the important component of the immune-system of the body which fights against the infection. These viruses start destroying the CD4$^+$ T cells. In normal healthy individuals CD4$^+$ T cells are around thousand (1000) and more. As the disease progresses there is an ongoing decease in CD4$^+$ T cell count. In the beginning, the patients may be asymptomatic but when the counts decrease to 300 or less, then the immunesystem of the body collapses and it opens the door of all kinds of opportunistic infections.

Most patients of HIV have a progressive decline in CD4$^+$ count and that may take many years to cause profound immunodeficiency which is futher manifested by opportunistic diseases. The important clinical findings which predict the disease progression in HIV infected patients are thrush, oral leukoplakia, unexplained fever, diarrhea and weight loss.

Factors Affecting the Risk of HIV

1. Quantity of blood exposure
2. Visibility of blood on the needle
3. Deep injury with hollow bore needle
4. Terminally ill HIV patient
5. Viral load of the patient
6. Duration of exposure.

The important diagnostic tests are ELISA (enzyme-linked immunosorbent assay) and the western blot. Both of these tests detect the presence of viral antibody. It is always necessary to demonstrate the HIV virus by detection of p24 antigen or HIV RNA (HIV viral load).

Indication for Initiation of Antiretroviral Therapy

• Symptomatic HIV infection regardless of CD4$^+$ count or viral load

• Asymptomatic HIV infection, CD4$^+$ cell count <200 regardless of HIV viral load.

Risk of Hepatitis B Infection

Hepatitis B is a major worldwide health problem. Percutaneous transmission through the use of any contaminated needle is the most important route of HBV infection and is common in intravenous drug abusers. Sexual transmission is another mode of infection and the incidence is higher in male homosexuals and heterosexuals with multiple sex partners.

Hepatitis B virus (HBV) exposure poses a far greater risk to the operating surgeon than HIV. The risk of seroconversion is 100 times higher with HBV than HIV. All surgeons should undergo immunization against hepatitis B. Risk after needle stick injury has been found to be related to HBeAg positivity. Hepatitis C virus is also transmitted through needle stick injury but the risk of transmission in cases of hepatitis C is higher than that of HBV or HIV viruses. About 70% of patients of hepatitis B virus infection are subclinical or anicteric phase and another 30% show the picture of icteric hepatitis. Incubation period is 1–4 months.

Remarkable advances have been made in the prevention of hepatitis B virus infection. In the past the prevention of hepatitis B virus infection was from passive immunization with immunoglobulin containing high titers of antibody to HBsAg. Currently the immunization may also be used in post-exposure prophylaxis. HBsAg containing vaccines has been developed with good safety and efficacy profiles. These vaccines are primarily used for pre-exposure prophylaxis but can be used in post-exposure settings along with immunoglobulin.

Treatment for the HBV is largely aimed at patients with chronic liver diseases. The two most important therapies are interferon and nucleoside analogue lamivudine. Many times the corticosteroid may also be used with additional benefits along with interferon.

Regimen of Hepatitis B Immunization

Engerix B 1 ml (deltoid muscle) three doses at 0 time, 1 month and 6 months

Response rate: More than 90% of healthy adults develop adequate antibody response and field trial shows 80–90% efficacy.

Revaccination: Revaccination of non-responders will produce response in 15–25% with one additional dose and 30–50% with three doses.

It has been observed that risk for exposure was highest when the operative procedure lasted for more than 3 hours, there is more than 300 ml of blood loss intraoperatively and in major surgical and gynecological procedures. At times it is advisable to do the screening of patients of high-risk group like homosexuals, history of drug abuse, hemophilics and partners of above.

In the background of the above facts it is of utmost importance that surgeons should have the understanding about the universal precautions to avoid getting infected with HIV, HBV and HCV. Under the universal precautions principle blood and body fluid from all the patients should be considered infected from the viruses. Universal precautions include:

1. *Wearing of gloves:* It should be worn to avoid contamination with infected fluid and should always be worn in following situations—putting of IV drip, while giving IV injections, dressing of open wounds, during all operative procedures. It is always preferred to have double gloves as it has been observed that skin contamination by glove perforation can be reduced to five-folds by wearing two pairs of gloves.

2. *Use of waterproof garments, masks and cap:* It is quite common in major operative procedures that body fluids from the patient soaks the surgeon. It is often seen that surgeons OT clothes get soaked if they do not wear waterproof garments. For this reason, gown should be water-proof.

3. *Eye protection:* One should always use the eye protection devices with side shields.
4. *Footwear:* Chappals should always be avoided as these do not protect the feet especially in endourological procedures. It is advisable to wear the gumboots to have better protection.

Needle Stick Injury

Needle stick injury poses the greatest risk for the transmission of viruses. Injury by a suture needle is considerably found to be less harmful than that by blood-drawing hollow needle.

Factors Minimizing the Risk of Viral Transmission

1. All persons with open wound should be prohibited from participating in the operation.
2. Surgical assistants should be kept to minimum and are instructed not to make unnecessary movements.
3. All the persons should follow the universal precautions.
4. One should avoid recapping the needles.
5. Suture needle should always be grasped by instruments and never by hand.
6. It is advisable to remove the needle before tying the sutures.
7. One should prefer to use the skin stapler than suturing to close the skin.
8. Use of electrocautery and scissors should be preferred instead of scalpel.
9. Transfer of sharp instruments should be done using a trey and never hand to hand.
10. All spills of infectious fluid should be decontaminated immediately. Antiseptics effective against HIV
    - Undiluted savlon solution
    - Chlorhexidine
    - Household bleach
    - Formalin 4%
    - Povidone-iodine 2%
    - Ethalonol 70%
    - Dettol solution—No effect.

Table 27.1: Regimens for 28-day postexposure prophylaxis for HIV infection.[1]

Regimen	Dose	Daily pill burden[2] (no)	Advantages	Disadvantages
Two-durg regimens				
Tenofovir-emtricitabine (Truvada)[3]	One tablet (300 mg of tenofovir with 200 mg of emtricitabine) once daily	1	Well tolerated; once-daily dosing	Potential nephrotoxicity
Zidovudine-lamivudine (Combivir)[4]	One tablet (300 mg of zidovudine with 150 mg of lamivudine) twice daily	2	Preferred in pregnancy	Twice-daily dosing; less well tolerated than tenofovir-emtricitabine (nausea, asthenia, neutropenia, anemia, abnormal liver-enzyme levels)
Three-drug regimens[5]				
Ritonavir-lopinavir (Kaletra) (plus either tenofovir-emtricitabine or zidovudine-lamivudine)	Two tablets (50 mg of ritonavir with 200 mg of lopinavir per tablet) twice daily, or four tablets once daily	5 or 6	Either once-daily or twice-daily dosing; one copayment; no refrigeration required; most experience in pregnancy; high genetic barrier to resistance	Gastrointestinal side effects such as diarrhea; may cause elevated liver-enzyme levels or hepatitis
Ritonavir plus atazanavir (plus either tenofovir-emtricitabine or zidovudine-lamivudine)	100 mg of ritonavir plus 300 mg of atazanavir once daily	3 or 4	Once-daily dosing; well tolerated	Ritonavir must be refrigerated; potential for asymptomatic jaundice, renal stones; may cause elevated liver-enzyme levels or hepatitis
Ritonavir plus darunavir (plus either tenofovir-emtricitabine or zidovudine-lamivudine)	100 mg of ritonavir plus two tablets, each containing 400 mg of darunavir, once daily	4 or 5	Once-daily dosing; high genetic barrier to resistance	Ritonavir must be refrigerated; gastrointestinal side effects; may cause elevated liver-enzyme levels or hepatitis

1 Tenofovir, emtricitabine, and lamivudine all have activity against hepatitis B. Patients with chronic active hepatitis B (i.e. patients who are positive for hepatitis B surface antigen) may have flares of hepatitis on withdrawal of these agents at the completion of postexposure prophylaxis treatment. Referral to a hepatitis specialist or serial monthly monitoring of liver-enzyme levels for up to 6 months after treatment should be considered.

2 The daily pill burden in the three-drug regimens depends on which two-drug regimen is chosen.

3 The dose of tenofovir-emtricitabine should be reduced to one tablet every 48 hours in patients with a creatinine clearance of 30 to 49 ml per minute. Tenofovir-emtricitabine is not recommended in patients with a creatinine clearance of less than 30 ml per minute or in patients who are undergoing hemodialysis; see the guidelines from the Department of Health and Human Services for considerations regarding doses of individual agents in patients with advanced renal dysfunction.

4 Zidovudine-lamivudine is not recommended in patients with a creatinine clearance of less than 50 ml per minute; see the guidelines from the Department of Health and Human Services for considerations regarding doses of individual agents in patients with renal dysfunction.

5 The boosting agent ritonavir is not considered to be an active drug in tabulating the number of agents in the three-drug regimen.

Table 27.2: Laboratory tests generally recommended for persons after exposure to HIV.[1]

Test	Recommended during treatment		Recommended at follow-up		
	Baseline	Symptom-Directed[2]	4–6 wk	12 wk	24 wk
ELISA for HIV antibodies	Yes	Yes	Yes	Yes	Yes
Creatinine, liver function, and complete blood count with differential count	Yes	Yes	No	No	No
HIV viral load	No	Yes	No	No	No
Anti-HBs antibodies	Yes[3]	No	No	No	No
HBsAg	Yes[3,4]	No	No	No	No
HCV antibodies	Yes	No	Yes	Yes	Yes
HCV RNA[5]	No	Yes	Yes	Yes	Yes
Screening, including rapid plasma regain test, for other sexually transmitted infections[6]	Yes	Yes	No	Yes	No

1 Patients who receive zidovudine plus lamivudine-based regimens should have a complete blood count and measurement of liver-enzyme levels at 2 weeks of treatment, irrespective of the presence or absence of clinical symptoms. Tenofovir plus emtricitabine-based regimens generally involve few side effects, and symptom-directed assessment of serum creatinine or liver-enzyme levels should be considered. The addition of a ritonavir-boosted protease inhibitor should be followed by symptom-directed assessment of liver-enzyme levels, serum glucose levels, or both. Anti-HBs antibodies denote hepatitis B virus surface antibodies, ELISA (enzyme-linked immunosorbent assay), HBsAg (hepatitis B surface antigen), and HCV (hepatitis C virus).

2 Symptom-directed tests are for signs or symptoms of toxic effects (rash, nausea, vomiting, or abdominal pain) or HIV seroconversion (fever, fatigue, lymphadenopathy, rash, or oral or genital ulcers).

3 If tests for anti-HBs antibodies and HBsAg are both negative, a vaccination series against HBV infection should be initiated and completed.

4 If the patient is HBsAg-positive, he or she should have monthly follow-up of liver-function tests after discontinuation of postexposure prophylactic regimens containing tenofovir, lamivudine, or emtricitabine; referral to a specialist in viral hepatitis should be considered.

5 HCV RNA testing may identify early HCV seroconversion; early detection and treatment during acute HCV infection may avert or ameliorate chronic disease. Data are from Dienstag and McHutchison.

6 Rapid plasma regain testing and testing of urethral-swab and rectal-swab specimens for gonorrhea and *Chlamydia* and of pharyngeal-swab specimens for gonorrhea should be performed as appropriate, according to the patient's sexual risk-taking behaviors and the type of exposure to HIV.

Exposure to Infectious Fluid

Postexposure prophylaxis should be initiated as rapidly as possible after exposure to HIV. Greater benefit of postexposure prophylaxis is seen when it is initiated within 6 hours after exposure. Postexposure prophylaxis should be continued for 28 days (Flow chart 27.1, Tables 27.1 and 27.2).

Immediate measures on exposure
- Thorough wash with soap and water
- Flush exposed mucous membrane with water
- Use of disinfectant in open wound
- Eyes should be irrigated with clean water
- Antiretro viral therapy.

Follow-up of Exposed Cases

- Baseline HIV testing
- Follow-up testing at 6 weeks, 3 months and 6 months by ELISA
- Role of HIV DNA PCR—if unclear (must be confirmed by ELISA)

Recommended post-exposure prophylaxis for exposure to HBV			
Vaccination and antibody response status of exposed workers	Treatment		
	Source HBsAg positive	Source HBsAg negative	Source unknown or not available for testing
Unvaccinated	HBIG × 1 and initiate HB vaccine series	Initiate HB vaccine series	Initiate HB vaccine series
Previously vaccinated			
Known responder	No treatment	No treatment	No treatment
Known non-responder	HBIG × 1 and initiate revaccination or HBIG × 2	No treatment	If known high risk source, treat as if source were HBsAg positive
Antibody response Unknown	Test exposed person for anti-HBs 1. If adequate, no treatment is necessary. 2. If inadequate*, administer HBIG × 1 and vaccine booster.	No treatment	Test exposed person for anti-HBs 1. If adequate, no treatment is necessary. 2. If inadequate*, administer vaccine booster and recheck titer in 1–2 months.

*A non-responder is a person with inadequate levels of serum antibody to HBsAg (i.e. anti-HBs <10 mlU/ml).
Source: MMWR, June 29 2001, vol 50, RR-11, p22

Flow chart 27.1: Post-exposure prophylaxis

Percutaneous injury e.g. with needle stick injury or cut with sharp object

More severe injury, e.g. deep puncture, needle used in patients artery or vein

Less severe, e.g. solid needle or superficial injury

Infection status of source

Asymptomatic HIV or known low viral load < 1500 copies/ml — Recommended expanded 3-drug regimen PEP

Symptomatic HIV, AIDS, acute seroconversion or known high viral load — Recommended expanded 3-drug regimen PEP

Source of unknown HIV status — Generally no PEP warranted, consider 2-drug PEP for source with HIV risk factor

Unknown source — -Do-

HIV negative — No PEP warranted

Infection status of source

Asymptomatic HIV or known low viral load < 1500 copies/ml — Recommended expanded 2-drug regimen PEP

Symptomatic HIV, AIDS, acute seroconversion known high viral load — Recommended expanded 3 drug regimen PEP

Source of unknown HIV status — Generally no PEP warranted, consider 2-drug PEP for source with HIV risk factor

Unknown source — -Do-

HIV negative — No PEP warranted

Index